WOMEN
AND
HIV/AIDS

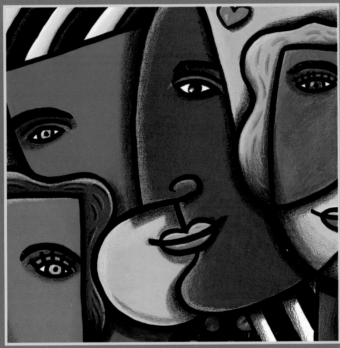

AN INTERNATIONAL
RESOURCE BOOK

Information, action and resources on women and
HIV/AIDS, reproductive health and sexual relationships

MARGE BERER
with Sunanda Ray

MARGE BERER is a writer and editor, and has been working for women's reproductive rights internationally since 1979. She is the editor and one of the founders of *Reproductive Health Matters*, a new international journal, and lives in London.

SUNANDA RAY is a medical doctor and women's health activist, living and working in Zimbabwe as a public health physician and lecturer. She is a founder member and chairperson of the Women and AIDS Support Network, Zimbabwe.

This book has been published in association with **Reproductive Health Matters** and **AHRTAG (Appropriate Health Resources and Technologies Action Group)**, both based in London.

Reproductive Health Matters is a new international journal by and for women's health advocates, health service providers, researchers and policy-makers. It contains papers which explore reproductive health needs from a women-centred perspective and how these can best be met through empowerment of women, education, policy and services. It aims to promote increased communication and collaboration between women's health and advocates and professionals in the field.

AHRTAG, an international health information agency, produces newsletters and special publications on HIV/AIDS, diarrhoeal diseases, acute respiratory infections, disability issues, and primary health care, and runs a resource centre and enquiry service for health workers.

All royalties from this book will be used to subsidize its distribution in developing countries.

All materials received will be kept in the AHRTAG Resource Centre.

WOMEN AND HIV/AIDS

AN INTERNATIONAL RESOURCE BOOK

Information, action and resources
on women and HIV/AIDS, reproductive health and
sexual relationships

Written and edited by

MARGE BERER

with Sunanda Ray

Pandora
An Imprint of HarperCollins*Publishers*

Pandora Press
An Imprint of HarperCollins*Publishers*
77-85 Fulham Palace Road,
Hammersmith, London W6 8JB

Published by Pandora Press 1993
10 9 8 7 6 5 4 3 2 1

ISBN 0 04 440876 5

Typeset by Harper Phototypesetters Limited,
Northampton, England
Printed in Great Britain by
Butler and Tanner, Frome, Somerset

Dedication

If we want to end the epidemic of HIV, a virus which has, above all, taken advantage of how all of us, across the world, live our sexuality, it is our relationships that we must start to question and transform.

Having only one lifetime partner is not necessarily possible nor even desired by all of us. However, no matter how many partners women have had or why, we want to be valued sexually and as women and treated with respect, integrity and care.

Whether our experience in sexual relationships has been positive or negative, we are taught not to reveal it. Perhaps if we begin to name our experience openly, we will help each other find the strength to value ourselves and our own needs more, and to take more pride in ourselves as women. Perhaps, then, more of us will be able to seek what we want, refuse what we do not want, and express our sexuality instead of hiding it where it cannot be exposed and destroyed. Only then can our relationships become safe for us, and only then will sex begin to be safe for us as well.

This book is dedicated to all the women who are trying to make sense of their experience of sexuality and relationships, to have more control over their lives, and to support each other.

Contents

Acknowledgements

Sunanda Ray's knowledge, perspectives and experience helped to form and transform this book. Our discussions, her suggestions, questions, ideas, support and encouragement throughout, and especially her co-editing, were invaluable.

AHRTAG agreed to support the publication and distribution of this book both before they had seen a word on paper and after. Kathy Attawell read and edited several drafts. She and Nel Druce did a terrific amount of work to help to make this book available.

The following readers gave many excellent editing comments and encouragement: Michael Tan, Esther Rome, Charles C.J. Carpenter, James Chin, Barbara James, Toni Belfield, Jane Urwin, Claudia Garcia Moreno, Sue Lucas, Debrework Zewdie, Elvira Lutz, Alan F. Fleming, T.K. Sundari, Hilary Hughes, Nel Druce, Christopher Castle, and D.J. Oshry.

Barbara James helped to write to groups and authors, compile and edit the list of groups and resources, typed many papers, gave constant support and assistance and an endless amount of practical advice.

Blanca Fernandez, Ruth Mahnen, Philip Bickle and Graham Fletcher did translations from Spanish and French.

Sara Dunn, Margaret Busby, Karen Holden and Lucy Allen put a lot of effort into this book for Pandora Press.

We have been overwhelmed throughout by the willingness of hundreds of generous and dedicated professionals and activists to contribute material of every description, all of it valuable, in order to share it with colleagues throughout the world. There is an enormous network here, willing to be of use to each other. Their contributions have made this book the rich resource we had hoped it would be.

Family, friends and colleagues have given tremendous personal support.

Sponsorship

Many thanks to Agnete Strom and the Women's Front of Norway, Judy Norsigian and the Boston Women's Health Book Collective, Janita Janssen and the Women's Health Action Foundation in Amsterdam, and Kathy Attawell and AHRTAG, who sponsored this project and took responsibility for the funding. Without their support, it could not have been funded.

Funding

This project was funded by the Norwegian Agency for Development Cooperation, the European Economic Community, the Netherlands Ministry of Foreign Affairs & Development Cooperation, the John D. and Catherine T. MacArthur Foundation (USA), Oxfam UK, and the Population Council (USA).

Many thanks to Kar-Olaf Wathne, Robin Gorna, Fineke van der Veen, Elizabeth McGrory, Carmen Barroso, Claudia Garcia Moreno, Judith Bruce, Beverly Winikoff and Christopher Elias.

This funding was not only a commitment of money but also of support for work on women, reproductive health and HIV/AIDS.

About the Contributors

DARIEN TAYLOR is an AIDS activist, co-founder of Voices of Positive Women in Toronto, Canada, and co-editor of *Positive Women: Voices of Women Living with AIDS.*

JUDITH WASSERHEIT was chief of the Sexually Transmitted Diseases Branch, National Institute for Allergy and Infectious Diseases, and is now director, Division of STD/HIV Prevention, US Centers for Disease Control, Atlanta, USA.

CHARLES C.J. CARPENTER is professor of medicine, Brown University, Providence, USA.

CARMEN ZORILLA is an associate professor, School of Medicine, Department of Obstetrics & Gynecology, University of Puerto Rico, San Juan, Puerto Rico.

BROOKE GRUNDFEST SCHOEPF is an independent scholar and carried out medical research and training as director of *Projet Connaissida* in Zaïre from 1985 to 1990.

SUSAN ALLEN is with the Center for AIDS Prevention Studies, University of California, San Francisco, and works with the *Projet San Francisco*, in collaboration with the Ministry of Health, Rwanda.

JON UNGPHAKORN works with Access, an AIDS counselling organization in Bangkok, Thailand.

JANET L. MITCHELL is chief of Perinatology, Department of Obstetrics & Gynecology, Harlem Hospital Center, New York City, and a member of the National Minority AIDS Council, USA.

SANDRA DICK is midwife responsible for HIV services and women using injection drugs at St Mary's Hospital, Paddington, London, England.

M. TEMMERMAN and co-authors are from the WHO Collaborating Centre for Research and Training in STDs, and various medical departments of the University of Nairobi, University of Manitoba, and the Institute of Tropical Medicine in Antwerp.

ANN B. WILLIAMS is a family nurse-practitioner and assistant professor of community health nursing at Yale School of Nursing, USA, where her clinical practice has focused on substance abuse and AIDS.

CHRISTINE OBBO is Ugandan and an associate professor of anthropology, Wayne State University, Detroit, Michigan, USA.

MARY T. BASSETT and MARVELLOUS MHLOYI are

researchers at the University of Zimbabwe in Harare, Zimbabwe.

JOHN HUBLEY is honorary lecturer at Leeds University, England, author of *The AIDS Handbook*, and freelance consultant specializing in health education in developing countries.

SUSIE BRIGHT is former editor of *On Our Backs*, San Francisco, USA.

BARBARA JAMES is an HIV/AIDS researcher at the Institute for the Study of Drug Dependence and active in the Women and HIV/AIDS Network, London, England. PATRICIA WEJR is publications/newsletter editor at Women's Health, London, England.

ELVIRA LUTZ is director of education at the Family Planning Association of Uruguay, an active member of the Uruguayan Sexology Society, and on the Advisory Board of the Latin American & Caribbean Women's Health Network.

JANET HOLLAND and co-authors are lecturers and researchers at universities in England, and members of the Women, Risk and AIDS Project (WRAP) team, c/o Institute of Education, University of London, London.

ERIK CENTERWALL is a sex educator, author and freelance journalist in Sweden.

VICKIE M. MAYS is director of Black C.A.R.E., associate professor at UCLA and a clinical psychologist. SUSAN D. COCHRAN is co-director of Black C.A.R.E., professor at California State University, Northridge and UCLA, USA. They are currently conducting a study of young heterosexual and lesbian women's risk of HIV infection.

MINDY THOMPSON FULLILOVE and co-authors researched the paper reprinted here as part of the Multicultural Inquiry and Research on AIDS, a project of the Center for AIDS Prevention Studies, University of California, San Francisco and the Bayview-Hunter's Point Foundation, USA.

SOPHIE DAY is honorary senior research fellow at St Mary's Medical School and lecturer in anthropology at Goldsmith's College, London. HELEN WARD is honorary lecturer in public health at St Mary's Medical School, London, England.

CAROLE A. CAMPBELL is an assistant professor of Sociology, California State University, Long Beach, USA, and has written a number of papers on women and AIDS.

L.M. BARUGAHARE is director of the AIDS Information Centre, Kampala, Uganda.

ANNA STREBEL is at the Department of Psychology, University of the Western Cape, Cape Town, South Africa.

MARIE MARTHE SAINT CYR-DELPE formerly worked for the Women & AIDS Resource Network and the Haitian Coalition on AIDS, and is currently deputy director of Community Relations, NYC Commission on Human Rights, New York City, USA.

ROSAMAE BAIN is nursing officer Grade I, nurse epidemiologist, Community Health Services, Ministry of Health, The Bahamas.

GRUPO PELA VIDDA is a support group for people affected by HIV/AIDS in São Paulo, Brazil, sponsored by the Brazilian Interdisciplinary AIDS Association (ABIA).

ANONYMOUS wrote to the *Guardian* in the UK.

MISHA wrote to Association Aspasite, a group concerned about and supporting better conditions for sex workers in Geneva, Switzerland.

JACQUELINE REVOCK left the Union County Jail in late November 1991 and entered a residential treatment centre.

THERESA KAIJAGE is one of the founders of and works with WAMATA, Dar es Salaam, Tanzania.

KARI HARTWIG is with Family Health International, AIDS Prevention and Control (AIDSCAP) Project, Arlington, USA.

ADEPEJU A. OLUKOYA is senior research fellow, Institute of Child Health and Primary Care, Lagos, teaches medical students and other health professionals, conducts research in primary health care, and provides primary health care services in urban and rural communities in Nigeria.

I.S. GILADA is the honorary secretary of the Indian Health Organization, Bombay, India.

WERASIT SITTITRAI is with the Institute of Population Studies, Chulalongkorn University, and the Program on AIDS, Thai Red Cross Society, Bangkok, Thailand.

KATE THOMSON formerly worked full-time for Positively Women and is now coordinator, International Community of Women Living with HIV/AIDS in London, England.

JANE WILSON is a senior clinical psychologist at the Muirhouse/Pilton Drug Project in Edinburgh, Scotland.

ANA MARÍA HERNÁNDEZ CÁRDENAS is coordinator of the Women, Sexuality and AIDS Programme, Salud Integral de la Mujer (SIPAM), Mexico City, Mexico.

JUDITH B. COHEN is director of the Association for Women's AIDS Research and Education (AWARE), San Francisco, USA.

ELLEN SPIRO is a journalist in the USA.

HELEN SCHIETINGER was formerly director of the Shanti AIDS Residence Program, Shanti Project, San Francisco CA, USA, and a consultant to the World Health Organization when she wrote the paper reprinted here.

AIDS COUNSELING AND EDUCATION ORGANIZATION is for women in the Bedford Hills Correctional Facility, New York, USA.

KAREN HECKERT was AIDS health education specialist in the Pacific for the WHO Western Pacific Regional Office, Suva, Fiji. She is on sabbatical for doctoral studies.

MRIDULA SAINATH was formerly medical officer in charge of the STD Clinic, Suva, Fiji, and is now in private practice.

DI SURGEY is coordinator, Women Talk about AIDS Project, and is now developing information resources for sex workers from non-English speaking backgrounds for the Prostitutes' Collective of Victoria in Melbourne, Australia.

Introduction

How this book came about

Like many other women, I became an activist in reproductive rights and more recently in HIV/AIDS work because of personal experiences. Women with HIV, women who are involved in AIDS work as professionals and activists, as well as women involved in women's health and reproductive rights work, have long been aware of the effect of the epidemic on women, but during the 1980s were isolated voices.

HIV/AIDS as a major women's issue has only been officially acknowledged by concerned international agencies since a meeting in Paris in November 1989, given adequate public recognition with World AIDS Day on 1 December 1990, and begun to receive adequate professional attention at the eighth International Conference on AIDS in Amsterdam in July 1992. Only since the late 1980s have HIV/AIDS research, public education and prevention and care projects focusing on women begun to multiply. What was growing slowly and quietly behind the scenes is now developing at a faster and faster pace, and there is much more hope for the future.

I decided in mid-1990 to start this book because there were major gaps in the published information about women and HIV/AIDS. What was available in any one country was so fragmented and limited that most women had more questions than answers and were becoming increasingly vocal about the need to know more. I was also very concerned that the majority of those active in the reproductive health field internationally were still not taking the implications of HIV/AIDS on board or incorporating it into their perspectives or work. At the same time, it seemed to me that many women in AIDS work had few links with the broader women's health movement and were not taking advantage of the perspectives and experience that have been gained there.

My hope was and still is that this book will help to bring the two sets of issues and the two, often distinct groups of women together. For that to succeed, an international focus and the voices and knowledge of many women and men were necessary. I started the project by sending out more than 500 letters to everyone I knew in the reproductive health field and to as many groups and organizations whose addresses I could find in women and HIV/AIDS work. I asked them to send me anything and everything that they were willing to send on the subject, and any further groups they knew of whom I could contact. I also began to read and collect published material about HIV and

AIDS of all kinds, for, as I soon realized, I knew next to nothing of what there was to know.

The response to my letter from all corners of the globe was overwhelming. So many people sent material that I did not know what I was going to do with it all, and I began to feel as grateful to those who had not responded as to those who had. The fact that World AIDS Day in 1990 was about women and HIV/AIDS meant that there was a sudden explosion of publications about women. Many were short articles and overviews, and most were national in scope. Some had also begun to delve more deeply into the outstanding questions. Most called for more information.

As I began to put together what I had collected and received, it became clear that I could easily produce a book of a thousand or more pages if it were to include everything I thought was important and valuable. I had to cut a third of my original outline in order to cover reproductive health and sexuality adequately.

I wanted the book to try to answer the questions women with HIV were asking about the effects of the virus on their own health and lives. I also wanted the book to address those who are involved because they are aware of how much everyone is affected by this virus, those who know they ought to become involved and have not yet done so, and those who do not yet realize that they need to be involved. Central to this have been the voices and experiences of women who know they have HIV and/or AIDS.

I decided on a format in which most chapters would consist of a summary of the issues, written by me, with relevant papers and materials by others at the end of each chapter. I also reserved several chapters for papers and materials prepared by others. The process of working on the book has consisted almost entirely of cutting and honing the original, mammoth manuscript. I found I could only summarize and reference most papers and

include longer excerpts only from a small number of others. Even with hundreds of references, two-thirds of what I collected could not be included.

Sunanda Ray became involved in the midst of this process and has had a major influence on the content and perspectives of the book, and on what has finally been included. Between London and Harare, we have worked together almost entirely by phone and letter. Although both of our perspectives on the issues dominate the book, we depended heavily for their insights on everyone else whose name and work appears in this book and the many more we could not include, and this cannot be acknowledged enough.

Many of the people working at AHRTAG also became involved in the editing, publishing and distribution of the book, starting in late 1991. They not only brought a fresh perspective and a critical eye, but almost daily personal support and suggestions for difficult editing, funding and publishing decisions. All the materials received for this book have been donated to their resource centre.

The groups and resources section has probably been the most problematic to work on, and has had the least editorial time and attention. In April 1992 Barbara James and I sent out about 450 questionnaires to update and increase the information we had hoped to put in this section. We got many replies, and when Barbara typed it up, there were about 100 pages.

We had several dilemmas – there was not enough space for the information we had, some groups had sent much more than others, some groups had not replied and there were others with whom we had had no previous contact but whom we knew should also be included.

We compromised by including a broad selection instead of everyone or no one. A thoroughly researched directory of everyone involved in women and HIV/AIDS work and

What are HIV and AIDS?

HIV is a new virus. Much remains to be learned about its effects, especially in women, and there are many unanswered questions. If this book often says that something 'may' be true, it is because no one has been able to show if it is or not. We are having to act without always having certain knowledge. Much remains to be thought about and discussed before it can be acted upon effectively.

On the other hand, HIV is not the first virus in the world, nor the first sexually transmitted disease, nor the first potentially fatal one. All the issues which AIDS raises about sexuality and relationships, women's health and health care, pregnancy, birth control, and women's personal and professional lives were already there. HIV and AIDS merely add a new dimension which must be taken into account.

AIDS was killing women before it had a name and before a cause for it had been found. It had become the leading cause of death among women of reproductive age in many parts of the world by the second half of the 1980s. Yet it was only on 1 December 1990 that World AIDS Day called the whole world's attention to the extent of a problem women had been living with and dying from for more than a decade.

Not all women are equally vulnerable when it comes to illness and its consequences, and HIV and AIDS are no exception. Poor and marginalized women are being hit worst all over the world. All of the inequalities and injustices that affect women's health and access to health care also occur with HIV and AIDS.

However, HIV does not recognize gender, race, class or national borders. Because of how it is transmitted, all of us are potentially vulnerable. We and those close to us may personally be at risk or already have HIV. Given the extent of this epidemic worldwide, we should not imagine that we are divided into those who have HIV/AIDS and those who do not. In fact, we are divided into those who know they are affected by HIV/AIDS and those who do not know.

This virus and its defeat belong to all of us. We can only act once we recognize that all of us are living with HIV and AIDS – for as long as some of us are.

One of the central lessons of working in the international women's health movement is that despite the differences between us, we have much in common and can share what we have learned. We may have different ways of seeing and approaching our problems, and cannot always copy each other's solutions. But we can adapt what others have to offer, and get the strength of knowing we are working for the same goals.

Many thousands of women, children and men have died and many more are becoming ill and dying from AIDS-related causes. To prevent the millions more deaths that are predicted, many more of us need to act. This is a challenge that women and women's health advocates cannot ignore.

What is HIV?

HIV stands for human immunodeficiency virus. HIV is a sexually transmitted disease. Like some other sexually transmitted diseases, it can also be transmitted through blood and during pregnancy. Like herpes, it is a virus. Like syphilis, it affects the whole body, can take few or many years before it causes serious damage, and can be fatal.

HIV cannot live on its own, or in the air or water. People can get a cold, the flu or pneumonia just being near someone who has them. People can get hepatitis A or salmonella from contaminated food or water, and malaria from being bitten by mosquitoes.

People do not get HIV in any of these ways. People do not get HIV from living in the same house or room with someone who has HIV. People do not get it from being at school, at work or socializing with someone who has HIV. No one has been known to get HIV from kissing.

HIV is mainly transmitted through:

- unprotected sexual intercourse, both vaginal and anal;
- infected blood or blood products given by transfusion or injection;
- sharing or re-using injection drug equipment containing infected blood without cleaning it between uses;
- pregnancy and possibly childbirth.

In the coming years, 90 per cent of new HIV infections will occur through unprotected sexual intercourse. Heterosexual, bisexual and homosexual women and men are all at risk of infection in this way. Preventing HIV transmission is the key to the solution of the AIDS epidemic. The rest of this book is about how difficult a problem that is proving to be.

HIV is a new virus

In the late 1970s doctors began to recognize that a new pattern of illnesses was occurring in a growing number of people and that a new type of infection was spreading. AIDS was recognized as a syndrome of illnesses in 1981, and HIV, the virus which causes it, was identified in 1983.

HIV is a new, complex virus. No one knows how it evolved into its present form. Before anyone knew it existed, it was being passed from one person and country to another and had spread worldwide.

The earliest cases of people who died of HIV-related illnesses were identified in the 1980s from stored samples of tissue and fluids. They include a seafarer from England, who died in 1959[1]; a teenage boy from the USA, who died in 1969[2]; a sailor, his wife and their youngest daughter from Norway, who began to develop HIV disease in the mid-1960s and had all died by 1976[3]; and a blood donor from 1959 in Zaïre. Sporadic cases of AIDS in people who had contact with West Africa date as far back as the mid-1960s.[4] No one understood at the time why these people had become ill and died.

'It is not unusual for new viruses to [appear suddenly], nor is HIV the first virus to cause a serious epidemic. For example, the Spanish Flu virus in 1918–19 killed 20 million people in a widespread epidemic, and then appeared to die out. The appearance of new viruses, and the occurrence of new forms of disease, are natural events.

Viruses easily change or mutate, and two viruses may combine to produce a new one.

HIV itself has at least two major strains (HIV-1 and HIV-2) with numerous variations. In the search for a vaccine or cure, it may be helpful to know how the virus developed into its present form, and whether it came from another species of animal. This might provide clues for tackling the problem medically. However, for most of us these questions are not important in a practical sense. It is not the question of where the virus came from, but where it is going to, that should be of most concern.'[5]

How does HIV infection occur?

A person may be exposed to HIV only once or many times before infection occurs. The more often exposure occurs, the more likely a person is to become infected.

HIV has to enter the bloodstream for infection to occur. In the bloodstream, HIV attacks the immune system. The immune system protects the body against disease by producing various cells in the blood to fight it. Among these are T4 cells, whose role is to identify the intruder and to authorize other cells to produce antibodies to kill it. If HIV gets into the bloodstream, it enters and lives inside T4 cells. It replicates by changing the genetic structure of a T4 cell and making it into a 'virus factory'.[6]

In the first weeks after infection, the virus rapidly reproduces itself. Then, antibodies to HIV start to kill the virus, reducing it to minimum levels.[7] These antibodies do not seem to be able to eliminate HIV from the body entirely, however, possibly because some virus is 'hidden' inside T4 cells. There is much about the disease process that is not yet understood.

Even after someone has become infected, protection from repeated exposure remains important, because repeated exposure increases the quantity of HIV in the bloodstream.

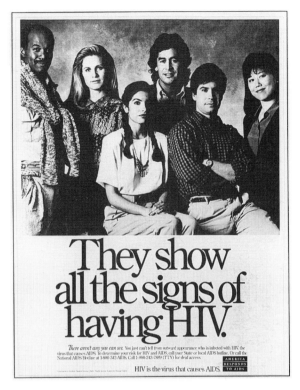

Department of Health and Human Services, Public Health Service, Centers for Disease Control, Atlanta, USA

Do people know they have been infected?

Most people with HIV have no idea when they became infected. Many get no sign whatsoever. Some get symptoms that last for a few days or weeks after infection. The most commonly reported are fever, swollen glands, sore throat, skin rash and aches. These almost always disappear, though swollen glands may persist.[7] Because these are common symptoms of colds, flu and other illness, people usually do not realize what has happened.

Nor can people find out that they have been infected immediately, even if they are tested. The HIV test that is currently used measures antibodies to HIV in the blood, which indicate the presence of HIV infection. It takes from about two to six months, and sometimes longer, for the blood to produce enough antibodies to HIV for a blood test to detect them. This is called the 'window period'. A person with HIV can transmit it to others during this period, even though an antibody test may be negative.

Hence, protection from infection is important for everyone.

What happens after HIV is in the bloodstream?

From the bloodstream, HIV travels to other parts of the body. HIV has been isolated in cells in the gastro-intestinal tract, kidney, lungs, bone marrow, certain brain cells, adrenal glands, eyes, heart, joints, liver, skin, and thymus.[8] However, HIV does not necessarily enter all possible tissues. This may explain why some people get certain HIV-related illnesses and others get different ones,[8] and why women and men do not always get the same ones.

In men, HIV has been isolated in the prostate and testes.[8] It is found in varying amounts in the semen of infected men,[9] in some cases at much greater concentrations than is usually found in blood.[10] HIV has also been detected on sperm cells, where it may be able to replicate.[11,12] There is strong evidence that sperm may contribute to replication of HIV in the lining of the female reproductive tract, especially in the presence of inflammation.[12,13]

In women, HIV has been isolated in cervical tissue,[8,10,14] cervical and vaginal mucus, in the lining of the vagina, in menstrual blood,[15,16,17] and in the placenta of pregnant women.[8] In the small numbers of women who have been studied, HIV was only sometimes found in these sites, in small quantities, and not in all the women.

The higher the amount of HIV in the semen or vagina of a person who is infected, the more likely it may be that they can transmit the virus sexually.

Although HIV has sometimes been isolated in very low quantities in other body fluids, only blood, sperm/semen and vaginal mucus are considered generally infectious in everyone who has HIV.

How can HIV cause illness?

HIV is a slow-acting virus. Low levels of HIV may remain quietly in the body for years and appear to cause few or no problems.

Over time, other organisms that can cause illness will get into the bloodstream, and the immune system is activated. T4 cells are also activated, and those containing HIV produce more HIV. New HIV virus can then enter more T4 cells. This is why maintaining health and getting early treatment for any illness is important for people with HIV.

The more the immune system is activated to fight infections or disease, the more HIV replicates.[6] HIV also slowly seems to prevent the blood from producing new T4 cells. It is not clear whether HIV directly destroys the immune system or provokes the immune system into self-destruction.[18] As fewer healthy T4 cells remain to fight infection, a cycle of HIV-related illness begins. Certain potentially fatal organisms, which would normally be controlled by the immune system, are able to cause illness. These infections are called 'opportunistic' because the failing immune system gives them the opportunity to take over.

What is AIDS?

AIDS stands for acquired immune deficiency syndrome. Immune deficiency means that the immune system is being prevented from functioning. A syndrome is a group of symptoms or illnesses originating from one cause, in this case HIV.

If HIV reduces immune function to a certain level, and/or when one or more serious illnesses related to HIV occurs, a person is said to have AIDS.

Immune function can be measured by testing for the number of T4 cells (also called $CD4^+$ lymphocytes) in the blood. Immune function is considered to be at an advanced stage of impairment when this count goes below 200 per cubic millimetres of blood.

Almost all HIV-related illnesses can now be treated if the resources are available. People with HIV do not necessarily feel ill at all, and people with AIDS do not necessarily feel seriously ill, or not all the time.

AIDS may develop more quickly if a person is exposed to HIV repeatedly.

Does everyone with HIV become ill or die?

Some people have had HIV for more than twelve years with no sign of illness. Their bodies may have developed effective self-protective factors, and they may never become ill. Researchers may be able to learn from them how to prevent everyone from becoming ill from HIV.

The majority of people with HIV do get HIV-related illnesses, and these can occur irregularly over many months or years. Minor symptoms and illnesses are more likely to appear first, but some people get a serious illness as their first sign of HIV infection.[19] Some people get more than one serious illness, and their health can decline quickly.

Unfortunately, all the signs suggest that the longer a person is infected, even if they feel well, the more likely they are to lose immune function, become seriously ill and die.[19]

Different patterns of wellness and illness may occur because certain strains of HIV are more virulent than others, and the virus may also become more or less virulent over a period of time in the same person.[7,8] Overall state of health can also make a major

difference. Treatment can prolong both life and health substantially. Improvements in treatment and care, where available, are making HIV infection a chronic disease that can be controlled for increasing periods of time.

Survival with HIV and AIDS

Studies of the natural history of a disease indicate what to expect over a period of time, how to intervene with care and treatment and, it is hoped, how to prevent and cure it. With a slow-acting virus like HIV, such studies require more than ten years. The information from these studies is also changing as treatment helps people to live longer, and different patterns of health and illness occur.

Very few women have been followed for ten or more years, compared to men, because it was assumed that HIV would act in the same ways in both. Data about small numbers of women exist, but longer-term data will only become available from the mid-1990s.

In a large group of adult gay men with HIV infection in the USA, followed for twelve years:

- Fewer than 1 per cent developed AIDS in the first two years after infection.
- 15–20 per cent developed AIDS within two to five years after infection.

Overall:
- 50 per cent developed AIDS within ten years of infection.
- 25 per cent had symptoms of illness after ten years of infection, but did not have AIDS.
- 25 per cent had no signs of illness after ten years.[19]

It is estimated that in developed countries, the median time from infection with HIV to developing AIDS is 10–13 years.[20]

A five-year study in 200 women in the USA found that progression of HIV disease was comparable to that in larger groups of men studied, and did not differ according to how the women had become infected.[21]

Other studies in the USA and Brazil have found that women survive a shorter time with AIDS than men. In the former, the women lived an average of 6 months after diagnosis with AIDS, while the men lived an average of just over a year. This does not indicate how long they had HIV, nor how long they had AIDS. Lack of treatment was thought to have made the biggest difference to their survival.[22] In the latter, the men with AIDS lived just under 17 months and the women just under 6 months. Women who used injection drugs fared worst.[23]

Factors other than gender may have been involved. Shorter times between HIV infection and first signs of illness, and shorter survival times with AIDS have been shown in African and Caribbean countries in comparison to developed countries. A study in Kampala estimated a median period of seven years between infection with HIV and progression to AIDS. Gender did not influence progression of illness.[20]

Of 123 women sex workers with HIV in Nairobi, all had signs of HIV disease in less than three years, and the median time to development of AIDS was only 40 months.[24] It is likely that frequent exposure to HIV and other diseases, poor health and a lower level or lack of treatment were all major factors affecting survival time.

Living longer with HIV

Once someone learns that they have HIV, they can take steps to protect themselves and others from repeated exposure, seek early treatment for any illness, and take other steps that help to prolong life and health.

Staying healthy longer with HIV is possible. A 16-month study in Switzerland among injection drug users with HIV infection, both men and women, found that stopping the use of injection drugs slowed the progression of HIV disease.[25] Other studies have shown that cigarette smoking, poor diet, stress and severe depression all have an adverse effect on the health of people with HIV.[26,27] Learning of their HIV infection has often been a catalyst for people to make positive changes.

It also makes a major difference if social and psychological support, health care, resources and essential drugs are available. A comparison of two small groups of inner-city women with HIV disease in the USA found important differences in survival time from diagnosis to death. These were related to the kind of support and care they received after diagnosis. The women attending a specially designed HIV clinic were screened for medical and gynae-cological problems, had access to a nurse educator, social worker and psychologist on the premises, and specialist care and treatment as well. They lived an average of about 71 weeks after diagnosis, with a range of 5–196 weeks. The women who were hospitalized when required, but had no outpatient care or support, lived an average of about 28 weeks, with a range of 0–114 weeks.[28]

Infection with HIV is not necessarily an early death sentence, and certainly not an immediate one. People with HIV are living full lives, often for many years, if the resources to help them are there when needed.

Testing positive

by Darien Taylor

AIDS is a woman's issue. Gone are the days when we believed that we lived safely on the outside of this epidemic. We grieve and mourn the loss of friends and family members. We offer support and care. We educate and counsel. AIDS forces us to re-evaluate basic patterns in our lives, particularly how we express ourselves sexually. And increasingly, women are testing positive to HIV.

Since November 1988, a support group for HIV-positive women has met weekly in Toronto. Since its inception, approximately twenty women have attended, some continually, some once or twice. These women have concerns which are unique, and existing support groups, which were largely composed of gay men, could not meet their needs. Aside from testing positive to HIV, most of the women have little else in common.

They tell the stories of lovers, wives, mothers, sisters, friends and daughters, of productive working lives, fulfilling relationships and rewarding studies. Stories of physical violence, sexual abuse and racism. Stories of poverty, addictions, eating disorders and destructive relationships. These stories remind us that the health of most women hangs in a precarious balance.

Most women who have attended the group were infected by a bisexual partner. In many cases they were unaware of their partner's bisexuality. Some were infected by a heterosexual partner from an area where HIV infection is widespread. A smaller number trace their infection to injection drug use. They were sharing needles and also having sex with a partner who was an injection drug user. One was infected by a blood transfusion. A few are not sure of the source of their infection.

Many have chosen celibacy as their response to positive HIV status. Roughly a third have male partners and a similar number have children, some as single parents. In all cases where the woman's partner is HIV-positive, he has an advanced infection. In the past few months, two of the women have lost their partners to AIDS. None of the women has a child who is HIV-positive.

Three women of colour have attended, all of them immigrants. Some of the group members are bisexual, but none considers herself to be a lesbian. Most participants are healthy and asymptomatic, though five have significant symptoms of immune impairment, such as shingles, pneumonia, chronic diarrhoea or significant weight loss. None of the women have died.

At first the support group served the very basic but extraordinarily important function of bringing HIV-positive women together for the first time. Most women who receive a positive HIV antibody test do not know any other women in the same situation. Lacking a community in which to share their fears and grief, HIV-positive women remain isolated, secretive, and fearful. In a society which does not produce or reflect accurate images of women living with AIDS, the support group offers them the reassuring opportunity to meet other HIV-positive women, hear their stories and realize they are not victims but survivors.

Many HIV-positive women are not well informed about their medical condition so they look to the support group to help them get this information. They are often not prepared for a positive test result and have not thought about the possibility of having AIDS. Many do not know how to manage the various aspects of serious and unpredictable illness. They are often not provided with useful or accurate information by their physicians or health care workers, who may not perceive them as 'at risk'. Their symptoms of HIV infection are usually attributed to other causes and they are often discouraged from taking an HIV test.

The mainstream media also contribute to women's ignorance of their condition by representing HIV in women either with sensational accounts of sex workers, which incorrectly scapegoat them as 'reservoirs of infection', or with sentimental stories of 'innocent victims'. Women who test HIV-positive do not fit these stereotypes.

As long as HIV-positive women are not provided with an accurate model of their infection, they will continue to ignore its symptoms and AIDS will diminish our lives unnecessarily. HIV-positive women will continue to seek treatment when significant damage to their immune system has already taken place. If we change the model of AIDS and AIDS education to include women and begin to value women's lives, we prevent the spread of AIDS. For those women who do get it, we will know how to manage the illness better and survive longer.

Women in the Toronto support group are learning about the broad physical and social contexts of HIV and its management and their own experiences are voiced and validated. An atmosphere of mutual support and self-help has been nurtured.

As the confidence of HIV-positive women grows, many have begun to see the need for more accurate representations of themselves.

Some now feel that it is part of their personal agenda to educate and inform various audiences about women's experience of HIV. Some have begun writing projects such as diaries, magazine and newspaper articles or correspondence with other support groups for HIV-positive women. One woman has appeared on television and in an educational film, identifying herself as an ex-sex worker living with AIDS. Others have spoken out publicly at forums, conferences and demonstrations.

Every woman who has attended the Toronto support group, even for a short time, has shown a great willingness to put aside her personal beliefs, moral judgements and prejudices to listen to the stories of other HIV-positive women and to offer sympathy, advice and support. Inevitably, even the greatest goodwill does not support women whose lives are in crisis or who feel marginalized by age, race, culture or lifestyle. HIV tends to bring women together but other circumstances can set them apart. Thus, an ex-sex worker, whose lifestyle is different from other women in the support group, stayed until her drug addiction pulled her away. An immigrant woman who may have felt uncomfortable because no one else shared her language, ethnic background or strong religious beliefs, attended until her childcare arrangements broke down. A battered woman left the group in the midst of her attempt to break with her abusive partner. All of these women faced problems beyond HIV. These are often difficulties that the support group is unable to contain.

Patterns of membership and attendance in the group point to the need for a variety of outreach services for women. In practice, wide-ranging membership is difficult to maintain. The support group cannot be responsible for breaking addictions or intervening in an abusive relationship. It cannot force women to confront issues they are reluctant to face.

For many women, a pre-condition to dealing

with HIV is getting other areas of their life in order. HIV provides a very strong impetus to confront such things as addictions or abusive relationships. But the will to change is not enough; our social services must be ready to facilitate these changes. Yet there are still too few childcare places available, too few beds in women's shelters, too long a list of people waiting for addiction treatment and affordable housing and never enough money. These are problems central to women's lives, made more extreme by HIV. Though services exist to help women whose health is jeopardized in these ways, these services are over-taxed, under-funded and scrambling to deal with the implications of HIV. Under these circum-stances, some women with HIV find it difficult to cope.

These pressing needs of women must be met, before HIV-positive women will be free to explore alternative treatments.

For women living with HIV it is a time of uncertainty and hesitation, of coming to terms with who we are and what we want as women and as HIV-positive women. We will be stronger to demand these things that will help us to manage our infection. We will also benefit from greater integration within the AIDS community and from access to an increased number of groups which deal with HIV in a way which allows women to be included.

HIV-positive women are moving out of their isolation to develop connections with each other and with other people living with AIDS. They are making important and caring decisions about the way they want to live and, should it happen, the way they want to die.

Here are some women who have attended the Toronto support group:

- A young woman, infected nearly ten years ago by one of her first boyfriends. She is currently enrolled in a clinical trial of DDL, a promising anti-viral drug. Her employers have noticed her physical deterioration and are complaining about her job performance. She believes that her job is the key to her survival but fears she may be fired without notice and lose her medical insurance plan.

- An older woman from Eastern Europe whose husband recently died of AIDS at home amidst their extended family. When their adult children learned about what was happening to their parents, they purchased a large house so that they could all live together during this time of crisis.

- A diabetic woman caring for her partner, an ex-sex worker and injection drug user. They live on family benefits and she is responsible for managing most aspects of their daily life, including waking her partner for his medication.

- A health worker with three children who did not know of her husband's bisexuality until he developed AIDS. She arranged for his admission to a residence for people with AIDS and moved with her children.

- A young wife grieving for her husband who died of AIDS during the preparation of this article. Her two-year-old daughter is healthy, but was born since her mother has been HIV-positive. This woman, who seldom speaks during group discussions, has written 85 pages of an autobiography detailing her experience of living with AIDS.

- A black woman from the West Indies infected during a blood transfusion, who was initially told by her doctor that she was HIV-positive because she came from Africa.

- A woman with AIDS-related disease who is an ex-sex worker and an injection drug user. She held a dinner for other group members at her apartment and then never returned to the group. After a clean year, she is back on the streets.

- A young student who tested positive during her first year of law school and who is about to begin practising in a prestigious law firm.

- The woman who wrote this article.

HIV/AIDS-related illnesses, effects on women's health, treatment and care

If someone is afraid they have signs of HIV infection, they should be encouraged to get counselling and an HIV test and/or medical advice. Self-diagnosis and jumping to conclusions can cause a lot of unnecessary fear and harm.

Only a confirmed HIV-antibody test can indicate with certainty that a person has HIV. However, in those countries that cannot afford enough testing kits, the only option has been clinical diagnosis of those who are already ill, using the *case definition* of AIDS.

Case definition of HIV/AIDS

The case definition of AIDS is a list of the minor and major illnesses which, alone or in combination, are most likely to indicate that a person has AIDS and not something else. Its purpose is for all countries to collect comparable statistics on the number of cases. Only people who fit the definition are counted.

Patterns of HIV/AIDS-related illness are not universal. Certain illnesses have been more or less common in certain sub-groups of people and certain regions. The presence of different organisms in the environment in different regions means that different opportunistic

infections may be more or less common. Certain illnesses tend to occur mainly in people surviving longer with AIDS.

The case definition has been revised as more has been learned about HIV and AIDS, and has been modified for North America, Africa and Latin America.[1] The lack of a universal definition has caused as many problems with statistics as it has with diagnosis. To try to get round this, in early 1992 the US Centers for Disease Control proposed to change the case definition of AIDS again, as follows. A person would be considered to have AIDS if:

- they have a confirmed positive HIV test, plus
- one or more of 23 life-threatening infections and cancers that are HIV-specific,
- and/or a T4 cell count of less than 200.[2]

A positive test result and a T4 cell count would give a universally applicable definition. However, not all countries have the resources to do HIV testing and T4 cell counts. In addition, statistics about who has AIDS would be greatly altered. In the USA, for example, it is thought that the number of people considered to have AIDS would double overnight, because there are many who have confirmed positive HIV tests and T4 cells counts below 200 but no AIDS-defining illnesses.[2] Because of such criticisms, this proposed definition may not be accepted and other changes in the case definition may be proposed.

Diagnosis of HIV in women

HIV can manifest itself through a range of illnesses and effects on women's health, some of which are specific to HIV/AIDS and others not. The case definition of AIDS is not enough as a guide to diagnosis and treatment of people with HIV. Certain illnesses that affect people with HIV are not included in the case definition because:

– they are common in people who do not have HIV as well as in people who do, so their presence may not be an accurate indicator of HIV infection;
– not enough is known about their precise association with HIV. [2,3]

Cervical cell abnormalities, vaginal thrush, herpes and human papilloma virus are all examples of these.[3] Although they are often not related to HIV at all, frequent and severe vaginal thrush and herpes were the most common first symptoms of HIV that women were aware of in a large US study.[4] For early diagnosis and treatment of HIV in women, clinicians need to know about these and other effects. Otherwise, a woman's request for an HIV test may be dismissed as unnecessary, or she may not get the most appropriate or timely treatment.[5]

Gender differences in the manifestations of HIV/AIDS

There are gender differences in the manifestations of many diseases, for example with sexually transmitted diseases such as gonorrhoea and chlamydia.[5] There is also evidence that certain HIV-related illnesses can appear earlier or later, or with different frequency and severity in HIV-positive women than in HIV-positive men.

Yet more is known about regional differences with HIV/AIDS than those relating to gender. HIV-positive women in developed countries have been calling for more gender-specific research on HIV/AIDS in women since the mid-1980s. The scientific community has been slow to respond.[6]

These inadequacies were acknowledged in a meeting on research priorities relating to women and HIV/AIDS at the WHO Global Programme on AIDS (GPA) in November 1990.[7] Now, greater awareness within the scientific community, along with pressure from outside, is needed to ensure that the research is undertaken.

HIV-related illnesses and effects on women's health

Effects on mental health and wellbeing

'Once you are told you are HIV-positive, there is no such thing as being asymptomatic. You may not have physical symptoms, but your life is forever changed.'[8]

Most personal testimonies by women describe how much they are affected by learning they have HIV or AIDS, and the difficulties of coming to terms with this knowledge. They question their whole lives, they worry about the future and about what will happen to them, their close relationships and families, particularly their children. Many women become angry with or blame themselves, no matter

Living with HIV and AIDS: psychological adjustments

People with HIV/AIDS who were asked about their anxieties listed the following:
- the risk of infection they presented to others;
- social, occupational, domestic and sexual hostility and rejection;
- being abandoned and left alone in pain;
- an inability to alter their circumstances;
- how to make sure of the best possible physical health in the future;
- the possible appearance of repeated or new infections;
- the ability of their lover/partner/family/friends to cope with their problems;
- the outcome of their infection/disease in the short and long term;
- the availability of appropriate medical and/or dental treatment;
- the possible loss of privacy and confidentiality;
- a declining ability to cope in the future;
- the loss of physical and financial independence.[9]

how the infection occurred. Many feel isolated and alone.

Uncertainty is possibly the most difficult aspect of infection or disease to manage.

Fear, stress, depression, isolation and feeling unable to cope adversely affect physically healthy people, and more so people who are ill or find themselves in situations where they feel they have no control or may become ill at any time.[9] Women are particularly susceptible to stress and depression, or at least seek help for these more often than men. The rejection and discrimination experienced by many people with HIV/AIDS can exacerbate these problems. Fear of rejection can be even worse and often stops women from telling anyone or seeking help.

Psychological factors, including people's vulnerability to stress and anxiety, and their ability to manage these factors, play an important role in determining the physical response to infection and the likelihood of developing AIDS. There are also parallel findings in research on patients with other chronic diseases, such as cancer. Thoughts of suicide are a common response. Actual suicide

is a rare phenomenon – people with HIV and AIDS want to live!

Overcoming the problems that arise is a tremendously difficult challenge and becomes a central part of women's lives. Many women describe the potential for personal growth and change involved, though it is never easy. Fighting uncertainty means learning as much as possible about HIV/AIDS and treatment options, recognizing that stress and anxiety are normal reactions, learning how to manage them in the situations where they arise, and accepting and taking responsibility for what happens next.[9]

'Taking responsibility is possibly a major factor separating those who live effectively and even enjoyably, from those who become wretched and miserable. Many people I have seen with HIV and AIDS have initially felt that their medical circumstances would be from now on the centre of their lives, around which all other issues would revolve. This is not true at all. It might be at times, if serious illness intrudes, but certainly not all the time.'[9]

Minor signs of HIV infection

No gender differences have been described in the frequency, severity or time of appearance of minor signs of infection. However, as women's health advocates note, medical professionals may interpret symptoms in women differently from in men. For example, many early symptoms of HIV infection may be attributed to depression, stress or overwork. Women themselves may not view their own symptoms as seriously as they do the symptoms of others. Often, mothers who are obviously ill go to a clinic only when their children are ill, and may not expect attention for themselves.[5]

The minor signs of HIV infection are:

- Unexplained enlarged or swollen lymph glands in the neck, armpit or groin for more than three months, felt as painless lumps (generalized lymphadenopathy).
- Chronic or severe tiredness, lack of energy, and general weakness.
- Unexplained weight loss of more than 10 per cent of body weight. Women generally have more body fat than men, so weight loss may be ignored or misinterpreted as something desirable in women in some cultures.
- Unexplained fever lasting more than one month, chills and night sweats.
- Itchy skin or skin rash.
- Infections of the skin – fungal, bacterial or parasitic.
- Muscle and joint pains.
- A viral infection on the tongue which appears as white marks (oral hairy leukoplakia). This may come and go and is not thought to be infectious. It is very rare except with HIV.
- Loss of appetite, nausea and vomiting.
- Shingles (herpes zoster virus). Shingles is a recurrence of childhood chicken-pox and is very infectious. It used to be seen mainly in elderly people and sometimes in those with

other illnesses that cause immune deficiency.[5,10,11,12]

Effects on menstruation and fertility

Many women with HIV have reported changes in menstrual patterns, most commonly irregularity of periods.

A USA study compared 17 HIV-positive and 20 HIV-negative women with similar histories of injection drug use. Loss of periods was reported by 24 per cent of the HIV-positive women and 13 per cent of the HIV-negative women. Bleeding between periods was reported by 18 per cent of the HIV-positive women and 6 per cent of the HIV-negative women. Drug use was probably not the primary cause of these differences.[13]

A controlled study in Uganda found loss of periods and possible lower fertility to be more common in several hundred women with HIV. Five per cent of the HIV-positive women had no menstrual periods, compared to two per cent of the HIV-negative women. The HIV-positive women had an average of four living children compared to five in the HIV-negative women, though their ages and other factors were comparable.[14]

A study in Rwanda reported that the fewer children women had, the more likely they were to be HIV-positive, but did not examine this as a fertility issue.[15] A large, controlled, three-year study of women who had just given birth in Zaïre found reduced fertility in each year in HIV-positive women compared to HIV-negative women. The biggest difference was among the women with AIDS. Figures were adjusted to take account of use of birth control.[16]

If women with HIV stop having unprotected intercourse, which is not uncommon, fertility as measured by number of pregnancies will be reduced. This is different from possible adverse effects of HIV on the reproductive organs, which may affect the ability to become pregnant. None of the studies described here took account of this distinction.

Loss of periods, menstrual changes and effects on fertility could be caused by sexually transmitted diseases, frequent use of heroin, weight loss, the effects of immune deficiency on hormone production, or damaging effects of HIV itself on sperm, ova, or the reproductive organs. There may also be an association with specific AIDS-related diseases.

Ovarian cysts associated with cytomegalovirus were found in a woman who had died of AIDS, and this had previously been reported in two other women with other causes of immune deficiency.[17] As HIV disease advances, the number of mature sperm and sperm cells in the male testes declines. In a small group of men who died from AIDS, no sperm at all were found.[18]

Other anecdotal reports of reduced fertility exist. For example, a man and woman, both with HIV, who had both previously had children with former partners, unsuccessfully tried for a pregnancy for several years. Investigations indicated that the woman had ovarian cysts and the man had abnormal sperm. Her immune function was at the lower end of normal, while his was somewhat lower.[19]

Although this evidence is sketchy, all major illnesses cause fertility to decline.[20] Whether and how quickly this may occur with HIV infection is relevant to women's decisions about pregnancy, and more research is needed.

We also need to ask if there are adverse effects on the breasts, uterus, fallopian tubes, ovaries or ova in women with HIV or AIDS.

Interaction between HIV/AIDS and pregnancy

Does HIV or AIDS in pregnant women increase the risk of maternal morbidity and mortality? And does pregnancy have an adverse effect on immune function and progression of illness in HIV-positive women? These questions have to be answered together, because any such effects would not occur independently of each other.

In general, if a woman with HIV is well or has only minor symptoms of infection, has not been infected for a long period, and has a low risk of other pregnancy-related morbidity, few if any adverse effects up to two years after pregnancy have been found in studies in the USA, Scotland and Sweden.[21,22,23]

Effects do begin to appear with longer periods of follow-up and infection, but these may have occurred in the absence of pregnancy. Of 54 pregnant HIV-positive and 55 pregnant HIV-negative women in Uganda, all of whom were healthy, it was found after five years that 41 of the HIV-positive women were still healthy, 8 were ill and 6 had died. Among the HIV-negative women, there were no deaths.[24]

A Swedish study followed pregnant HIV-positive women who were similar in age, clinical status, and immune status at delivery. HIV-related disease progression and increased immune deficiency occurred after pregnancy in 46 per cent of the women. The affected women had generally had HIV infection for a longer period of time, and were also more likely to have an infected child, than the women whose health was unaffected. Follow-up was for a mean of just under three years.[23]

Adverse effects appear to be worse in women of low socio-economic status, especially in developing countries,[25] as with other maternal mortality and morbidity. At Harlem Hospital Centre in New York City, women with HIV are often the same women who have poor outcomes with sexually transmitted diseases, pelvic inflammatory disease, ectopic pregnancy, low birth weight, maternal complications and infant mortality.[26]

Where a woman's health is already compromised or poor, HIV in pregnancy may exacerbate her condition, and this is more likely if previous pregnancies have affected her health, if she has had HIV for a longer time, or is at more advanced stages of HIV-related illness.[21],[23],[27],[28],[29]

Few effects on the rate of maternal complications in HIV-positive pregnant women have been investigated in developing countries, where these are most likely to occur. The risk of miscarriage in HIV-positive women was double that of HIV-negative women in a large Malawi study.[30] The risk of stillbirth was higher for HIV-positive women in one Kenyan study[31] but lower in the Malawi study.[30]

Specific AIDS-related illnesses may lead to complications during pregnancy or birth. The rate of emergency caesarean section deliveries to HIV-positive women in the Swedish study was not significantly higher than in the general population. But of seven emergency caesareans, one was because the woman had pneumocystis pneumonia. She also had shingles, herpes and cytomegalovirus, and she died.[23]

Long-term, comprehensive and controlled studies of the interaction between pregnancy and HIV are few. Most have only included small groups of women and infants, and more attention is generally given to outcomes for infants. No two studies have measured the same outcomes in women, used similar (if any) control groups, involved the same follow-up period, or looked at the same (if any) co-factors. Many have not controlled for age, number of pregnancies, socio-economic status, other risks of maternal mortality and morbidity, reproductive tract infections or injection drug use, all of which can influence outcomes. Many questions remain unanswered.

Studies would need to compare similar groups of HIV-positive women, some of whom get pregnant and some not, with control groups of HIV-negative women. Asymptomatic women with little or no immune deficiency and women at different stages of illness and immune deficiency would have to be included.

Because most women have more than one pregnancy, studies should follow them throughout childbearing. Infants could be followed at the same time. All of this is difficult, not least because women cannot be asked to refrain from becoming pregnant for the sake of a study. It would be possible, however, if global protocols were developed and if data were pooled regionally, so that enough women could be included.

Interaction of HIV and reproductive tract infections

Reproductive tract infections (RTIs) affect both men and women and require treatment in both. RTIs can be frequent and sometimes chronic, with or without HIV.

They include a variety of bacterial, viral, and protozoal infections of the lower and upper reproductive tracts. Most RTIs are sexually transmitted by intercourse. Women also get infections from the use of unclean menstrual cloths; insertion of agents into the vagina to increase a male partner's pleasure, prevent pregnancy, induce abortion, or treat infection; unsafe childbirth or abortion techniques; and other harmful practices such as female circumcision. Some infections are due to the overgrowth of organisms that are normally present in the reproductive tract.

Female RTIs originate in the lower reproductive tract (external genitals, vagina and cervix) and in the absence of early treatment they can spread to the upper tract (uterus, fallopian tubes and ovaries). The risks of upper tract infection rise dramatically during procedures such as IUD insertion, abortion, and childbirth when instruments are introduced through the cervix.[32]

Little is known about the extent of RTIs in women, particularly in developing countries. One of the first community-based studies in a developing country, in two villages in rural

India, found that 55 per cent of the women had specific gynaecological complaints, but only 8 per cent had ever had a gynaecological examination. On examination, 92 per cent actually had one or more infections or disorders, with an average of 3.6 per woman. Half of these were infections. There was a lack of information among the women and a belief that many conditions were 'natural' and therefore not the subject of treatment. Many of the women were unwilling to attend a clinic because women doctors were not available. After the study, 1,300 men from the villages signed a petition stating that they had reproductive tract infections too and wanted to be treated.[33]

HIV and many RTIs may interact and greatly amplify each other:

- The presence of RTIs may greatly increase the chances of getting and transmitting HIV sexually.
- The presence of HIV may increase the chances of getting and transmitting some RTIs.
- The presence of HIV may make some RTIs more serious and difficult to treat.
- HIV disease may progress more quickly if certain RTIs are present.[34]

The following RTIs have been investigated in relation to HIV:

Vaginal and genital thrush (candidiasis, yeast infection)
One-quarter to more than one-third of women with HIV infection may develop vaginal thrush.[35] Two studies in the USA found recurrent vaginal thrush to be the most common first symptom of HIV infection in women,[3,36] yet in the latter study, in no case had HIV been suspected or tested for. This latter study considered vaginal thrush to be indicative of possible HIV infection if it occurred at least four times in a year and two

times more often than in the woman's past experience.[36]

Men with HIV may also get thrush on the glans (tip) of the penis and foreskin.[37]

Herpes simplex, chancroid, and syphilis
These are often called genital ulcer diseases, because they cause ulcers or sores in the genital and anal area, and in the vagina. There is widespread evidence that all three greatly facilitate transmission of HIV, affect immune function, and are more severe and difficult to treat in people with HIV.

A number of USA studies have found that herpes occurs more frequently in more than one area and can be more severe in women with HIV than in HIV-negative women. Some have found herpes to be one of the most common early signs of HIV infection.[3,36,38] One of these studies found herpes to be more common in women than men. It considered herpes to be indicative of possible HIV infection if sores occurred at least eight times in a year and two times more often than in the woman's previous experience.[36]

Chlamydia, gonorrhoea, and pelvic inflammatory disease
Preliminary data suggest that chlamydia and gonorrhoea increase the risk of transmission of HIV.[32] Some clinicians in the USA and Zambia have reported that pelvic inflammatory disease (PID) occurs more frequently and severely in women with HIV, and requires longer hospitalization and more frequent surgery for treatment of abscesses.[38,39] In contrast, a USA study[36] did not find an increased risk of PID.

A study in Zimbabwe found that genital ulcers and urethral discharge in men, and genital ulcers and PID in women were associated with and may have been partly responsible for HIV disease progression.[40]

Vaginal trichomoniasis and bacterial vaginosis
These are the most common RTIs in women. Preliminary data indicate that trichomoniasis

may increase the risk of HIV transmission. If so, the impact may be substantial.[41]

Genital warts and lesions caused by human papilloma virus

Women with HIV seem to be susceptible to unusually aggressive lesions and warts from human papilloma virus (HPV).[38] Three of the many strains of HPV (16,18,13) are also associated with an increased risk of cancer of the cervix, vulva, vagina and anus in women, and of the penis and anus in men. HIV may increase this risk further.[42,43,44]

Cervical and genital cancers

Cervical cancer usually develops gradually over a number of years, starting with abnormal cells and progressing through several distinct stages prior to invasive cancer. Preventive screening, early detection and treatment have greatly reduced the incidence of cervical cancer in developed countries.

In developing countries, cervical cancer is frequently the leading cause of cancer deaths among women, occurring most often among poor rural women over age 35. There are about half a million new cases per year internationally, 77 per cent in countries where preventive screening and early treatment is not available to most women.[45,46]

Many studies have shown that women with HIV have a significant risk of abnormal cells of the cervix, vagina, anal and genital area, and a higher incidence of pre-cancerous abnormal cervical cells (cervical intraepithelial neoplasia, or CIN). Abnormal cervical cells have been found to occur at a younger average age in HIV-positive women, and progress to more serious stages more quickly if untreated. These risks become higher in the presence of reproductive tract infections and as immune deficiency increases.[36,38,47,48,49]

Among 1,060 Zaïrian women, 18.5 per cent of the HIV-positive women had evidence of CIN on Pap smear compared to 6.7 per cent of the HIV-negative women. The risk of CIN increased in women with a diagnosis of AIDS and with T4 counts of less than 200.[49]

In another USA study of 114 women with pre-invasive and invasive cervical cancer, those women who were HIV-positive had more advanced cervical disease. Among those with advanced cervical disease, the median time to recurrence was one month in HIV-positive women and 9 months in HIV-negative women. The median time to death was 10 months in HIV-positive women and 23 months in HIV-negative women. Of ten HIV-positive women with advanced cervical disease who died, nine died of cervical cancer and only one of an AIDS-defining condition.[48]

These findings are a major source of concern. In 1986, based on data from Europe and North America, the International Agency for Research on Cancer recommended that cervical screening should start some years before the age of 35, be aimed principally at women aged 35–60, and be done every three years or less. Screening every five or ten years offered appreciably less protection, but was better than nothing.[50]

Also in 1986, the World Health Organization (WHO) recommended two alternatives to reduce the number of cervical cancer deaths in developing countries:

(i) those countries with the least resources should screen women aged 35–40 once, and try to include all of them;
(ii) those countries who can afford it should screen all women aged 35–55 every five years.[45]

These policies need to be reviewed in the light of the effects of HIV on cervical disease patterns. Screening at an earlier age and greater priority on screening and treatment services are called for. The US Centers for Disease Control and some clinicians in the USA and Europe suggest annual cervical screening for women with HIV.[48] Some clinicians suggest that screening should be done every six months in HIV-positive women, especially those at risk of other reproductive tract infections.[5,36,48]

The incidence of anal and other potential cancers of the reproductive tract in HIV-positive women needs further investigation. All countries need to assess whether their services reach and meet the needs of HIV-positive women.

Major and life-threatening signs of HIV/AIDS

Oral and oesophageal thrush (candidiasis, yeast infection)

Thrush can appear on the tongue, all surfaces of the mouth, in the throat, the oesophagus and the gastro-intestinal tract. Throat and oesophageal thrush can be very debilitating. They can cause loss of appetite and difficulty eating and swallowing, which can lead to serious weight loss and be fatal if not treated effectively. These thrush infections have been the most frequent opportunistic infections observed in groups of North American, Haitian and Central African women with HIV.

A US study in women[36] found that the appearance of oral thrush indicated greater immune deficiency than vaginal thrush, while oesophageal thrush tended to be a sign of even more advanced immune deficiency. Oesophageal thrush was more common as a first AIDS-defining condition in women in this study than in larger groups of men with HIV, and this has also been found in other studies.[4,36,51]

Chronic diarrhoea for more than one month and wasting

Diarrhoea is one of the most common health problems in developing countries. In addition to other causes, diarrhoea with HIV infection may be associated with opportunistic infection in the gastro-intestinal tract. It requires treatment.

In advanced HIV disease, severe diarrhoea and fever are life-threatening and can lead to a rapid wasting away of the body. In Uganda and Malawi, wasting due to AIDS is very common. Ugandans call AIDS 'slim disease' referring to the severe weight loss. One US study found that ten per cent of women with AIDS had wasting syndrome, compared to three per cent of men with AIDS.[52]

Bacterial infections

An increased incidence of bacterial infections, including pneumonia and other lung and gastro-intestinal infections, have long been reported in people with HIV/AIDS in the USA and Europe. Evidence that bacterial infections are a serious problem in sub-Saharan African patients with HIV/AIDS has been reported more recently. The type of bacteria can differ between regions, depending on what is present in the environment.[53] Infections that are usually self-limiting, like shigella or non-typhoid salmonella, can be dangerous for people with HIV/AIDS.[54] Early diagnosis is vital.

A study in the USA found bacterial pneumonia to be the most common bacterial infection in women, occurring in 15 per cent.[36] In HIV-positive women in Canada and the UK bacterial pneumonia has also been found to be common.[55] Preventive treatment can be given.

Tuberculosis

More than seven million new cases of tuberculosis (TB) occur in developing countries each year, affecting all age groups. An estimated 2.6 million people die from TB each year, mostly in developing countries.

The interaction between TB and HIV is making this worse.[56] In Africa and the USA, it has been found that latent TB infection may be re-activated by HIV infection. In some developing countries, more than 60 per cent of adults have latent TB infection.

Studies from Burundi, Tanzania, Zaïre,[57] Malawi,[58] Zambia,[59] Uganda and the USA,[60] all show an increase in the numbers of people with active TB. Among these, depending on the country, between 10 and 67 per cent also have HIV infection. In Malawi, most TB cases used to be in people over the age of 45. Due to interaction with HIV the majority are now age 25 to 45.[58]

Tuberculosis may present in the lungs, where it is infectious to others through coughing, in the lining of the lungs and heart, and other areas. In women, an increase in pelvic tuberculosis due to HIV is predicted.[61]

A previously rare form of TB caused by mycobacterium avium intracellulare (MAI) is becoming a common form of TB with HIV.[10]

Anyone with HIV infection and latent TB is at risk of active tuberculosis. Anyone under the age of 45 with active TB should be considered at risk of having HIV infection.[62,63] In developed countries, preventive anti-TB treatment is presently recommended for everyone who has HIV and latent TB. The aim is to protect both the affected person and their contacts. However, the costs of preventive anti-TB treatment may be prohibitive in poorer countries[57], and in many places, TB has become drug-resistant. Careful strategies are needed.[64]

Pneumocystis carinii pneumonia (PCP)
PCP is a rare pneumonia, occurring only in people with immune deficiency. It can be fatal quickly and requires immediate treatment. Signs are: persistent dry cough, shortness of breath, difficulty taking a deep breath, and chest pain.[12] It can be passed from one person to another only if the other person is also immune deficient.[65]

In the USA the majority of men and women with HIV have developed PCP at some stage.[3] One USA study found that the incidence of PCP in women was less than in men.[36] Even so, in the 1980s it was the leading cause of death in women with AIDS in the USA.[3]

PCP is much less frequent with AIDS in Africa, but this may be because people are not surviving other AIDS-related illnesses long enough to get it.[66] In Belgium, PCP occurred in 27 per cent of African AIDS patients and 44 per cent of Belgian AIDS patients.[25]

Improved diagnosis and quick treatment have greatly reduced deaths from PCP,[67] but up to 40–60 per cent of those who recover develop PCP again within one year. Mortality after two or more episodes is higher. Preventive treatment can be given.[68]

Infections of the central nervous system
Infections such as toxoplasmosis, cryptococcal meningitis, and cytomegalovirus attack brain cells or the lining of the brain and are life-threatening if not treated.

Cytomegalovirus can cause visual defects leading to blindness, weakness in the legs and difficulty in walking, lower-back pain, difficulty urinating, peri-anal and limb numbness, neck stiffness, and constipation.[69]

Symptoms of the other infections in this group range from memory lapses and headache to major interference with thought, emotion, awareness and behaviour, impaired mental function, coma, fits, peripheral and central paralysis, and lack of coordination.

Treatment of the responsible infection can reduce the effects. Preventive treatment has been suggested for anyone with advanced immune deficiency.

AIDS-dementia, the most severe form of central nervous-system disease, may occur in the late stages of AIDS. Treatment for AIDS-dementia has not yet been found.[70]

Kaposi's sarcoma
This slow-developing and mostly benign form of tumour is endemic in tropical Africa, among European Ashkenazi Jews and some Mediterranean populations, especially in older

> # AIDS Attacks the Body
>
> # Prejudice Attacks the Spirit
>
> **One is caused by a virus.
> One is caused by ignorance.**
>
> ## BOTH CAN KILL

The incidence of HIV-related KS decreased in the USA during the 1980s in all groups, while it is increasing in both women and men in Uganda. In Uganda and France, KS has been found to be more aggressive and more quickly fatal in women than in men with HIV.[72,74]

Lymphomas
The risk of cancer of the lymph nodes, skin, gastro-intestinal tract and brain is about 100 times greater in people with HIV than in people who do not have HIV.[12] Chemo- and radiotherapy may be used as treatment.

Inflamed joints
Disease in the joints, including severe arthritis, especially in the knees and legs, has been reported. At late stages of AIDS, this can contribute to a rapid ageing process, a common feature of AIDS in people just before their deaths.[75]

Heart disease
Heart disease seems to be more common in people with AIDS than was first recognized, and may shorten survival time. It may be caused by many of the opportunistic infections described above, by HIV itself, or by drugs used to treat opportunistic infections. A joint US-French study found cardiac symptoms more often in women with AIDS than in men and more often at later stages of disease.[71]

men.[12] In people with HIV, it is more aggressive, covers more of the body and can be fatal. It appears as a purple or red/brown patch and is often associated with swelling. It is a tumour of small blood vessels and can also occur in the mouth, lungs, heart,[71] gastro-intestinal tract and on the genitals.[72]

In developed countries, Kaposi's sarcoma (KS) occurs most commonly in homosexual and bisexual men with HIV. Very few women with HIV get KS. Those who do are more likely to have been infected sexually by a bisexual man. Theories that KS may be caused by a distinct virus, and that it may be sexually transmitted, have been put forward but not proven.[73,74] Women with HIV in some countries in the Caribbean, Central America and Africa have a higher incidence of KS than women in developed countries, but still much less than in men.[73]

Treatment and care for women with HIV/AIDS

Early treatment for any illness, HIV/AIDS-related or not, is important for anyone with HIV, in order to maintain overall health. Screening and treatment for all reproductive tract infections and disease are especially important, both to help prevent HIV transmission and HIV-related disease progression.

Early stages of infection

Women may or may not know their HIV status when they attend for health care. Asymptomatic women who are healthy may attend a clinic for antenatal, family planning, infertility, pediatric or other reasons. They may have conditions that fail to respond to treatment, e.g. a reproductive tract infection, or following minor surgery, or may have a poor pregnancy outcome due to underlying HIV infection.

Management of the majority of asymptomatic patients and those with minor HIV-related conditions by primary care clinicians and other health-care providers is no more difficult than management of the other illnesses treated by clinicians every day.[38] Many people with HIV may need little or no treatment for long periods of time, but HIV-positive patients may require more medical attention on average than others in their age group.

Decisions have to be made about what conditions can be cared for at which levels of a health system. With the addition of only a few drugs, treatment of some manifestations of HIV can be decentralized to a lower level, provided staff are given guidelines, training, and appropriate quantities of drugs.[39]

Women's first approach for care

Few studies indicate which parts of health services women first approach with HIV-related complaints. In one health district in London, of the 81 HIV-positive women who presented for care up to 1990, the majority first went to an STD clinic or drug dependency unit specifically to ask for an HIV test, or had been tested at an antenatal clinic during pregnancy. The remainder had complaints that indicated possible HIV infection – mainly reproductive tract infections, swollen lymph glands, flu-like illness and general malaise – though they were not necessarily aware of the link. They went to a private or hospital gynaecologist, STD clinic, chest clinic, or general hospital clinic. Two had an HIV test prior to blood donation, and one was tested when her baby was found to have HIV at a post-natal clinic.[76]

In Zimbabwe, both rural and urban women present mainly through primary health centres with babies who are failing to thrive, or when they themselves have reproductive tract infections, swollen glands, shingles or chronic diarrhoea. Most do not ask for an HIV test but have it suggested to them by senior staff. Women who go to district hospitals or infectious disease hospitals are likely to present initially with TB. Many women travel to urban centres when they are chronically ill, because their partners work there and because they believe, often mistakenly, that treatment will be better.[77]

Such studies are valuable because they indicate how early after infection women seek medical care. This information can be used for educational campaigns to encourage women to seek medical advice as early as symptoms occur. They also help health services with planning, to ensure that at each level of care, health workers are aware of what kind of complaints women with HIV first come with and which parts of health services they are likely to present to.

Later stages of infection

Patients with one or more AIDS-related conditions require hospital and/or home care. Temporary cure of most major infections is possible, but patients often relapse or require lifelong treatment. Complex treatment is often required by those with advanced illness, whose health may fail unexpectedly and repeatedly. In many cases, outpatient and home-care teams could reduce hospital stays and provide pain relief, care and treatment.

For patients who are terminally ill, hospital,

hospice or supported home care are options.[39] Caregivers at home will need simple training in handling of blood and body fluids, hygiene and how to cope with problems like diarrhoea.

It should be remembered that people may be living in overcrowded conditions with poor sanitation and that the women (and men) who are assumed to be providing daily care at home may well be ill themselves. Some patients have no one to care for them at all, let alone a place in which to be looked after.

Volunteers who support the work of professionals, families, partners and friends have been invaluable in helping to provide basic care, practical and emotional support. This improves quality of life for people who are ill and for their caregivers.

Effects on health services and patients

Everywhere HIV is prevalent, health services have faced major increases in patient numbers and counselling services have had to be developed, often for the first time.[39] There are often not enough trained staff, beds, drugs or facilities.

While treatment benefits everyone except those near death, many poorer countries are having to decide how to use limited resources. Resources are being concentrated on illnesses where treatment is more successful, with symptomatic relief and comfort, as well as psychological and social support, at late stages of illness.

Protocols to prevent shortages of essential drugs for all patients need to be drawn up and discussed widely among those treating HIV/AIDS patients. Such protocols could address treatment, the types of drugs to be used, but also give advice on counselling, HIV testing and diagnosis, and what to tell patients. The committee responsible for drawing up such guidelines should be broad-based, with representatives from hospital(s), surrounding health facilities, clinical officers, nurses and relevant community members.

A sense of helplessness and frustration on the part of medical and nursing staff may be expressed in requests for 'high-tech' solutions or sophisticated drugs and test kits, or in burn-out. Realistic, feasible treatment guidelines and protocols can reassure staff that they are doing as much as can be expected for their patients. Consistency across hospitals would reduce 'shopping' for care and the resultant double counting of cases, since treatment would be approximately the same in most places.[39]

Drugs

Drugs have an important role to play at all stages of HIV-related illness. Many symptoms can be managed adequately and much relief and comfort provided with inexpensive essential drugs. Planning is required to ensure that supplies of drugs for patients who will benefit from treatment are not exhausted.

Specific drugs and supplies, for the most part, are the same essential drugs provided (in kits) for primary health care, including antibiotics, antifungals, antidiarrhoeals, oral rehydration salts, anti-cancer drugs, anti-TB drugs, analgesics, antiseptics and supplies, particularly gloves. The more routine essential drugs are required in large quantities.

Adequate supplies of condoms in all clinics should be a high priority. Condoms were added to the WHO Model List of Essential Drugs in December 1987.

The more complex and expensive drugs require diagnostic, nursing, laboratory and management skills that may be available only at major hospitals. Unless they are purchased in quantities that can be used properly at the appropriate levels of care, the economic impact of the purchase of these drugs could be overwhelming.

The WHO Drug Action Programme has developed a simple computer model for estimating the additional requirements for some of the most basic drugs.[39]

Support and care

Women with HIV/AIDS have multiple and complex needs. When health begins to fail and when there are children and probably other adults to care for, women often do not have the strength or ability to travel from one source to another for treatment and support. They may experience periods of illness more often and be unable to go on working. They may increasingly need financial, childcare and household support.

In Rwanda, discussions with HIV-positive women were held to identify what kind of help they would like to receive. Many of the women were single and had little in the way of family, social or economic support. Sixty per cent said they would not be able to rely on a husband or family. Support from self-help groups, especially with an income-generating component, was very relevant to them. Housing and employment assistance were a high priority for the women who were asymptomatic, though preparing for the future in the event of illness or death was also important. For those who were ill, childcare, food and funeral services were major areas of concern.[78] These needs are universal.

Integrated treatment and care

Integrated programmes have been shown to be the most effective in meeting women's needs.

In Chicago, USA, one hospital offers the following integrated care programme for women: internal medicine, pediatrics, obstetric/gynaecological care, preventive drug treatment, drug dependency counselling and treatment, individual and peer counselling, case management, physical and occupational therapy, childcare support and foster-care arrangements, home nursing and housekeeping support, family support and legal services.

This model is based on continuity of care, active community outreach and prevention education. It is both family-oriented and community-based wherever possible, and provided to women by women.[79]

In Agomanya, Ghana, the only clinic has 35 beds, mostly for maternity cases. There is free antenatal care, a child-welfare clinic and a daily outpatient clinic. Patients pay a small sum for drugs, unless they have AIDS. There was no doctor until 1988. The woman doctor who came in 1988 divides her time between community health and the clinic.

Most patients with HIV or AIDS are women. HIV testing and counselling are provided. There is no special AIDS clinic, but everyone is seen when they need treatment. One day a week there is a TB clinic, which anyone with AIDS is invited to attend, to see the doctor and collect food and medicines. Only basic drugs such as antibiotics, gentian violet and oral rehydration salts are available. For a short period, two herbal treatments from Korea and Zaïre were given as part of a research trial, but the supply ran out.

Condoms are provided free and anyone suffering from malnutrition is given cassava flour or rice. Two health workers make home visits twice a week to people too ill to come to the clinic, and medicines and food are given to them if needed. Health education and support in caring for the sick are also provided.[80]

With training, community-based groups can also provide some of these services, as The AIDS Support Organisation (TASO) in Uganda is doing. TASO provides clinical diagnosis and treatment, referrals for specialist care, counselling, teaches families how to care for people who are ill, makes sure that nutritious food is not lacking, home drugs and remedies are available, school fees can be paid, and childcare support is provided.[81]

Self-care and home care

'The long-term survivors with HIV disease, as of other life-challenging illnesses, are those who attempt to empower themselves and use all the tools they can find to try to strengthen and heal themselves.'[82]

Treatment for some minor HIV-related symptoms can be achieved with simple home remedies. For example, gentian violet may help to dry sores and reduce secondary infection from herpes and shingles.[12] Loose-fitting cotton underwear or no underwear at all will reduce dampness in the genital area and may help herpes sores to disappear. Warm salt-water baths may also help.

Gentian violet can be painted inside the mouth for oral thrush[83] and on the external genitals for genital thrush. For vaginal thrush, a tampon can be dipped in gentian violet and inserted in the vagina overnight for three nights, using a sanitary towel or equivalent to prevent leaking.[84] Precautions to protect clothes and bedclothes from staining are needed.

Superficial skin infection may clear with adequate cleaning with mild soap and clean water,[12] and soaking for ten minutes in clean water several times a day can help. Soothing preparations such as calamine lotion, aqueous cream or E45 emollient cream can be used for itchy skin rashes.[12]

With minor diarrhoea, oral rehydration therapy can help to prevent dehydration. For adults, 750ml of boiled, cooled water with six teaspoons of sugar and half a teaspoon of salt can be taken after each loose bowel movement. Severe diarrhoea requires medical attention.[84]

Although self-medication is extremely common, use of any drug without medical advice to treat infection in anyone with HIV should be avoided. Not only can the wrong drugs be ineffective and still hide symptoms, but infections can become resistant to treatment. In the end, people may become more seriously ill and even die unnecessarily.

Diet and nutrition

It is important to maintain both health and weight with HIV infection. A balanced diet with emphasis on foods high in both protein and calories is generally recommended. Protection against infection-causing bacteria in food and water is important for people with HIV/AIDS. Water should be boiled if it is not clean, and food should be protected from contamination. Handwashing is suggested before eating and preparing food and cooking, and eating areas should be kept clean.

HIV infection may cause vitamin and mineral deficiencies, even in people with a healthy diet. Taking a single multi-vitamin/mineral tablet may be useful, but is not a substitute for food. It should be considered only if vitamins are free or affordable in addition to food.

Although studies are lacking, there is no evidence to support taking large doses of any specific vitamins or minerals without medical advice. Individuals may have specific needs, e.g. women with anaemia will require iron and folate supplements.

People with symptomatic illness may have vomiting, difficulty eating or swallowing or may eat less because of lack of appetite, illness or the adverse effects of medication. People should eat what they like best to help overcome this.

For loss of appetite, small, frequent meals may help. High-calorie foods, frequent snacks and nutritious liquids are all suggested. For nausea, small meals and eating slowly can help. Fluids taken in small amounts can help against vomiting. For sore mouth or nausea, a straw may make swallowing easier. For diarrhoea, plenty of fluids should be drunk in small, frequent amounts and eating continued.[85,86]

The role of traditional healers

Many people in developing countries go to traditional healers first if they feel ill. Reliable practitioners of traditional medicine do not claim to be able to cure AIDS or prevent HIV-related illness, but they do help people come to terms with illness by giving spiritual comfort. In many African cultures, illness is blamed on disharmony among ancestral spirits. Rituals that appease those spirits may not cure the illness, but will satisfy patients and their families that the correct measures have been taken, allowing acceptance and support for the patient by the family.

Traditional healers can give health and hygiene education, recommend condom use, and give preparations that may help someone to feel better psychologically. They can also encourage anyone with symptoms of HIV infection to see a doctor. Cooperation between traditional healers and health services will greatly benefit the people with HIV who rely on both, as with other illness.

Alternative and holistic treatment

Treatments such as homoeopathy and acupuncture, which have biomedical effects, may also be helpful to people with HIV/AIDS. More research into their use is needed, so that any effective treatments can be made widely available in tandem with other medical care.

'Holistic medicine emphasizes the integrity and inter-relatedness of mind, body and spirit, and the body's innate ability to heal itself. From this perspective, restoring health is not so much a process of destroying invading organisms as of strengthening the individual's resistance and recuperative ability from within, so that disease cannot maintain a foothold.

From a holistic point of view, any infection can be considered opportunistic, because it takes advantage of a weakened body. Symptoms are seen as the manifestations, however unpleasant, of how the body is trying to heal itself. Prevention and treatment are parts of a continuum. Ideally, disease is prevented before it occurs. If disease occurs, it is treated non-invasively by assisting the body to throw it off.

The alternative therapies available for treating AIDS are frequently the same or overlap with those used for other chronic disorders, because holistic medicine is basically not disease-specific. Instead, it is specific to the individual.

Holistic treatments are based primarily on indigenous healing traditions, such as Ayurvedic medicine; traditional Chinese treatments such as acupuncture; traditional Tibetan and Islamic medicine; African, Native American and European herbology and their eighteenth- and nineteenth-century offshoots of homoeopathy and naturopathy; and chiropractic.

These offer both comprehensive, individualized treatment and the use of specific techniques and substances to treat particular conditions. Attention to nutrition, stress reduction, mind-body connection through meditation or other techniques, and exercise and other health-promoting techniques are also often involved.

While the World Health Organization has emphasized the importance of investigating such traditional therapies as treatments for HIV/AIDS,[87] the response of the medical establishment is very slow. One problem is the difficulty of assessing the multiple treatment protocols used by holistic practitioners through standard research methods such as controlled double-blind studies. A more useful type of research methodology that is gaining scientific support is called outcomes research.

Some holistic practitioners are not waiting for official support, but are conducting their own clinical trials. In a study in Zaïre, two groups of men and women with HIV were given conventional drug therapy, but one group was given concurrent homeopathic treatment. The group receiving both treatments fared much better.[88] This and other studies have shown that people experience weight gain, a decrease in opportunistic infections, and decrease in or resolution of symptoms such as night sweats, fatigue, chronic diarrhoea, skin rashes, respiratory infections and gastro-intestinal problems with these therapies.[89]

Alternative and holistic therapies remain a controversial medical issue in many countries. They are rarely offered in tandem with western medicine nor covered by medical or health insurance, whether state or private. It remains up to individual practitioners to treat people, and where possible to treat low-income patients on a low or sliding-scale basis. In these circumstances, these therapies remain restricted mainly to the privileged and knowledgeable few.'[82]

Anti-HIV drugs

The search by people with HIV and AIDS for cures of all kinds has been intense. Many can not afford it and false hopes have been created. There is no vaccine against HIV nor drugs that specifically target HIV, though many are being investigated.

People with HIV and AIDS have organized in the USA and Europe to demand entry into drug trials at earlier stages and in larger numbers, and have called for drugs to be made available more quickly than set protocols normally permitted. In the USA, this has led in some cases to protocols being altered. It requires great care to try to accommodate people's needs and still protect the value of information obtained in trials.

Zidovudine, commonly called AZT, was originally developed for treating cancer. It kills but does not specifically target HIV. In 1986, AZT was shown to make the T4 cell count rise for up to six months, improve wellbeing, lead to weight gain, decrease the frequency and severity of opportunistic infections, and increase survival time in those with advanced immune deficiency. In developed countries, zidovudine began to be widely prescribed in high doses for people with advanced disease.[90]

With more advanced disease, the advantages of AZT usually outweigh the disadvantages. AZT in high doses could have serious adverse effects: nausea, vomiting, diarrhoea, insomnia and headaches for up to six weeks after it is started, damage to vital organs, and anaemia, which, if severe, requires regular blood transfusion. Regular attendance at a specialist clinic for monitoring was required.

Now, much lower doses are being given. These are equally effective, cost less and greatly reduce adverse effects, though regular monitoring is still needed. If someone finds that the drug makes them feel worse instead of better, they can stop taking it.

In developed countries zidovudine is now prescribed more widely, in some cases to any HIV-positive patient who wants it. Others have been more cautious, as trials in those with no or minor signs of infection have so far given short-term results only.

HIV develops a resistance to zidovudine in most people with symptomatic disease who have taken it for six months or more. In asymptomatic people, this also occurs but more slowly. If people who are well take it for several years, it may be of no use to them once they begin to get ill and side effects in someone who feels healthy are not desirable.[91]

However, zidovudine has been found to delay progression to AIDS and delay a fall in T4-cell counts in people who are asymptomatic or have early signs of infection. Delays in progression to AIDS and improved survival time in people who had started zidovudine by the time an AIDS-defining illness was diagnosed have both been found. Other treatment, especially preventive treatment against PCP, was also thought to be important.[92,93,94]

Zidovudine appears to be as helpful for women as for men. Imperfect though it may be, its beneficial effects have become more impressive as data has accumulated.[95]

Very few women have been recruited to participate in zidovudine or anti-HIV drug trials to date. Three reasons have been given: the drugs were initially contra-indicated in pregnancy because of potentially toxic effects on the foetus; researchers said they did not have access to women with HIV/AIDS; and effects in women were assumed to be the same as in men. Some researchers are now actively recruiting women, and women with HIV and AIDS are being encouraged to volunteer for trials.

Researchers have begun to ask whether non-toxic doses of zidovudine and other drugs during pregnancy could help to protect a foetus from infection or at least delay HIV-related illness in an infected infant. There are no firm answers yet. Two Italian studies involving fewer than ten pregnant women each found that toxic effects of AZT in the infants did not occur or were moderate and reversible, including anaemia. Rate of infection needed longer follow-up.[96]

Anecdotal reports from the USA indicate that some doctors offer zidovudine to pregnant women with advanced illness in order to prolong the women's lives, not knowing whether the foetus may be damaged as a result. In spite of fear of criticism from the anti-abortion lobby, this ought to be done openly so that knowledge could be gained to help pregnant women with HIV/AIDS and their babies.[97]

A range of other drugs that kill HIV are in the development and trial stages of research. A drug called DDI (didanosine) has been licensed in some countries, as an alternative for people who cannot tolerate zidovudine.[10]

Zidovudine and DDI are both very expensive, though DDI is somewhat cheaper than zidovudine. Their cost, and the resources needed to monitor them and treat adverse effects, prevent the vast majority of people from having access to them.

The future

The many people who have made themselves available for the trials and studies described here and in so many publications deserve acknowledgement and thanks for making it possible for everyone to benefit.

Research to find a vaccine that can prevent HIV infection or a targeted drug that can kill HIV with fewer adverse effects is going on all over the world. There is continuing hope that researchers will find better alternatives or the vaccine everyone is waiting for. Each year, this looks more possible as more is learned about HIV.

The biggest priority globally is to make preventive and curative treatment available to people with HIV/AIDS in developing countries, who are bearing the brunt of this epidemic and benefiting least from existing knowledge, research and treatment.

The costs of reproductive tract infections in women

by Judith Wasserheit

Some of the most commonly cited reasons given by the international health community for not addressing reproductive tract infections (RTIs) are:

- they are not fatal;
- they are too expensive and too complicated to treat;
- they are related to sexual behaviour, which is very difficult to study and to change;
- they are likely to stigmatize programmes.

These arguments reflect the perception that the individuals at risk for RTIs are primarily relatively small numbers of sexually promiscuous women, such as prostitutes, rather than significant numbers of the general population of sexually active women. I would like to challenge these perceptions.

Biomedical costs

The diagram below provides an overview of the biomedical costs of RTIs in women. Either directly, or through the development of upper tract infection, lower tract RTIs cause numerous, potentially devastating outcomes. These occur in both industrialized and developing countries. In the latter, because of

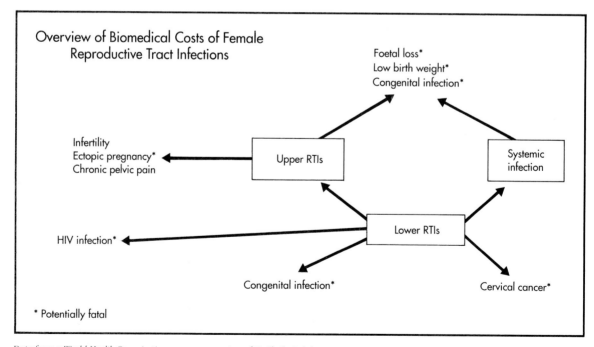

Data from a World Health Organisation summary, courtesy of Dr Sheila Lukehart

cultural barriers to seeking care for RTIs, lack of availability of care, and because of antibiotic resistance patterns, these outcomes are more common yet. In view of the impression that RTIs are not fatal, I want to emphasize that six of the eight complications of RTIs shown here can result in death, particularly in the developing world.

If we are concerned about the quality of life and productivity of women, then the impact of non-fatal outcomes such as infertility must be considered along with the impact of cervical cancer, foetal loss or HIV infection.

In non-pregnant women, the complications of pelvic inflammatory disease (PID) are frequent and usually irreversible. In Western countries, infertility occurs in 17 to 25 per cent of women following PID, and a potentially ectopic pregnancy is six to ten times as common in this group as among women who have never had upper tract infection. Chronic pelvic pain and recurrent infection each develop in roughly 20 per cent of women who have had pelvic infection.

In pregnant women, both sexually transmitted and endogenous pathogens may play a role in foetal loss, low birth weight, and congenital infection in infants. The impact of infection on pregnancy depends on the organism involved, the stage of gestation during which infection occurs, and how chronic the infection is.

Foetal loss occurs in as many as 25 to 50 per cent of pregnancies in acutely infected women. Low birth weight or prematurity complicates roughly 25 to 50 per cent of acutely infected pregnancies. This means, for example, that women with acute chlamydial or gonoccocal infection are three to five times as likely to deliver a low birth weight or premature infant as are uninfected women.

Congenital or peripartum infection of the infant may result in transient illness, permanent disability or neonatal death. Vertical transmission occurs in approximately 30–70 per cent of mothers infected with common reproductive tract pathogens.

Current evidence also suggests that human papilloma virus infection (subtypes 16, 18 and 31) of the cervix is associated with at least a three- to ten-fold increased risk of cervical neoplasia.

Finally, data continue to demonstrate an association between those RTIs that result in breaks in epithelial barriers or that elicit strong inflammatory responses and an increased risk of transmission of HIV.

Psychological, societal and economic costs

In much of the developing world a woman's status within her family and her community remains tied to her role as a wife and mother. In such a context, the impact of RTIs goes far beyond the biomedical consequences.

The societal costs may include an impact on use of birth control. RTIs may create the perception of a contraceptive side effect as well as a fear of limiting fertility in the face of possible infertility resulting from complications. In either case, one might argue that care for RTIs is an essential component for the success of family planning programmes, rather than stigmatizing them.

As for the economic costs, treatment of RTIs need not be expensive. In fact, particularly in resource-poor settings, public health planners too often forget that the most efficacious, least expensive treatment for upper tract infection, infertility and ectopic pregnancy is timely diagnosis and treatment of lower tract infections.

Few data are currently available estimating days lost from work, potential years of reproductive life lost, or annual comprehensive costs for these diseases in the Third World. But they are judged to be very substantial for the individual and the health system.

Prevalence of RTIs in developing countries

These infections are common in most of the developing countries in which they have been investigated. Although data are much more limited for Asia and Latin America than for Africa, in general the prevalence of each infection is greater in African women studied. Little is known about the prevalence of chlamydia or bacterial vaginosis, despite their severe consequences.

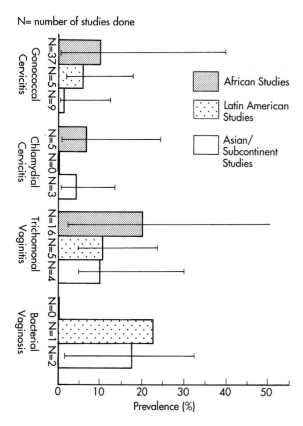

Median Prevalence of Lower RTIs Among Non-Prostitute, Non-STD Populations of Third World Women by Continent

N= number of studies done

Genital ulcers are also common in non-STD clinic populations in much of the developing world. The following table, for example, shows the prevalence of syphilis in antenatal popula-

tions in Africa. It is estimated that, at a prevalence of 10 per cent, between 1 in 20 and 1 in 12 pregnancies that survive beyond 12 weeks will result in foetal death or the birth of an infant with syphilis.

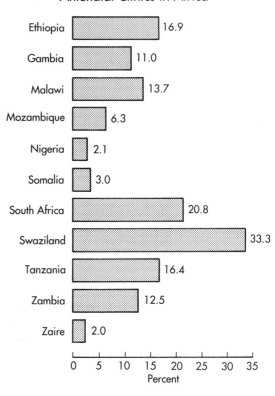

Syphilis Seroprevalence* in Antenatal Clinics in Africa

Ethiopia	16.9
Gambia	11.0
Malawi	13.7
Mozambique	6.3
Nigeria	2.1
Somalia	3.0
South Africa	20.8
Swaziland	33.3
Tanzania	16.4
Zambia	12.5
Zaire	2.0

*TPHA/FTA –abs

Data from a World Health Organisation summary, courtesy of Dr Sheila Lukehart

In spite of the importance of the sequelae of these infections, especially those that lead to upper tract infection, very few prevalence studies have been done worldwide.

There is a terrific amount of work to be done, including social action and education, modifications in ongoing primary health care, family planning, maternal and child health and STD/HIV programmes, as well as technology development and research.

HIV infection in North American women: experience with 200 cases and a review of the literature

by Charles C. J. Carpenter, Kenneth Mayer, Michael Stein,
Bryan Leibman, Alvan Fisher and Theresa C. Fiore

This study took place in Rhode Island, a northeastern state of the USA with a relatively high incidence of HIV infection in women. It looked at the natural history of infection, clinical manifestations and social aspects of having HIV for women. Two hundred women participated for a period of 12 to 60 months between 1986 and the end of 1990.

As in other parts of the country, black, Hispanic and Native American women were disproportionately affected by HIV and AIDS. Among the women in this study, 53 per cent were white, 28 per cent black, 16 per cent Hispanic and 2 per cent Native American. The mean age at diagnosis was 33 years, and 94 per cent of the women were between 17 and 40 years old.

Source of infection

Sixty-three per cent of the women had a history of injection drug use. All of them had shared needles with between 3 and 500 people. The sex workers had had a median number of 5,000 clients/partners since 1978. All of the sex workers except one had a history of injection drug use. Ninety-four per cent of the sex workers had been in prison because of drug use and/or sex work.

Overall, 35 per cent of the women became HIV positive through heterosexual intercourse. Hispanic women were the most likely to be sexually infected by male partners. But the proportion of women infected through sex with male partners rose from 23 per cent at the start of the study to 60 per cent by the end, making heterosexual transmission an increasingly important route of infection.

The women infected through sex with male partners had had a median number of only three sexual partners since 1978. Their number of partners was no different from women in the general population. Seventy per cent of the women infected heterosexually, and 33 per cent of the women infected through injection drug use, were in stable relationships and were monogamous. Other studies have shown a similar pattern. Hence, it was not the number of partners, but a monogamous relationship with an already infected partner that put most of the women infected sexually at risk.

Seeking diagnosis

Of the 200 women, 168 perceived that they were at risk and requested HIV testing for themselves. Most of the others had had mandatory tests on entry to prison or as a requirement for starting methadone treatment. The majority of the women entering the study in 1989–90 were still asymptomatic when they were tested, more than those entering in previous years. This is a positive indication that community educational efforts about HIV are increasingly reaching women. Women drug users were more likely to be asymptomatic at the time of diagnosis than women infected sexually.

Clinical manifestations

Of the 117 women who developed HIV-related symptoms either before entering the study or after, thirty-eight per cent had recurrent vaginal thrush as the most common initial clinical sign of HIV. Yet in no case did thrush prompt HIV testing. Because vaginal thrush is common in women with or without HIV, the authors of this study defined thrush as HIV-related when there were four distinct episodes in a year and when the frequency had increased at least two times compared to the woman's past experience. There is similar evidence from other studies that vaginal thrush is a common first sign of HIV infection.

Better educational efforts among both women and health care professionals is needed, so that recurrent vaginal thrush becomes recognized as a marker of HIV infection in women who have no other symptoms.

Most of the 117 women had minor symptoms such as thrush or oral hairy leukoplakia for many months or years before a serious opportunistic infection occurred. Swollen lymph glands were the second most common initial sign of infection in 15 per cent of the women, followed by bacterial pneumonia in 13 per cent.

Of all the HIV-related symptoms recorded during the study, vaginal thrush dominated the list, followed by oral/throat and oesophagal thrush, herpes, bacterial pneumonia, and PCP. Because herpes is also common with or without HIV, it was defined as HIV-related if there were eight episodes in a year and two times more than in the woman's past experience.

Oesophagal thrush as a first AIDS-defining condition was more common in this group of women than in larger groups of men with HIV,

which has also been shown in other studies. The incidence of PCP was much lower than in men. Men were much more likely to have Kaposi's sarcoma. These are the main gender differences the study found in HIV/AIDS-related illness. The authors suggest that this may have something to do with the hormonal differences between men and women, but this is still uncertain.

Gynaecological conditions

After vaginal thrush, venereal warts were the most common genital infection found, but it is not clear if these were more common than in women without HIV. Syphilis was only found in a few women and there was no evidence of chancroid, in contrast to women in Central Africa. The comparative absence of these genital ulcers may explain why the female-to-male transmission rate in Rhode Island is very low compared to other places. Herpes was the only type of genital ulcer found, affecting 20 women, all of whom had previous histories of herpes.

Bacterial vaginosis and trichomonal vaginitis were found in 28 and 18 women respectively. Only four women had episodes of pelvic inflammatory disease, though 32 women had had PID in the past.

Abnormal cervical and vaginal cells were found in 25 per cent of the women and acute inflammation of the cervix and vagina was found in 36 per cent, the latter usually related to other reproductive tract infections. A history of exposure to other sexually transmitted diseases and not HIV alone were thought to be responsible for this. However, these particular data are for only 65 women in this study and may not be representative of all 200 women.

Enough evidence of cervical and vaginal cell abnormality and inflammation was found to warrant annual smears for women at lower risk of other STDs and 6-monthly smears for those at higher risk. None of the women developed invasive cancer, as prompt treatment was given.

Pregnancy and children

Ten women became pregnant during the study. Two had abortions. Eight had normal pregnancies with no evidence of decline in immune status or life-threatening opportunistic infection. One woman had twins, and one baby was born slightly prematurely. Three infants were seronegative, two were seropositive at more than 15 months, and four were too young for their status to be certain.

Of 161 women in the study, 95 per cent had children, mostly two or three each. Four had living children with HIV infection, aged 2–11 years old. Three had children who had died of AIDS. One woman was a grandmother whose daughter and granddaughter both had HIV infection.

More of the women infected heterosexually had been in a stable relationship with a partner and children for the three years previous to diagnosis of HIV. Ninety-two per cent were caring for their own children, while a grandmother or other relative was caring for the children of the others. Of the women infected through injection drug use, only 5 of 102 had been in a stable relationship with a partner and children for the three years previous to their diagnosis of HIV. Twenty-five per cent were caring for their own children, while grandmothers were caring for 21 per cent, other relatives for 17 per cent, and foster parents for 36 per cent. The majority of the women in this study were single parents and often provided the only source of income for their children.

Survival

During the course of the study, 18 women died of an AIDS-related condition, one from another illness, and one was murdered.

Overall, these women are surviving with relatively good health, and at least as long as men, in contrast to findings in earlier studies. Socio-economic status and access to earlier diagnosis and care may be better in this group of women than in others studied. But this study indicates that with appropriate care and support, women need not become ill or die of AIDS faster than men.

3

The epidemiology of HIV/AIDS in women

The epidemiology of HIV/AIDS has broadened its focus in the last decade to include four interdependent aspects:

- links between who has HIV and AIDS, where they live and how they became infected;
- the specific circumstances and behaviours that expose people to infection;
- the biological factors that increase the risk of infection if exposure occurs;
- the effect of social, economic and political factors. [1]

Limited understanding of AIDS in the 1980s

Who had AIDS first vs who has HIV

Epidemiologists were initially concerned to determine who had AIDS first and where. It took time to understand at a global level how fast HIV was spreading and how. The long latency period of HIV was not yet clear. Only those who are ill or thought to be at high risk have been tested in most countries. The vast majority of people who may have HIV are not ill, and very few have been tested.

By 1988, the World Health Organization had discerned three distinct patterns in who first had AIDS globally, based on reported cases of AIDS in each region. These patterns made it look as if only those groups in those regions were at risk. The reality has turned out to be much more complicated.

Disease has never been equally distributed globally, and many factors have contributed to a more rapid spread of HIV in some parts of the world than in others. Overestimations of how many people had HIV/AIDS in Africa before the mid-1980s, and the rapid spread of HIV in the region after that, led many to believe that HIV came from Africa. This not only fed racism and discrimination against Africans. It also caused denial and a delayed acknowledgement that HIV/AIDS were a global problem. [2] In countries such as Brazil, Thailand and India, the extent of HIV infection has only emerged since the late 1980s.

Some deaths have not been identified as AIDS-related, which can affect statistics and the information they provide. In the New York City area the number of deaths among women aged 15 to 44 from unusual causes such as pneumonia, tuberculosis, septicaemia, and rare parasitic infections increased dramatically from 1981 to 1986. These were not seen to be related to AIDS at the time, [3] but a later review confirmed that they were related. Under-reporting of AIDS deaths in men was also found.[4] Under-reporting has also occurred because relatives and others may not want anyone to know why someone has died, to avoid stigma.

In many countries, the actual incidence of infection is still unknown. Governments are failing to do or permit studies, or findings are being kept secret for political reasons. In Pakistan, for example, in 1991 a public health official denied at a public event that there were any cases of AIDS there, although 104 cases of HIV infection had been officially reported and a number of people are known to have died of AIDS.[5]

Information about who has HIV is limited where testing is restricted to specific groups. In India and the Philippines, figures to 1989 show that more women than men had HIV, but only because the vast majority of tests had been done among women sex workers.[6]

In the Philippines by the end of 1990, almost 150,000 sex workers had been tested, compared to only 2,500 gay and bisexual men, 1,000 returning overseas workers, and almost 4,000 blood donors. In absolute numbers, more sex workers were found to be infected, but the prevalence among sex workers was not as high as in some of the other groups tested.[7,8]

The belief that HIV and AIDS are restricted to particular, apparently well-defined, and often marginalized groups, has reinforced stereotypical views and prejudices about sexual identity and immoral sex, rather than emphasizing what is common to all sexual behaviour.[1]

Being among the first to become infected, gay men, sex workers, and injection drug users were mistakenly seen to embody the threat of AIDS and the fear associated with AIDS reduced society's tolerance of them.[1] In Morocco, for example, an opinion poll found that people thought one measure was essential for stopping the spread of HIV – the imprisonment of all sex workers.[9]

Many sexual relationships and much sexual behaviour are not admitted. There has been widespread denial of the extent and risk of sexual transmission of HIV through heterosexual intercourse.[1]

Lastly, it has taken time to identify the biological, social and economic factors influencing transmission, and much remains to be learned.

Limited information has probably been an important contributing factor in the spread of HIV. Certain circumstances and behaviour put people at risk, whether they are young or old, rich or poor, rural or urban, married or single, men or women. Some are more at risk than others. A lot of public education is still needed to get individual people to think about themselves and HIV in these terms.

How people become infected *vs* who they are

The terms used to describe the main routes of adult HIV transmission – heterosexual, homosexual/bisexual, injection drug use, and blood products – have also been used in statistics to describe the people who were infected by that route. This gives an inadequate picture of how they might transmit HIV to others.

There is a hierarchy in the list of routes of transmission, and each person is listed under only one of them. The hierarchy for women is: injection drug use, blood products, heterosexual, and not identified. The hierarchy for men is the same except that bisexual/homosexual is listed above heterosexual.[10] This reflects understanding of risk in the USA in the 1980s. Heterosexual transmission is low on the list for both men and women.

Multiple-risk exposures are not accounted for. People who may have been infected through injection drug use or blood products have sexual relations as often as everyone else. Whether they were infected one way or the other, or both, they will be listed only under injection drug use or blood products, because these are higher in the hierarchy. Sexual transmission may appear to be less frequent than it is.

Effective education about HIV/AIDS can alter risk factors, but because of the hierarchy, changes may not be reflected. A USA study in 1990 found that women drug users were sharing equipment more often than men, but were also disinfecting it more often than men. Because there was a low rate of condom use with their drug-using partners,[11] the women might have become more at risk sexually than through sharing drug equipment.

Much epidemiology has not been gender-specific in the past, and gender is often unclear in HIV/AIDS statistics. Figures often do not state whether people infected through heterosexual intercourse, injection drug use or blood transfusion are men or women. This has helped to make risks among women less visible, even where many women are known to have HIV.

It is also rare to see figures about children which are broken down by gender. Unpublished data from Zambia show that in 1986, girls under the age of 15 with HIV outnumbered boys. Some of the infected girls also had other STDs. Among those under the usual age of consent, infection through sexual abuse is strongly suggested.[12] Evidence of HIV infection through sexual abuse has also been found in young girls in North America.[13] Combined figures to 1990 for cases of AIDS in children up to age 14 in Argentina, the Bahamas, Barbados, Haiti and Honduras indicate that more than twice as many girls as boys had HIV.[14]

Sexual identity and route of sexual transmission are often not distinguished. Bisexual/homosexual in figures refers only to men, not women. Because bisexual men are grouped together with homosexual men, there seems to be an assumption that infection came from other men, when this may not be true.[15] Further, there is an implicit assumption that homosexual men may transmit HIV only to other men. Yet a large minority of men who identify as homosexual, sometimes have sex with women. And men who identify as heterosexual sometimes have sex with other men.[16]

Neither homosexuality nor bisexuality is openly acknowledged in the majority of countries. Transmission by these routes may be underestimated in all regions. In Haiti, for example, a high proportion of early AIDS patients were not open about having homosexual relationships. They identified themselves as heterosexual, partly because of cultural taboos and partly out of fear of difficulties with the US authorities, where homosexuality is an excludable category under immigration laws. Many were sex workers catering for gay clients from North America and Europe, some of whom had HIV. Many also had women sexual partners and the rapid spread of HIV to Haitian women was the result.[17]

Lesbians have been among the most invisible as women who may be at risk. In the USA, 79 women with AIDS to 1990 identified themselves as lesbians. Of these, 75 got HIV through injection drug use and 4 through blood transfusion. Of 103 women who identified themselves as bisexual, 79 per cent were injection drug users, 16 per cent had had male sexual partners with HIV or at high risk of HIV infection, and 4 per cent had histories of blood transfusion.[18] These figures are not published. Because sexual transmission between lesbians is rare, lesbian and bisexual women with HIV have been listed under heterosexual or other transmission categories. In most countries, such information will not be recorded at all.

How these shortcomings have affected women

Epidemiological descriptions of HIV/AIDS in women have suffered from a contradictory mix of too much and too little visibility of women, to women's detriment.

The stereotype of the good woman and the bad woman have heavily influenced public thinking about women and HIV. Because high rates of infection in women sex workers have been found in some countries, it has been thought that infection is concentrated in sex workers, though much of the evidence is to the contrary. For example, The first recorded AIDS case in Nigeria was a 13-year-old girl.[19] The first woman diagnosed with AIDS in Mexico was a 52-year-old housewife. Her only known risk behaviour was having unprotected sexual intercourse with her husband.[20]

Many people consider HIV to be a 'promiscuous women's disease', along with all sexually transmitted diseases,[8,9] particularly men who are looking for someone else to blame. Early AIDS posters warn men to beware of 'those women', as posters have done in the past with regard to other sexually transmitted diseases, e.g. during the last World War.[21]

Few questions have been asked about who infected women sex workers to begin with. Studies of HIV in sex workers usually fail to ask whether they got HIV from their clients, their partners, sharing of injection drug equipment or a transfusion, though these have all been found to occur in significant numbers. And it is rarely acknowledged that the men who have

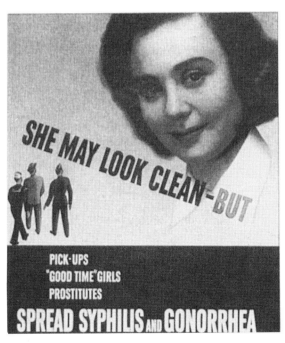

World War II poster USA once more explicitly blaming women

National Library of Medicine, USA

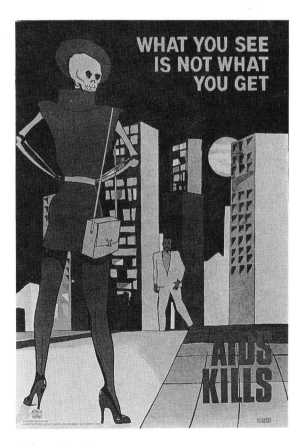

Aids poster, Kenya

Rob Cousins, Panos Pictures, London

infected sex workers are also likely to put their other partners at risk.

Stereotypes continue to prevail in many places. Although the extent of HIV among women who are not sex workers is known, many education and prevention efforts have not focused on women generally.

Much concern centres on the risk to infants. Although most women get their infection from men, it is women and not their male partners who have been seen as the source of pregnancy-related infection of infants. Studies in infants rarely indicate whether fathers are also infected. Women often learn they have HIV during or after pregnancy. Thus, women's partners and their partners' families, previously unaware of the man's own infection, often blame the woman for infecting him as well as the infant.

As a result of all these factors, women are often held responsible for spreading HIV, whether as sex workers, wives and sexual partners, or mothers. Preventing women from transmitting HIV has often had higher priority in policy and programmes than preventing women from getting HIV.

Epidemiology of HIV/AIDS in women

Women become infected with HIV through all the known routes of transmission. Women are most at risk through unprotected sexual intercourse with an infected man – whether vaginal or anal; whether with a husband, steady partner, occasional partner or sex client; and whether he became infected through injection drug use, blood transfusion, or sex with another man or another woman. Sharing of unsterilized injection drug equipment and infected blood transfusions also continue to put many women at high risk.[16]

AIDS has become the leading cause or one of the major causes of death for women of reproductive age in major cities in the Americas, western Europe and sub-Saharan Africa.[22]

By 1992 four to five million women in the world were thought to have been infected with HIV, mostly women of reproductive age. More than three million of the women thought to be infected were in sub-Saharan Africa. Five to six million men and up to a million children were also thought to have HIV by 1992.[23]

Table 1. Estimated number of women aged 15–49 with HIV infection by 1990

Region	Number per 100,000 women	Number of women
Former Soviet Union/East Europe	less than 5	< 4,000
North Africa	20	10,000
Asia	30	200,000
Western Europe	70	60,000
Oceania	70	< 4,000
North America	140	100,000
(New York City	580)	
Latin American/Caribbean	200	200,000
Sub-Saharan Africa[23,24]	2,500	> 2,500,000

Figure 1.

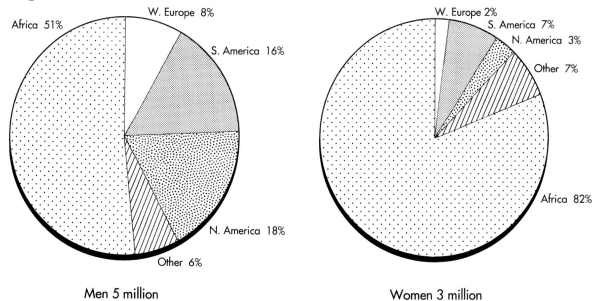

Men 5 million   Women 3 million

World Health Organisation

From Current and Future dimensions of the HIV/AIDS Pandemic, A Capsule Summary Sept 90 WHO GPA SFI/90.2 Rev 1

Table 2. Main routes of HIV transmission

The following are estimates by the World Health Organization of the distribution of HIV infection by route of transmission up to 1990:

Source of exposure	% of total
Sexual intercourse	75
Vaginal	(60)
Anal	(15)
Pregnancy-related	10
Injection drug use	10
Blood transfusion[25]	5

A few examples show just how different the picture can be with gender-specific figures:

Source of exposure in women	% of total		
	Europe	Brazil	Mexico
Injection drug use	57	32	0.5
Heterosexual	27	34	31
Blood transfusion[14,26]	12	18	66

Since 1990, 90 per cent of new cases of HIV infection in adults globally have occurred through heterosexual transmission.[22] How fast the rate of heterosexual transmission can rise is evidenced in Haiti. In 1983, 22 per cent of Haiti's AIDS cases were ascribed to heterosexual transmission. Two years later, this had risen to 72 per cent of newly reported cases.[16]

Sexual transmission has been responsible for the large majority of cases of HIV infection since the epidemic began, and unprotected sexual intercourse is now the most common way women are getting HIV infection.

What does the risk of HIV infection mean?

Transmission of HIV through sexual intercourse, blood and pregnancy are interconnected events. Blood donors, blood recipients and injection drug users have sexual relationships. Getting pregnant can only happen through unprotected intercourse. It does not matter how people become infected. What matters is that risk-related conditions and behaviours exist at community and public level, which makes it more likely that HIV will be transmitted.

Talking about HIV transmission means talking about risk. No definitive statements can be made that are true for everyone. People may or may not realize or admit to themselves that they are at risk of HIV infection. People with HIV may not know they have it or that they are putting others at risk. The overwhelming majority of people with HIV never intend or want to infect other people, just as no one wants to become infected themselves. There are only a rare few who purposely try to infect

other people, a phenomenon of all epidemics.

Most people who know they have HIV try to protect others, though there may be limits on how much they can do so, including the limits placed on them by their own circumstances, by those same others and by factors outside their individual control. There may be conflicting needs that are hard to overcome. Recognizing these limitations and problems is the first step towards finding ways to reduce risk and prevent infection.

Being exposed to HIV does not necessarily mean being infected, as this table shows:

Exposure	Likelihood of infection per exposure
Blood transfusion	> 90%
Pregnancy-related	20%–40%
Sexual intercourse	0.1%–1.0%
Injection drug use	0.5%–1.0%
Other needle type[25]	< 0.5%

The vast majority of people are at risk through these main routes of transmission. The media often devote a lot of space to reports of rare forms of transmission, because of their very rarity. People often become frightened out of all proportion by these, perhaps because rare events emphasize that everyone is vulnerable.[27] This can make people forget what the real risks are about.

With all forms of exposure, although the relative risk differs, one exposure can lead to infection and each repeated exposure carries the same risk. In general, the more virus per exposure and the more times a person is exposed, the more likely it is that infection will occur. Multiple exposure increases the risk. Re-infection through continuing exposure after infection also occurs and may contribute to disease progression.

Social, economic and political factors that increase risk for women

HIV has to be present or introduced into a community before it can be transmitted. The more people who become infected in that community, the more others are at risk, because there is more opportunity to be exposed.[23] The specific conditions that help HIV to spread are found in every local area, country and region, though to different degrees.

Socio-sexual factors

Each year, as the proportion of cases due to heterosexual transmission increases, proportionally more of those infected are women. The increase in infection among women can be shown by looking at the changing ratio of men to women with HIV/AIDS in particular countries or regions over time.

Infection of a woman by a man is biologically more likely than infection of a man by a woman, that is, per exposure and if other risk factors are equal. If men generally have more sexual partners than women, then more women will be exposed to HIV by infected men than vice versa.[28]

Age

Women are getting HIV infection at a younger age than men all over the world, in line with socio-sexual norms. This fact is easily overlooked if gender and social factors are not taken into account.

Women tend to have sexual relationships with men at least a few years older than themselves, whether inside or outside of marriage. In some cultures, men marry women up to ten years younger than themselves for childbearing and other patriarchal reasons. Married men often have extra-marital relations with younger women. In polygamous marriages, second and third wives are often much younger than the husband.[39]

In each such relationship, the men have had more chance to be exposed to HIV, both because they are older and because they are likely to have had more sexual relationships. Their women partners are then more likely to be exposed at an earlier age.

A particular area of concern in this respect is that some men have begun to look for younger partners in the hope that they will be uninfected. They feel that they will avoid infection themselves if they only sleep with virgins, who will inevitably be much younger than them.[39]

Early childbearing and unwanted pregnancy

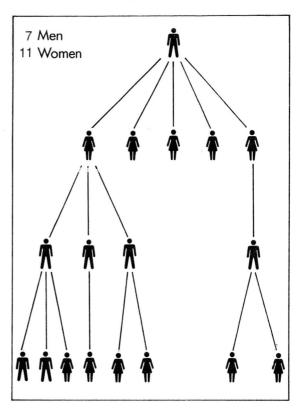

7 Men
11 Women

This chain of transmission could occur in one month or over a ten-year period.

The increasing proportion of women with HIV/AIDS

In Uganda, a review of reported AIDS cases has shown almost equal numbers of clinical cases reported in men and women. In three population-based studies, however, women were consistently found to have a higher infection rate – 1-to-1.4 men to women.[29]

In the Caribbean, of the adult cases reported in 1986, 34 per cent were due to heterosexual transmission. This proportion rose to 59 per cent in 1989. This pattern was recorded in all the Caribbean Epidemiology Centre member countries except Guyana and Bermuda. The male-to-female ratio in member states changed from 5.4-to-1 in 1983–5 to 2.1-to-1 by 1989.[30]

In the Bahamas, AIDS was affecting men and women at a ratio of 1.5 men to 1 woman in 1990.[31]

In Brazil, the male-to-female ratio of HIV infection changed from 120-to-1 in 1984 to 8-to-1 in 1989. Among injection drug users the male-to-female ratio changed from 7-to-1 in 1985 to 3-to-1 in 1989.[32]

Combined figures for Argentina, the Bahamas, Barbados, Haiti and Honduras showed a 2.5-to-1 ratio of men to women with AIDS in 1991.[14]

In Thailand, the male-to-female sex ratio changed from 17-to-1 in 1986 to 5-to-1 in 1990.[33]

Some countries exhibit more than one pattern of transmission. In Canada, for example, in 1990 the male-to-female ratio among the white population was 22-to-1, among the black population 2-to-1, and among the native population 3-to-1.[34] The majority of the black population in Canada with HIV are from the Caribbean or are recent immigrants from or have contacts with countries where heterosexual transmission is high.[35] The male-to-female ratio in the native Canadian community was thought to reflect a high rate of sexually transmitted diseases and injection drug use.[34]

In the USA, the male-to-female ratio among people with AIDS was 9.2-to-1 in 1989. However, a national survey of almost 80,000 primary health care outpatients showed a male-to-female ratio of those with HIV to be 4-to-1.[36] Nearly 50 per cent of adolescents with AIDS in New York State are young women.[37]

In 1985 in 16 European countries the male-to-female ratio of total AIDS cases was almost 10-to-1. In 1989, the ratio was 6.5-to-1. The percentage increase in new AIDS cases in women has exceeded that in men for every year since 1984.[38] The male-to-female ratio among injection drug users was 3.3-to-1 in 32 European countries in 1990.[13]

where abortion is clandestine can also pose a risk for young women in countries where the blood supply is not safe, since there will be a risk of infection through transfusions in cases of maternal complications at delivery or abortion. Comparable risks do not exist for young men.

As a result of these factors, most women with HIV are most likely to have been infected in adolescence or their early twenties, and to have HIV/AIDS-related illness by the time they are in their late twenties.

AIDS prevention education needs to start at primary school age and continue through adolescence, well before women are likely to become sexually active or marry. As one doctor said: 'I would prefer to be guilty of educating unnecessarily than of letting people get infected.'[16]

However, older women are also at risk. In the

Evidence of earlier infection in women than in men

In 16 European countries, for each year up to 1989, the largest number of AIDS cases in women were in the age group 25–29. Of the cumulative female cases of AIDS, almost 65 per cent were between the ages of 20 and 34. Over 78 per cent of male AIDS cases were found in the age group 25–49.[38]

In the Copperbelt Province of Zambia, the peak age of incidence of HIV-related disease in men was 30–34 and in women 20–24. In the same province, among HIV-positive STD-clinic attenders with no clinical signs of HIV disease, the men were on average aged 24–28, while the women were predominantly below the age of 21.[12]

In Zimbabwe, from 1987 to mid-1990, numbers of people infected in the 15–19 age group were low, but there were ten times more young women than men. In the 20–29 age group, 1.4 times as many women were infected as men. Beyond 30 years of age twice as many men were infected. Figures were predominantly from urban areas. Men are often in the towns while their wives stay in the rural areas, but all the reasons why age makes a difference still pertain. Updated figures in 1992 show the trend continuing.[39]

Older women at risk too

'An elderly woman is carried into the clinic by her daughters. She is wasted by chronic diarrhoea which, compounded with severe peripheral neuropathy, has left her unable to walk. She has been tested for HIV but not informed of her diagnosis. In privacy, she is told she has AIDS and that her prognosis is poor. Does she want to go home or come into hospital? 'I will go home,' she says. Should we discuss the diagnosis with her children? 'Are they in danger?' she asks. No. Then she will keep it to herself. And her husband? Well, he comes around only now and then, and she is staying with her elder daughter. What does he do for a living? He is a long-distance truck driver. 'He provided well for the family,' she says, 'driving up and down and bringing us money and bringing us AIDS.' She thanks us for explaining what is happening to her and goes home.'[40]

combined figures for Argentina, the Bahamas, Barbados, Haiti and Honduras, the age distribution of cases of AIDS in girls and women is:

Age	% of total female cases
0–14	7.6%
15–24	24.3%
25–34	30.1%
35–44	28.6%
45–54	6.2%
55+	3.3%

Almost 40 per cent of total cases of AIDS in these countries were in women aged over 35.[14] This is also true in Europe where, up to 1990, almost 35 per cent of the total cases in women were aged over 35.[38]

Migration, travel and social disruption

The extent and pattern of migration and travel – whether international, inter-urban, urban-rural or rural-rural – combined with sexual behaviour, other risk-related conditions and the prevalence of infection, determine how quickly HIV will spread, where and to whom.

In many countries, infection has been identified or reported first in urban areas, but it may or may not have started spreading in or been confined to urban areas. Many from rural areas go to cities or abroad to work and return home periodically or permanently. Although in many countries HIV/AIDS is mainly an urban problem,[8] it may well become a rural one too, as in Thailand, Zambia and Zimbabwe.[41]

In Uganda, HIV spread rapidly in the 1980s and reached high levels of prevalence early in some rural areas in the north and south, due to civil war and the movements of government and rebel fighters. In Mozambique, people affected by war, migration of internal refugees, disruption of society and the break-up of families had almost three times more HIV infection than those not affected.[12]

In contrast, poor roads and lack of transport discourage travel. Rates of infection in urban Zaïre are high, but in the rural province of Equateur, over a ten-year period up to the late 1980s, the prevalence of HIV remained low. Contact in the towns was the only identified source of risk, and was infrequent.[12,41] And in Nicaragua, thousands of Contra troops returning from rural Honduras did not bring HIV with them. Of 6,000 men demobilized in 1990 and an equal number of their relatives who returned, only three were HIV-positive, and all three were among the few who had high-risk contacts in the capital, where the prevalence of HIV was higher.[42]

Some countries have made ill-conceived attempts to stop foreign visitors or migrants from bringing in HIV, by requiring an HIV test for a visa. While HIV has to be introduced from somewhere, any country's nationals may travel and return without an HIV test, and they will be as much a risk as foreigners. HIV cannot be stopped through border checks, restrictions on travel, sending foreign nationals with HIV/AIDS home, or locking up people with HIV/AIDS. The WHO Global Programme on AIDS have opposed such restrictions. These violate human rights, are totally ineffective and usually indicate a denial that HIV is an internal and global problem.

Social class and social situation

HIV has affected all social classes, but not equally, and those affected may change over a period of time. HIV infection will continue to affect the upper and middle classes, but it is also another of the diseases of poverty.[43]

Poor and ethnic minority women are disproportionately represented among cases of HIV/AIDS in women in developed countries. In the USA, affected women and their partners are more likely to be poor, from an ethnic minority and from a drug-using community. In New York City, affluent areas have much lower HIV prevalence rates than areas dominated by poverty.[37] A clear association in Canada between lower socio-economic status and HIV infection among women in Montreal was shown in 1989,[44] and in Toronto at around the same time it was found that the incidence of AIDS was growing fastest in the black, predominately Caribbean, community.[35]

In Mexico, AIDS cases in upper and middle social sectors have been diminishing proportionately, while cases among poorer socio-economic sectors have been increasing.[45] In 1985, some 70 per cent of Brazilians with AIDS had university degrees. By 1989 that figure had dropped proportionately to 30 per cent.[46]

In Zaïre, physicians and manual workers seen at a Kinshasa hospital were equally likely to be HIV-positive in 1984. In 1986, the prevalence among the manual workers had doubled, while the level among the physicians had remained constant.[43] Shifts like these will be reflected among the women partners of these men as well.

Women's economic and social situation in themselves may increase vulnerability and therefore risk of infection. The risk of syphilis and HIV infection in Ethiopian women, for example, was almost three times higher in women earning less than US$25 per month than in women earning more than US$200. Infection was 6.5 times higher in single women, 9 times higher in divorced women, and 23 times higher in women sex workers than in married women.[47]

The future

In 1985, about half the people thought to have HIV lived in developed countries and half in developing countries.[48] In June 1990, the WHO estimated that by the year 2000, 15 to 20 million people would have been infected with HIV worldwide. Then, new information of higher rates of infection than expected began to come in, especially from Asia, Latin and Central America.[14,48] In 1992, about 65 per cent of cases were thought to be in sub-Saharan Africa, 10 per cent in Latin America, more than 10 per cent in Asia, and about 15 per cent in developed countries. Up to 30–40 million cases of HIV infection were predicted by the year 2000, 90 per cent in adults.[22]

Infection rates may have peaked in sub-Saharan Africa and developed countries in the mid-1980s. They will probably not peak in Latin America until the mid-1990s and in Asia and the Pacific until early in the next century.[49]

In most developed and some developing countries there is a lower or low prevalence of HIV infection so far, with a slow but steady increase in the number of new cases. In these countries, people in risk-related situations have a lower risk of exposure than they would have in countries where HIV prevalence is high, and people in low-risk situations have a low risk of exposure. But a false sense of security can itself have consequences.

Articles published in Australia,[50] Germany and Britain, and even in the USA, have said that the predicted AIDS epidemic has not happened in those countries, particularly among heterosexual people in low-risk situations. While current epidemiological data can be interpreted to support such statements, intense debate has centred on what this implies for the future, both for individuals and from a public health education point of view. Do most people in these countries have little to worry about, and therefore no cause to adopt safer sex practices, for example? Will they begin to ignore all public health messages if they are urged to worry about a risk that is negligible?

Is the so-called democratization of risk – treating everyone as at risk – an ill-conceived attempt not to stigmatize those who are definitely at higher risk? Does it represent an underlying anti-sex message?

Or is it better to err on the side of caution, and continue to encourage everyone to adopt safer sex practices? If so, for how long? Many argue that this epidemic is only beginning to show its full face. Complacency can make individuals more vulnerable and make those at risk unaware and invisible, especially women. It can also lead to a reduction in public education and services, and therefore potentially support the further spread of HIV.[50]

In countries with a high prevalence of HIV, public health debate centres on how to accomplish the task of getting enough people to change their risk behaviour in a short enough period of time to slow the spread of infection effectively. While the level of risk cannot be questioned, differentials between those at lower and higher risk remain, creating great uncertainty about how best to proceed.

While the debate in low-prevalence countries may appear to be academic, it is not academic for those already affected by HIV/AIDS. In high-prevalence countries, the urgency is obvious. One thing is clear: rates of infection, whether low or high, are becoming stable or decreasing among people who are taking preventive action. They tend to be increasing where nothing or not enough is being done to stop HIV from spreading.

The global increase in cases of heterosexual transmission of HIV is because heterosexual men and women have been doing least to protect themselves and each other. Protection of self and others is an issue for everyone, not just for people who know they have HIV. There is no need for anyone to stop living fully. Many people are aware and afraid of HIV and AIDS after a decade of public education, yet still have not translated information into personal, community and public action. We need to find ways to talk about risk reduction and prevention of HIV infection that do not make people feel powerless and helpless.

HIV/AIDS in women in Puerto Rico

by Carmen Zorrilla

In 1988, AIDS was already the eighth cause of death in Puerto Rico, and the principal cause of death for women aged 25–34, and men aged 25–44. As of November 1990, 17 per cent of AIDS cases were women.

Because cases are so concentrated, it is not only risk behaviour that places our women at risk, but also natural and accepted behaviour. The transmission of HIV to women in Puerto Rico is changing from mainly injection drug use to heterosexual transmission. In 1987, 28 per cent of women with AIDS acquired the infection by sexual contact. This increased to 43 per cent in 1990. By 1991, heterosexual transmission (58 per cent) had already become the most common risk factor for AIDS in women in Puerto Rico. In a place where there is a high prevalence of HIV, talking about risk behaviour is inconsequential to the young woman recently married to her first and only sex partner, who then presents to us with HIV infection discovered during her first pregnancy.

In 1986, we started a prenatal HIV screening programme in the Metropolitan Health Region. Roughly we have around 5,000 deliveries per year. More than 200 of these women and their children have been followed longitudinally. The HIV prevalence rate has been between one in 60 and one in 70 of all deliveries.

Eighty-two per cent of the HIV-positive women acquired the infection sexually. This included 6 per cent with seropositive partners who deny injection drug use; 6 per cent with multiple sex partners; and 55 per cent with partners who have used injection drugs. Only 15 per cent of the women have been injection drug users themselves.

Fifteen per cent had no risk factors upon interview. What we have realized is that it is very difficult to make a risk assessment in the health care setting. Imagine how difficult it is at the personal level, especially when a woman is psychologically, economically and socially dependent on her partner.

Most of the women are young, and about 12

per cent are adolescents, either married legally or by common law. A higher proportion of seropositive women were single (23 per cent) or in consensual unions (35 per cent) as compared to the control group, more of whom were legally married (70 per cent). Requiring the HIV test for a marriage licence will not identify the population at risk.

We also found a clear association with other sexually transmitted diseases – 25 per cent of HIV-positive women had a history of STDs, compared to three per cent in the seronegative group.

Only a minimal number of sexual partners was enough for many of the women to become infected. This group of women are not promiscuous, do not consider themselves at risk, yet they are still infected. As the spread of heterosexual AIDS becomes more prevalent, this is what we are likely to encounter in the future.

The social epidemiology of women and AIDS in Africa

by Brooke Grundfest Schoepf

In Africa, AIDS risk is not confined to any special group. It is not only a disease of poor women engaged in sex work and long-distance lorry drivers. Men and women in these occupations are at very high risk in the cities of Central Africa. However, they do not form bounded groups. Their social networks extend into virtually every social milieu and along the trade routes to all but the most remote villages. Since AIDS affects the general population of sexually active adults and adolescents, narrowly focused prevention strategies are not likely to stop the spread of infection.

Disease epidemics generally erupt in times of crisis and AIDS is no exception. Central Africa, like most other nations of the Third World, is in the throes of economic turmoil. Per capita incomes are ranked among the world's lowest. For example, in Zaïre in 1987 the average was estimated at $150 per year. Average figures mask wide disparities in wealth. Many families in Kinshasa eat only once a day and malnutrition is widespread.

Throughout the continent, poor women and children have experienced most severely the effects of structural adjustment policies; the deepening crisis contributes to the feminization of poverty and consequently to the spread of AIDS.

Slavery lasted well into the twentieth century and freed women worked for meagre subsistence. Throughout the colonial period, most wage labour was reserved to men, whose wages were too low to support families. Women were relegated to crop production and frequent childbearing. Women who escaped to the cities resorted to petty trade and selling services, including sex. While some were able to achieve substantial economic independence and social freedom in informal sector occupations, the majority were poor. Even following independence, few wage labour opportunities for women were created. At the same time, widespread insecurity, added to labour-intensive production techniques, low crop prices and gender inequality within households made the villages particularly unattractive to women.

Currently, Zaïre's cities contain as many women as men, but women constitute only four per cent of formal sector workers. An estimated 40–60 per cent of urban men are without waged employment. They, and the majority of women who are without special job qualifications, resort to informal-sector occupations: petty trade, food preparation, market gardening, sewing, smuggling, and prostitution. Trade and smuggling take place over long distances within Zaïre and across its borders. Multiple-partner sexual relationships regularly accompany such trade.

The already crowded informal economic structure is increasingly less profitable for many small operators. Moreover, many women who formerly could rely upon steady contributions from male partners or from their extended families report that both sources are dwindling because they too are hard-pressed to make ends meet. Women often seek occasional partners to meet immediate cash needs. As economic conditions continue to worsen, the social fabric is tearing apart and sexual strategies that maximize returns become increasingly important.

The presence of AIDS was identified in 1983. Infection is concentrated mainly in the cities, but is spreading along the trade routes. Not surprisingly, young urban women are at highest risk for AIDS in Central Africa. More than 90 per cent of women whose major source of subsistence comes from the sale of sex to multiple casual partners, are reported to be infected in several cities of Central and East Africa. In Kinshasa the rate among sex workers rose from 27 per cent of 287 women sampled in 1984 to 35 per cent of women attending a new screening clinic for STDs in 1988.

However, sex workers are not the only women at risk. Samples of women delivering in Kinshasa in 1986 found between 5.8 and 8.4 per cent to be infected. Nearly 30 per cent of infants born to seropositive women were infected and most died before the age of two years. Most of the mothers were married. Younger mothers age 20 to 30 years were most likely to be seropositive, while rates among unmarried women in this age group were higher still, with 16.7 per cent of hospital workers and 11.1 per cent of textile factory workers infected in 1986. Most were single and paid below-subsistence wages. In sum, many women of childbearing age are at high risk, as are young girls just becoming sexually active.

Both popular and biomedical discourse feature women as transmitters of HIV. Discourse about women and AIDS in Africa is amplified by racialist constructions of African sexuality.

The first two women described as probably having died of HIV infection contracted in Zaïre were a 'free woman' from Equateur Region, that is, a woman not living under the control of a father, brother or husband, and a surgeon from Denmark who worked in the same region in the 1970s. The contrasts in the implicit construction of these two women's lives in the biomedical literature are striking. The texts and their silences are evidence for cultural constructions of AIDS.

The Zaïrean woman is reported to have lived some years in Kinshasa, where she is assumed to have been a prostitute, supporting herself by selling sex to multiple partners. She then returned to the village, where her blood was collected in 1976 as part of a sample drawn by a team studying the new Ebola fever which erupted suddenly in a nearby village. This woman died several years later of AIDS-like disease, as did a 15-year-old youth. The blood of three other people tested also showed antibodies to HIV.

The Danish woman worked for several years at a mission hospital in the great forest. Since surgical gloves were in short supply, she often operated ungloved. Swollen glands without apparent cause were followed by a series of unusual infections, a cough, fever and constant fatigue. Too weak to work and worried by her inconclusive diagnosis, she returned to Denmark, where repeated tests failed to establish a cause or a name for the mysterious symptoms. Her condition was described by a physician-friend who observed her long illness. The anonymous African woman is mentioned in an epidemiological report.

Juxtaposing the two texts of these presumed cases from the pre-AIDS era allows us to compare their premises. The Zaïrean 'free woman' is assumed to have acquired and transmitted HIV infection to others as a result of sexual intercourse. The Danish surgeon (also a 'free woman' in the technical meaning of the term) is assumed to have acquired the disease from patients' blood. The report is silent about the possibility that she might have transmitted infection to others. Different characteristics, implicitly attributed to the women on the basis of gender, class and colour, emerge.

The resulting dichotomies are Cartesian in their simplicity: white woman/black woman, missionary/sinner; heroic work/dirty work; innocent victim/perpetrator; valued and named/unvalued and unnamed; good woman/bad woman. The possibility that an African sex worker might have acquired the infection from a blood transfusion is not entertained. The possibility that a white professional woman might have been infected through sexual intercourse is not entertained

either. The occupations of both women carry considerable risk. Nevertheless, either of them might have become infected in the manner assumed for the other.

In Kinshasa, not all sexually active people are at risk. Kinshasa includes an unknown proportion of mutally monogamous couples and celibate single people who live according to traditional or Christian tenets. Nevertheless, many types of multiple-partner relationships, with varying degrees of social recognition and legitimacy, exist among people of all social classes and ethnic origins. Even socially recognized relationships may be of relatively brief duration, leading, as in the West, to what has been termed 'serial monogamy'.

Some people report that they have changed their lifestyles in response to the AIDS danger. Monthly condom sales in Kinshasa and elsewhere in Zaïre have risen steeply, particularly due to social marketing. In 1989, they were used mainly by young men in casual encounters. Nevertheless, to effect more widespread HIV prevention there are some persistent obstacles to change which an effective programme must address. The constraints, common throughout the region, include many socio-cultural, economic and political forces that shape gender and sexual relations. Contextualized understanding is thus necessary to develop adequate prevention strategies and interventions that can lead to widespread change in sexual behaviour.

HIV infection in childbearing women in Kigali, Rwanda

by Susan Allen, Christina Lindan, Antoine Serufilira, Philippe Van de Perre, Amy Chen Rundle, Francois Nsengumuremyi, Michel Carael, Joan Schwalbe, and Stephen Hulley

In 1986, a nationwide seroepidemiologic survey of HIV-1 infection in Rwanda revealed a seroprevalence of one per cent in the rural sample and 18 per cent in the urban sample (30 per cent among 26–40-year-olds). A year earlier, the Rwandan Ministry of Health and the Red Cross had initiated one of the first and most effective blood-donor screening programmes in Africa. In 1986, these agencies, in collaboration with the Norwegian Red Cross, began an extensive AIDS-education programme using radio information and public health educators. A National AIDS Programme was established in 1987.

In 1986 the Projet San Francisco was established in Kigali. The goals were to study incidence and predictors of HIV disease in infected and uninfected urban women. An educational programme was developed, and studies of the acceptability and efficacy of condom and spermicide use in AIDS prevention are underway. This study has allowed a detailed examination of risk factors for HIV and their association with partner relationships and socio-economic variables in a large representative sample of urban women. This paper presents the women's responses to questionnaires administered at the time of enrollment.

In 1986 and 1987, a consecutive sample of 3,702 women aged 18 to 35 years who were attending the outpatient paediatric and antenatal clinics at the Centre Hospitalier de Kigali were screened for HIV infection. The prevalence of HIV was 29 per cent. From this group, two smaller representative groups were recruited, about 500 with HIV infection, and about 1,000 who were uninfected.

Most of the women in the study were 24–33 years of age, and 86 per cent had been married or in a common-law union for a mean of eight years. Seventy per cent were Catholic, 18 per cent were another Christian denomination, and 12 per cent were Muslim. There was no significant difference in prevalence of infection by religious denomination. The median number of living children per woman was three.

Two-thirds of the women had no income of their own and depended entirely on their partners for economic support. Almost half of the women had come to the city less than ten years before, and those who had been there for five years or less had the highest prevalence of infection.

Seroprevalence rates were highest among the youngest women aged 19–24 years (38 per cent HIV-infected). Women living with a partner had lower rates of infection than sexually active single, widowed, divorced, or separated women who were living alone. Women who were legally married were less likely to be infected than women in common-law unions. Partnerships with many children were also associated with lower risk of HIV infection. Women with partners with more education and income were more likely to be infected.

A striking finding was the high prevalence of infection among women who had been living with a partner for less than seven years (36–40 per cent). The risk of HIV infection declined markedly as the length of the relationship extended beyond seven years.

Men in Kigali become sexually active several years before they take a wife, and their sexual partners during this time are a small group of 'free women' (often single mothers) who have many partners. In this setting, men may acquire the infection before marriage or common-law union and transmit the virus to their partners.

The prevalence of infection in 'free women' in a similar Rwandan city was 88 per cent in 1983. If the rise in prevalence in this group increased rapidly in one or two years and peaked in 1982 and 1983, this would explain the high prevalence of infection in women whose steady partners had premarital sex in 1982 or later. This would also be consistent with the levelling off of infection for all those who entered unions after 1982. The pool of 'free women' was essentially saturated and the risk of premarital sex could not increase any further. A similar phenomenon was noted among homosexual men in San Francisco, California, where the prevalence of HIV infection rose rapidly between 1982 and 1984 and has been stable at about 50 per cent since that time.

Two-thirds of the women reported only one lifetime sexual partner, far less than that reported by women in the United States. Having more than one lifetime sexual partner and currently being in a non-monogamous relationship were strongly associated with HIV infection. Women with more than two lifetime partners had an HIV prevalence of 57 per cent.

However, the prevalence of infection among women who reported neither of these risk factors was still high – 21 per cent. Although some married women may underreport their own risk behaviour or underestimate that of their partner, the fact that their partners may have been infected before marriage results in significant risk even for women who have truly had only one currently monogamous partner.

Sex during menses, nonmenstrual bleeding during intercourse, and pain during intercourse were each associated with a higher prevalence of infection. (The latter two variables may indicate the presence of an STD and be related to this risk.)

Sexual intercourse near the time of delivery is common in Rwanda. Seventy-five per cent of women reported intercourse on the day of delivery of their last child. This is believed to ease the baby's passage. Forty-eight per cent reported intercourse less than two weeks after the birth, usually as part of the child's naming ceremony. These practices were not significantly associated with HIV seroprevalence.

Eighty per cent of the women's primary partners in this study drank alcohol, half of whom did so frequently according to the women. Higher frequencies of drinking by partners were associated with higher rates of infection with HIV in the women. Increased alcohol and drug use has been associated with high-risk sexual activity among both homosexuals and heterosexuals in the USA. Drug use of any kind is rare in Rwanda, and injection drug use is unknown. Drinking alcohol is very common for men in Kigali, however, and most drinking is done in bars where sex workers are readily available. Drinking by men, combined with the ability to pay for sex, were highly associated with HIV infection.

A history of sexually transmitted disease was associated with a high prevalence of HIV infection. It was similar between women who reported genital ulcers and women reporting only gonorrhoea. However, since much of the risk of STD was related to the behaviour of partners, we cannot conclude that ulcerative or non-ulcerative STD contributes independently to risk in the women in this study.

Use of oral contraceptives was not a risk factor for HIV infection in this study.

A history of blood transfusion, only in women or their partners who had been transfused between 1980 and 1985, was associated with a higher prevalence of infection.

Having a partner who travelled more than one week per month was not significantly associated with an increased risk of infection.

We conclude that the prevalence of HIV infection in childbearing women in Rwanda is high, especially among those in non-legal or non-monogamous unions, those marrying after 1981, and those reporting more than one lifetime sexual partner. However, most infected women are themselves monogamous and at risk of HIV infection as a result of the sexual behaviour of their steady male partners, behaviours that are linked to higher income and use of alcohol. These factors should be targeted in future educational interventions.

The impact of AIDS on women in Thailand

by Jon Ungphakorn

In Thailand, the rapid spread of HIV infection among most sectors of Thai society is centred on an illegal but powerful sex-service industry of huge dimensions, serving millions of Thai men and tens of thousands of foreign tourists. This is linked to the socially and culturally accepted practice among Thai men of all ages and social classes, whether single or married, of frequenting sex-service establishments. However, to place the root cause of the HIV epidemic solely on cultural factors would be misguided and unfair.

The main roots of the HIV situation in Thailand lie in the extremely successful national development policies of the past three decades, which have focused on rapid overall economic growth at the expense of all other considerations, and are pushing us towards becoming a newly-industrialized society. This has had a devastating impact in social, environmental and cultural spheres: bringing about widespread increases in economic and social disparities, rapid depletion of natural resources in the rural areas, and the wholesale disintegration and degradation of rural society with its traditional qualities of economic and environmental self-sustainability, family and community cohesion, and an in-built social welfare system. It has led to the loss of ability among rural communities to survive on agricultural income alone, accumulation of rural debt, physical and cultural disintegration of the family and community, and the forced migration of young men and women to the urban centres and foreign lands to sell their labour for much needed earnings.

Several hundreds of thousands of rural women are now employed in the sex-service industry, which flourishes throughout the country. At the same time, large numbers of young men from the rural areas are working in the cities, often separated from their wives and children. On pay-days, many visit sex establishments. In this situation, the rural population has lost all chance of immunity to the HIV epidemic, and will probably be hit even harder than the smaller urban population of the country.

Successive governments, unwilling to finance any social reforms or measures to cushion the impact on the rural population, have fuelled the sex-service industry by creating a ready supply of sex workers, promoting tourism at any cost, and implicitly supporting all forms of entrepreneurship regardless of ethical considerations.

Our society is presently being inundated by a third wave of HIV infection, with the fourth and fifth waves rapidly approaching. Once the fifth wave hits us, all sections of the population will have become affected.

The first wave of HIV infection swept through injection drug users. and by the end of 1989 had infected around 40 per cent of this mainly male group.

The second wave has hit sex workers, predominantly women. By the end of 1989 around ten per cent of low-income sex workers were infected, with the figures for some areas as high as 20–43 per cent. Infection among higher-income sex workers averaged at around two per cent.

The third wave of HIV infection has opened the door to the general population by striking at customers of the sex-service industry, probably numbering somewhere between three to eight million men in total. By the end of 1989, around ten per cent of male clients of government STD clinics were infected, with figures as high as 10–18 per cent in some areas. These would tend to be men visiting low-priced sex establishments on a rather frequent basis. More indicative of infection among sexually active young men in general would be the figures for blood donors, which averaged at almost one per cent, and reached as high as two to eight per cent in some areas (generally coinciding with areas having a high rate of infection among male clients of STD clinics). Army tests on new conscripts show that around two per cent have been infected, with infection as high as ten per cent in some northern provinces. A disturbingly large number of men have already been infected through sexual transmission.

It is not difficult to foresee the approaching fourth and fifth waves of HIV infection that will strike, with grim consequences, at married women and their future children. For married women, it has become high-risk behaviour to have unprotected sex with their husbands, unless they are absolutely certain that their husbands are not visiting sex establishments.

4

Blood-to-blood transmission

Transmission of HIV through blood is the source of infection whose prevention depends most on the public health services.

How HIV is transmitted by blood

Transfused blood and blood products

If blood products contain HIV, a person can get infected through a transfusion. Most reported cases of blood-to-blood transmissions of HIV have been through transfusions of infected blood and blood products.

Reused injection equipment and sharp instruments

If a needle/syringe that has been used to take blood from or give an intravenous injection to a person with HIV is reused within a short space of time on another person, small amounts of infected blood can be passed to the other person.

Repeated injections are more likely to lead to infection than one injection. Most cases reported have occurred through repeated sharing of infected needles by injection drug users who may share equipment more than once daily over long periods.

A few countries have reported clusters of

cases where injection equipment was reused repeatedly without sterilization on groups of hospital patients.

Some medical procedures and traditional practices using instruments on more than one person without sterilization may also lead to HIV transmission. Only a few cases have been reported.

Accidents in the health-care setting

A very small number of cases have been reported of HIV transmission through accidents involving blood-to-blood contact between health workers and patients, mainly needlestick injuries.

Organ transplants

Organs transplanted from an infected donor may transmit HIV. Testing of donors prevents this occurring.

Transfusion of infected blood or blood products

The likelihood of infection through transfusion depends on the quantity of blood transfused and how often, the prevalence of HIV among blood donors, and the efficiency of health services in excluding infected blood and blood products from use.[1]

This route of transmission has been reduced

as far as is feasible in developed countries and a growing number of developing countries since 1985, but further improvements and continuing vigilance are required. Some countries have only begun to tackle the problems and new cases of infection by this route are occurring and can be expected until problems are overcome.

Almost all countries are opening new blood-testing facilities and moving towards better controls, but not all have been able to implement needed measures uniformly. Rural services may suffer from a greater lack of resources.

Private blood banks are proving difficult to regulate or replace. In many parts of Latin America and Asia, payment for blood donation is common. Many paid donors are poor and susceptible to communicable diseases. Most are unemployed and sell their blood for a living as often as they are able and to more than one blood bank. Buying and selling of blood is a widespread and lucrative activity in some countries, including on the black market.

Brazil's blood supply has depended on a complex and secret network of blood-product suppliers and donors. Although the government announced its intention to screen all blood by mid-1988 and prohibited the sale of blood, in 1991 private blood banks were still not inspected by government and 40 per cent of blood donations were still said to be contaminated.[2,3,4]

In the Philippines, private blood banks using paid donors supply almost half the country's blood. They are inspected, but the government has no enforcement powers if conditions are below standard. There is evidence that these blood banks are not testing all the blood they get from donors, though they claim they are. Hospitals with laboratories often re-test these blood supplies, but not all hospitals have laboratories. No one knows if the blood supply is HIV-infected or not.[5]

Voluntary blood donation is practised throughout the world, and accepting donations only from groups at low risk of HIV infection is now recommended. In the developing world, however, rural hospitals and smaller blood banks often have to rely on relatives of patients, especially in an emergency. Relatives may recruit and pay donors without the knowledge of health professionals.[6] Blood testing may be done in batches, as this is less expensive. In an emergency situation, where there is no blood bank and someone donates blood at short notice, it may not be tested until after it has been transfused.

In Uganda in 1989, male volunteers in full-time education had among the lowest seroprevalence rates. In general, volunteer donors had a lower HIV seroprevalence (9–10 per cent) than relatives (15–22 per cent).[7]

In Mexico, paid donors had a seroprevalence rate of 7 per cent compared to 0.1 per cent in volunteer donors. Prevalence among donors was reduced to 0.04 per cent when prevention strategies were adhered to. But black-market problems and a lack of laboratories to test blood remained in 1989.[8,9]

Testing of blood donations is still far from universal. In Nigeria, for example, in 1990 less than five per cent of blood donations were tested for HIV. HIV testing had low priority at policy level, though there were signs that this was changing.[10] In Bolivia, hospitals were not testing donated blood in 1991 except at the request of the recipient or his/her family.[11]

High-risk practices

Topping-up

Topping-up means giving a transfusion as a routine measure to anyone in poor health or thought to be anaemic who is receiving other treatment. This practice used to be common in many developing countries. For example, women were topped up with transfusions when they had caesarean sections or were sections or were receiving other obstetric care, on the grounds that most of them were anaemic anyway.[12] Many countries have tightened up on this practice because of HIV/AIDS.

Pooling of untested blood

Donated blood is often pooled, e.g. to make blood products. This is not a problem if donors have been screened. In Gujarat state in India, some 430 of the 510 people confirmed as HIV-positive in 1989 were blood sellers.[13] The rate of HIV infection among them was so high because their blood was pooled without being tested. Then the donors were topped up for anaemia, using blood from the same pool they had donated to. It only needs one donor to have HIV for a whole group of recipients of the pooled blood to become infected.[12] This was also suspected to occur in Mexico.[9]

Why infected blood transfusions put women at particular risk

Most of the blood transfused in developing countries is for the treatment of anaemia in children and women, particularly pregnant women, and haemorrhage in women.

Anaemia and haemorrhage are major and contributing causes in the half-million maternal deaths internationally each year and morbidity in millions more women. Anaemia is caused by malnutrition, infection from malaria, hookworm and schistosomiasis, and blood disorders such as thalassaemia and sickle cell anaemia, and is aggravated by pregnancy. Haemorrhage can occur during pregnancy, from complications of childbirth and as a result of unsafe abortion practices.[6,15]

In 1988, for example, three-quarters of all adult blood transfusions in Uganda were given

---

The case of Romania

In Romania, surveys in 1990 among children under age four in orphanages, and children under age 12 living with their parents and with a history of in-patient hospital care, found HIV-seropositivity of about 8 per cent in both groups. Rates of infection as high as 21 per cent in institutions for very disadvantaged children were also found.

The complete spectrum of the modes of HIV transmission among the children is still not known. However, the majority had a history of multiple transfusions of blood or blood products and/or treatment with unsterile injections.

Topping-up was common from the mid- to late 1980s during the Ceausescu regime. Because of the acute food shortage, malnourished and sick children were given transfusions in order to 'support growth and natural defences against infection'.

In 1990, the Romanian Ministry of Health issued guidelines for the testing of all blood donations for HIV. Topping-up and the use of unsterile syringes and needles were prohibited. However, many district laboratories lacked HIV-testing equipment. At the end of 1990, only 60 per cent of all blood donations were being tested.

About one-third of the mothers of the children with HIV/AIDS were tested, and of these, 15 per cent were seropositive.[14]

This implies that a risk of blood transmission of HIV also existed for women, due to the Ceausescu policy of enforced pregnancy and illegal contraception and abortion. There was a high rate of morbidity from illegal abortions under Ceausescu and many women needed hospital treatment and transfusions. Women may have been as much at risk of HIV infection in hospitals as children.

to women, in most cases because of complications in childbirth.[16]

The need for transfusion for blood disorders varies greatly, from none at all to multiple transfusions. Women with blood disorders are at risk themselves, and the women partners of men with blood disorders are at risk sexually.

Evidence of transfusion-related infection in women

Rates of transfusion-related cases of HIV in infants and children are well studied compared to women.[15] In Africa, where the most women have had HIV/AIDS, there is practically no documented evidence.

A study in 1989 of risk factors in about 60 HIV-positive women in Guinea Bissau found that 55 per cent of the women had a history of blood transfusion, as compared to 8 per cent of HIV-negative women studied. This does not indicate how many of the women got HIV through a transfusion, only that it was clearly a risk factor. Blood is now screened in Guinea Bissau.[17]

In Rwanda, blood transfusion was associated with a high rate of HIV infection among childbearing women (45 per cent) from 1980–85 before blood screening was instituted, compared to a rate of 28 per cent among those who had never been transfused. However, less than five per cent of women reported a history of transfusion in that period. Of 3,702 women of childbearing age studied in 1986-7, 29 per cent had HIV infection. Of those, 8.4 per cent were associated with a history of blood transfusion.[18]

Many AIDS cases among Mexican and Brazilian women (66 per cent and 34 per cent respectively) are attributed to blood transfusions. Twenty per cent of cases among women in one study in Honduras were associated with transfusions.[19]

Sickle cell anaemia mainly affects people of African descent. In the USA, about five per cent of people with sickle cell are dependent on monthly routine transfusions. In one hospital in New York, 12–15 per cent of sickle cell patients who needed regular transfusions became HIV-infected before 1985.[20] In Africa, where care for sickle cell anaemia is more likely to be restricted to transfusions during crises, infection may have been more frequent.[1]

Thalassaemia mostly affects people of Mediterranean and southeast Asian descent. In the USA, people with thalassaemia receive transfusions of packed red blood cells twice a month, and 17 per cent of patients at the largest US thalassaemia clinic became HIV-positive before 1985. Almost all were women. No reason for the gender difference was known.[20]

Men with haemophilia require regular injections of Factor 8, a blood product made from pooled blood. In the USA and Europe, 80 to 90 per cent of men with severe haemophilia and 40 per cent of those with moderate haemophilia were seropositive by 1985.[20] In Brazil, about 85 per cent of haemophiliacs have HIV.[2] Factor 8 is now heat treated to ensure its safety.

Making blood transfusion safe

The following measures ensure safe blood transfusion services:

- Effective controls on or elimination of private blood banks, and sterilization of any equipment being re-used.
- Banning of paid blood donation and alternative employment for 'professional' donors.
- Public health campaigns to encourage low-risk volunteers to give blood.
- Use of low-risk volunteers in place of relatives where possible.
- Discreet, private and confidential enquiry to determine whether potential donors may be at risk of HIV infection. Anyone at high risk should be asked not to donate blood, and

donations should not be accepted. However, this precaution may not be effective enough where HIV prevalence is high, and other precautions are needed.[21]

High-risk behaviour may not identify everyone with HIV, especially anyone who may be in the window period. In Zimbabwe, the National Blood Transfusion Service is not accepting blood from high-risk donors and is concentrating on school-age donors over the age of 16. All new donors are tested and if they test negative, their blood is stored in dry packs. Only upon second donation, if the test is again negative, is the prior donation released for use, and the new donation stored.[22]

- Testing of all donated blood for antibodies to HIV.
- Using accepted heat treatment procedures to inactivate virus in all blood products, e.g. gamma globulin, Factor 8, and packed red cells.
- Prevention of the main health problems that require transfusion.
  Prevention of anaemia, pregnancy-related morbidity and provision of safe abortion should be the primary focus of prevention efforts centred on women. For example, more effective control of malaria, improved child health and better antenatal and obstetric care could reduce the need for many transfusions dramatically.[21] Treatment for disorders such as sickle cell anaemia can be improved so that they are not crisis-oriented and require fewer transfusions.[1]
- Use of alternatives to transfusion.
  Transfusions should only be given where it is thought that the patient will otherwise die or suffer permanent, severe disability, particularly if the blood supply has not been tested.

  In a hospital in Kinshasa, Zaïre, a study found that alternatives to transfusion could have been used in 13 per cent of cases of anaemia in children and 21 per cent in adults, because the anaemia was not severe. Under a new policy, transfusion for anaemia is given only if it is severe.[21]

  For women, proguanil prophylaxis against malaria in pregnancy is both safe and effective for prevention of malaria-related anaemia.[23] Plasma substitutes can be used as first-line treatment for haemorrhage.[24]
- In non-emergency cases, where it is known in advance that blood may be required, hospitals may take and store blood from the patient, a volunteer or a person known to the patient who is at very low risk, prior to operating.

  Where the blood supply is not universally tested, patients or their partners/relatives can try to insist that any blood used is tested.

Situations where blood transfusion should be given to save life, even when there is a high risk of HIV transmission:

- incipient cardiac failure
- imminent obstetric delivery crisis
- sickle cell disease crisis
- acute haemorrhage
- critical blood loss during emergency surgery
- critical neonatal jaundice.[1]

Sharing of equipment to inject illegal drugs

Illegal drugs like heroin, amphetamines, and cocaine are self-injected by the people who use them. Initially it was thought that injection of illegal drugs was causing widespread HIV transmission mainly in geographically clustered areas in developed regions, e.g. in New York City in the USA and in Italy and Spain in Europe.[25] But there are serious problems of illegal drug use in some developing countries. In Poland, Yugoslavia, Brazil, Thailand, Malaysia, Burma, Laos, India, and China, for example, evidence of high rates of injection drug use and increasing HIV infection have come to light.[26]

In São Paulo, users inject drugs in public toilets and use the water from the toilets to mix cocaine.[27] In Amsterdam, users often inject at night in the doorways of lighted houses, and in New York derelict houses are often gathering places for taking drugs. The conditions imposed by the illegality of these drugs are central to why so many drug users are at risk of HIV and other bloodborne infection, and why it is so difficult for drug-using communities to organize.[25]

Like blood, illegal drugs are big business and some economies depend on them, e.g. the economies of drug-using ghettos of most major cities, where unemployment is high.

Women and children in these communities may be supported by the drug economy, whether they are directly involved or not.[28]

In rural areas of countries like Colombia, Peru, Burma, Laos and Thailand, farmers survive by growing plants for drugs. In Thailand, the government has tried to develop alternative employment in these areas and growing of opium is said to have dropped. But the Thai ban on smoking opium backfired. Many users switched to injecting heroin instead, part of the reason why HIV infection among drug users is so high in Thailand.[26,29]

Injection drug use is often linked to the sex industry, which may be controlled by drug traders. It is in their interests to get sex workers dependent on drugs in order to control them. Drug users may travel to avoid high prices and police repression – e.g. from Ireland to London, from Germany to Amsterdam, and from Sweden to Copenhagen.[30]

Low social status, forced economic migration, high unemployment, low self-esteem, and racial prejudice may lead to drug use, especially where more than one of these factors pertains, as among young Surinamese in the Netherlands and black and Hispanic communities in the USA.[30] It has been argued that drug use can become a form of work where there is no other work, providing goals, a social network and meaning.[26]

Sharing scarce equipment is an act of friendship and loyalty, not an isolated,

---

How to clean injection equipment and sharp instruments
The following is the simplest and most effective advice for using and cleaning injection equipment or sharp instruments that could transmit infection:

- Do not share or re-use equipment if you can possibly avoid it.
- If you do share or re-use equipment, always clean or sterilize it between each use. Use one part bleach or alcohol to 10 parts of water. Rinse two–three times with this solution. Then rinse three times with clean water. At the very least, rinse all equipment with clean water. Dispose of the solution and the used water safely; do not inject them.

impersonal act. It is not uncommon for a drug user to allow a friend to share a recently used syringe filled with water to delay withdrawal symptoms until more drugs can be found,[28] and women often share equipment with their sexual partners.

Drug users form an often close, but not closed community, where members can get both emotional and practical support. Since 1984, risk reduction has been reported among some injection drug users in New York, New Zealand, San Francisco and the UK. The most common changes were increased use of clean needles and syringes and reduced sharing of needles. Fewer people were adopting safer sex practices, however.[25] Risk-reduction activities among black users in New York City were best predicted by whether their friends in the drug community were engaging in these activities.[28]

Safety and risk reduction for drug users

Wherever injection drug users are getting HIV, preventive measures are often discussed. They are at best only partially implemented.[25] More drug information and treatment programmes are needed, as well as more safer sex education, including in developing countries. Trained staff and programmes that offer treatment, psycho-social and practical support to drug users who want to stop using and rebuild their lives are crucial. HIV testing and counselling should be available.[31,32]

Stopping drug use requires a change of lifestyle and social network. For women, this may require help in dealing with low self-esteem, changing perceptions of peer-group norms, and beliefs about their ability to determine what happens to them. Feelings of powerlessness and the demands of poverty that underlie drug use may make women especially dependent on partners who may also be drug users. Stopping drugs may not reduce a woman's risk of HIV infection sexually unless she can influence her partner's behaviour or leave the relationship.[28,32]

Not all drug users want to or can stop using. In Italy, the Netherlands and Britain, among others, there is increasing emphasis on alternatives to injecting (such as smoking), safer sex for users and their partners, learning how to inject safely and clean equipment, and access to clean equipment as important risk-reduction strategies.[33,34]

Programmes for women are few in number or non-existent in most countries, particularly for pregnant women users, who may be motivated to give up drugs most during and after pregnancy. An antenatal programme in Scotland has shown this to be true. Contrary to popular medical belief, it is not dangerous to the foetus for women to stop using drugs during pregnancy.[34]

Other subgroups, including gay and lesbian users, young people experimenting with drugs, male and female sex workers, prisoners, and first- and second-generation migrants, also need more services. For many, the rate of HIV infection is already high.[31] Other risk-reduction measures are as follows.

- Doctors, health workers and HIV counsellors need training in sympathetic and informed contact with drug users, including those providing pregnancy care and birth control to women.
- Changes in legislation.
  Programmes may first require changes in legislation and policy agreements between public health and judicial departments. For example, needles and syringes may not be obtainable legally without a prescription. Programmes may bring drug users out into the open; cooperation with police is needed so that people are not arrested.[32]
- Provision of clean needles, syringes, and bleach or alcohol. All countries can follow the example of programmes in some European countries to provide clean needles/syringes and bleach or alcohol.[35]

These should be free or a very low price, preferably with exchange for old equipment, at sites accessible to users, in one or more of the following ways:

– Vending machines using tokens which have a place for safe disposal of used equipment, and dispense a package of needles, syringes, condoms, swabs, and a new token. Tokens may be picked up at a publicized site. This provides at least one contact with the user, during which training in cleaning techniques, counselling, drug rehabilitation and support may be offered. The UK, Norway, Denmark and the Netherlands all have vending machines on some sites.[35],[36]

– Buses can travel to where drug users are, providing methadone, clean needles, syringes, cleaning materials, and other drug-related health services, as is being done in Oslo and Amsterdam.[35]

– Certain approved public outlets could be supplied with equipment. Pharmacies (without a prescription), drug treatment centres, counselling and support agencies, hospitals, clinics, self-help and other organizations for drug users, and other sites in the community could be chosen. One London hospital has a store-front exchange scheme which gives out 9,000 syringes each month to about 257 drug users, with an 80 per cent return rate.[31],[35]

• Outreach and training
In the UK and the Netherlands it was found that women and young users are less likely to have contact with agencies. Hence, efforts must be made to reach users where they are. It is essential to do outreach and utilize the expertise and credibility of current and ex-users themselves, as no one else knows where to find users. Working with drug users as a community is more effective than working with individuals. Supporting self-organization by drug users may be the most

effective starting-point for outreach work.[32],[37]

• Disposal of old equipment
There has always been a danger from contaminated needles/syringes and sharps which are not disposed in a safe way in the community or at clinical and hospital sites. Most programmes give advice about this to needle exchange services and to drug users themselves. In Denmark, special bins are provided for disposal.[35]

Transmission of HIV in health care settings

Unsterilized equipment

In developing countries, health services often have a limited supply of sterile needles, syringes and other instruments. Sterilizers may not be available or may break down, with delays in repair or replacement. Manual sterilization procedures may be lax or non-existent. Hence, equipment is often reused. If it is not sterilized between uses, existing HIV and other infection in one person may be spread to others.

At the end of 1988, a woman living in Elistal, a city in Kalmykia (formerly USSR), was found to be HIV-positive when she donated blood for a friend. Almost at the same time, a child in a children's hospital was also found to be HIV-positive. The donor's child had died a few months earlier in the same hospital where the child with HIV was found. Tests among other children hospitalized at that time revealed that several were HIV-positive.

All the hospitalized children had been suffering from very serious infections or other diseases. Some were given multiple injections of various drugs. In a number of children, in order to administer the injections, a catheter was inserted into a vein for ten or more days.

After the drugs had been administered through the catheter, a small portion of blood was drawn into the syringe to verify that the catheter was still in the vein. Various injections were given to other children with the same syringe. Only the needles were changed.

In this way, HIV may have been transmitted to other children, whose stay in hospital partly overlapped with those who were already infected. Some children who had left the hospital became ill again and were hospitalized in other hospitals, where similar practices spread HIV further.[38]

At the time this chain of infection was discovered, the former USSR was producing only three per cent of the supply of disposable syringes they needed.[39]

In most developing countries, in addition to formal sector health care, there are informal practitioners and traditional healers who give injections, including traditional birth attendants, personnel in hospitals, health centres and outreach services, private practitioners, former medical corpsmen in the military, orderlies or janitors in the formal health sector, lay people supplementing their income from other work, village headmen, as a form of status, pharmacists or pharmacy staff, or travelling 'injection doctors' who specialize in giving injections. Such providers may not have the relevant knowledge to determine whether an injection is warranted or the equipment to administer it in a safe way.

Lay people sometimes possess their own syringes and needles. Based on their medical belief system and previous experience and advice, some will diagnose their own illnesses and respond with self-administered injections, e.g. for vaginal infections or sexually transmitted diseases. In some cases, neighbours will be asked to administer an injection.

In practice, there may be no clear division between the formal and the informal sector. Providers, as well as supplies of medicines, syringes and other equipment tend to flow continuously from the formal into the informal and traditional sector. As has been shown for Cameroon, it may even be in the interests of the formal sector to sustain the informal sector.[40]

Few countries have actively sought to eliminate informal injection providers, who may be the only source of non-traditional care in the more remote rural areas, for example. They are not only more geographically accessible, but also socially and status-wise closer to their clients than formal-sector health care workers. They may be more able to simplify the concepts of medicine or to fit these into a popular system for explaining disease.

For effective prevention of HIV transmission through unsafe injecting practices, isolated interventions will not work. The social, cultural and economic fabric of people's lives and the circumstances of health care provision must be taken into consideration. An integrated approach is necessary.[40]

Outreach, training and supplies for informal-sector injection providers and others involved in traditional practices in developing countries can be made part of new and existing training programmes, e.g. for traditional birth attendants.

Accidents

Infection of a patient by a health worker or of a health worker by a patient could occur because of accidents with injections or while taking and handling blood samples, during surgery or other internal procedures.

Health workers are often overworked, tired, in a hurry and under stress. Accidental needlestick injuries with a used needle are common. Blood from blood samples, splashes of blood during surgery or childbirth, contact when dressings are being changed, or with other visibly blood-stained body fluids from someone with HIV can get into cuts, eyes or mouth of health workers.

A worldwide literature review to February 1989 found almost 2,000 cases reported where such an accident occurred and where the patient was found to have HIV. Of these, 33 health workers (1.6 per cent) were found to be HIV-positive following the accident, though not all could be confirmed as work-related.[41]

Rates of infection among health workers have not been found to be higher than among their background communities.[39] Attributing infection to medical procedures is complicated by the fact that the HIV status of patients and health workers is usually not known, and one or both may well have been infected prior to an accident.

Considering how common these accidents are, this is an extremely small number of cases. Yet there is widespread fear of patients among health workers, many of whom have refused to attend or treat patients known or suspected to have HIV. This reaction is most common when health care workers know little or nothing about HIV/AIDS and have little or no experience of attending those affected. Health workers need to be trained in safe practices and counselled to overcome their fears, the same as everyone else.

Patients too have sometimes come to fear health workers, in spite of the lack of evidence of risk. In 1990 it was reported in a national newspaper in the USA that a prominent breast cancer surgeon had died of AIDS. So many of his former patients were upset by the sensationalist media coverage that all his 1,800 former patients were invited to be tested for HIV. No cases of infection were reported.

By the end of 1990, only one case of infection of three patients by a dentist who had AIDS had been documented in the USA. The way infection occurred was never proved, but it was thought to be invasive procedures where direct blood-to-blood contact occurred, if it occurred in the practice at all.[42]

Traditional practices

Communally-used instruments for tattooing, scarification, uvulectomy, tonsillectomy, cuts for mixing of blood for friendship and solidarity, blood letting and vein puncture, piercing of ears/nose/lips, shaving, extraction of milk teeth, and cutting of eyebrows to cure eye diseases may all have a role in the spread of HIV.[1,43]

Few studies have been reported. Two studies in Ethiopia found an association between skin piercing practices and hepatitis B infection, which has implications for HIV transmission. A recent study of the extent of these practices in Ethiopia found that many are still very widespread.[44]

Ritual scarification is being practised in Africa much less today than 15 or 20 years ago, but therapeutic scarification as treatment of localized pain and swelling is, if anything, increasing. HIV infection was correlated with scarification in one hospital study in Zaïre.[1]

Another study in a rural area of Senegal of 258 people, including 195 women, found that tattooing, scarifications, circumcision and clitoridectomy were not associated with HIV infection.[45]

In Brazil, the followers of the Afro-Brazilian religion Candomble often turn to houses of Candomble to solve their health problems. Religious rituals involve individual and sometimes mass scarification, done with a pocket knife. The leaders have prestige and a good reputation in the community. Meetings between a group of Candomble leaders and the Department of Health have discussed how to make these rituals safe and arranged training for other leaders.[46]

Safety in health care settings: universal precautions

Health workers have a right to expect their work situations to be as safe as possible. The risk of infection should not be ignored, understated or exaggerated.[47] Patients also have a right to health care that is provided in safe conditions.

Informed medical opinion has come down strongly on the side of universal precautions in clinical settings, that is, precautions to be used with all patients and invasive procedures, regardless of HIV status, which will improve safety for everyone. This makes HIV testing of staff and patients unnecessary except when this knowledge would affect the type of treatment provided to the patient.[47]

With universal precautions, there is a very low risk of HIV infection in the health care setting. Training is necessary to help health workers to adopt safe practices, many of which are not new and should always have been applied, taking account of actual conditions.

To do this in a hospital in Switzerland, nurses were asked to record all procedures performed, if and when gloves were worn, the number of times they experienced blood contact, and all injuries they sustained during a six-day shift. They were then told how to take precautions and given adequate supplies of gloves and needle-disposal containers. When they recorded the same information about

Follow the infection control rules
every hour... every day... every client

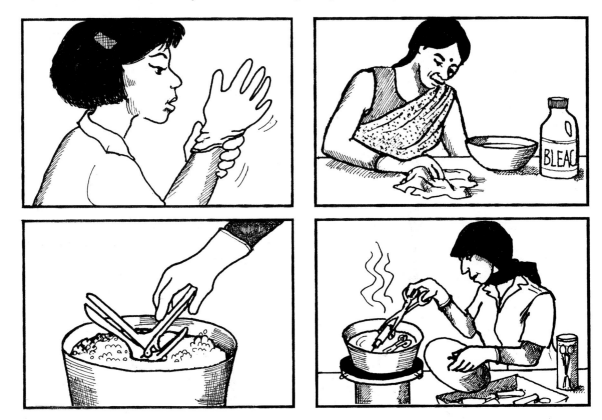

International Planned Parenthood Federation

their next shift, blood contact had decreased considerably, even though universal precautions were not always applied.[48]

Examples of universal precautions

Sterilization of equipment

Equipment and instruments used for surgery, injections and internal procedures should be sterilized between uses, with sterilizers or by hand. UNICEF provides a portable steam sterilizer, which was originally designed for use in immunization programmes.[49]

For women, unsterilized equipment for injectable contraceptives, cutting the umbilical cord, doing episiotomies, inserting and removing contraceptive implants, surgical abortions, laparoscopy, sterilization and assisted fertilization techniques, inserting IUDs, and speculums have all been implicated in spreading other infections and could be a risk factor for HIV transmission.

Non-reusable equipment

Syringes that can be used once only before they block have been developed by WHO and UNICEF in collaboration with manufacturers for immunizatlon programmes.[40]

Staff involved in immunization programmes are usually well supervised and trained in the formal sector. Immunization to prevent serious childhood illnesses continues to be strongly recommended for all infants and children by UNICEF and the World Health Organization.

The Programme for Appropriate Technology in Health (USA) and the WHO Special Programme on Human Reproduction have developed a non-reusable device for injectable contraceptives. It is also being used for other injectable drugs, such as prostaglandins for prevention of postpartum haemorrhage and vaccines. This new technology needs to be evaluated in the context it will be used.[50] While non-reusable needles/syringes are a sure way to prevent infection, they may increase the cost of drugs and equipment and make their use less accessible to those who already cannot

afford to replace what they have. This would be counterproductive: there may be attempts to reuse the equipment anyway.

In Somalia, some informal-sector injection providers now charge their clients more for new, unused syringes in the wake of AIDS-information campaigns. These may or may not be new, unused or sterile.[40]

Development of sturdier equipment that could be reused safely a number of times may make more sense, cost less and allow more equipment to be produced at prices developing countries can afford. HIV should not preclude efforts at safe recycling.

Protective equipment and procedures

In many cases, extra equipment and resources have to be made available before health workers can implement precautions, mainly rubber gloves, disposal bins and bags for needles and sharps, sterilizers, safety glasses where blood splashes may occur, and any specific protective equipment for specialists, e.g. surgical gowns and plastic aprons.

Thin, disposable plastic gloves are commonly used in obstetric, gynaecological and family planning practice for vaginal examinations. These gloves may tear easily and rubber gloves may be preferable.[51] However, disposable gloves are better than nothing.

Obstetricians and midwives should wear gloves that cover the lower arms to avoid direct contact with and to clean up the mother's waters and blood during and after childbirth, while cutting the umbilical cord and disposing of the placenta. Simple suction devices instead of mouth-to-mouth suction for removing fluids from newborn infants' mouths are also recommended.

A US study found that during 230 vaginal and caesarean deliveries involving 1,388 obstetric staff, there were 112 skin contacts with blood, 38 skin contacts with amniotic fluid, and two eye-splashes with blood. During episiotomy or repair of lacerations, there were four needlestick injuries. Knowledge that a

Body fluids to which universal precautions apply

semen	blood and other body fluids containing visible blood
vaginal secretions	amniotic fluid and placenta
tissues	cerebro-spinal, synovial, pleural, peritoneal, and pericardial fluids

Body fluids to which universal precautions need not apply (unless they contain visible blood)

saliva	sweat	tears	urine
nasal secretion	sputum	vomit	faeces

Centers for Disease Control, 1988[47]

woman had HIV, hepatitis B or was an injection drug user did not reduce incidents. This study indicates that the great majority of contacts involved only skin, which is extremely low-risk. No cases of HIV infection were reported.[52] Protective measures are needed but they can be kept quite simple.

In a hospital setting, disposal of placenta should be done according to the principles of safe practice in handling blood. If family members traditionally take the placenta home for burial, the practice can be continued. Addition of disinfectant or lime is unnecessary, but gloves or other means of safe handling should be used and burial should be deep enough that animals cannot dig the placenta up, leaving it exposed.[53]

Education and training

Rotation of staff, reduced workloads, compensatory career structures, and peer support are recommended to reduce stress and burnout that may lead to accidents.

HIV/AIDS education should be an integral part of initial and continuing training for health workers and professionals. Unions, professional associations or management could set up discussion groups or workshops for staff to confront their own attitudes, fears and misconceptions, clarify their own values and feelings, and consider the effects of these on people in their care. Such groups could also confront any overreaction regarding the need for safety or any refusal to care for patients with HIV/AIDS. Ongoing education programmes for all staff and specific education for areas such as obstetrics, midwifery and abortion are also recommend.[47]

Cooperation with and training for traditional practitioners recognizes their role in health care, including prevention of HIV/AIDS and sexually transmitted diseases.[54]

Traditional birth attendants (TBAs) are the least likely to have access to gloves for deliveries. No published study has examined whether the risk to these women is higher than for other health workers.[39] TBAs who work with their hands in rural settings may have cuts and grazes on them. Washing before and after the birth with a non-abrasive soap can be suggested. Scrubbing should not be so hard as to break the skin surface. Provision of gloves should be a priority, however.[55] TBAs use sharp instruments for episiotomy and to cut the umbilical cord. Those with training will have been taught to sterilize them against tetanus, and this should be reinforced regarding HIV.

Overall, there is much room for improvement.

Pregnancy-related transmission of HIV to women and infants

What is pregnancy-related transmission of HIV?

Pregnancy-related transmission of HIV can occur when a woman is trying to get pregnant, during pregnancy and possibly through breastfeeding.

The incidence of pregnancy-related HIV infection in infants directly depends on the number of women with HIV/AIDS. As long as the numbers and proportion of women with HIV keep increasing, so will the numbers of affected infants.

- It is not possible to practise safer sex and try to get pregnant at the same time. An unquantified number of women may have become HIV-infected when they were trying to become pregnant.
  A few cases of pregnancy-related transmission of HIV to women have occurred when women have been trying for pregnancy through inseminations from donors who had HIV. In 1985, four of eight Australian women became infected in this way, from one donor.[1] A few other cases have been reported anecdotally.
- Pregnancy-related transmission of HIV from mother to foetus can occur at some point during pregnancy or birth.

Terms for this form of transmission – perinatal, mother-to-infant and vertical transmission – are all inaccurate. Worse, they implicitly hold only women responsible. It takes two to get pregnant. Men with HIV are also responsible, and their role must be made visible, both prior to and during pregnancy. Where pregnant and birthing women have become infected through unsafe blood transfusions, possibly also infecting their infants, the public health services are directly implicated too.

Outcome of pregnancy in infants of HIV-positive mothers

HIV infection in mothers may or may not affect their infants. The mother's health status generally affects an infant's vulnerability to illness and may play a major role.

HIV in the mother may have a negative effect on the birth weight of an infant, but not always. In a Zambian study HIV-positive women were almost four times more likely to have low-birth-weight babies than HIV-negative women.[10] In the European collaborative study, however, the difference was not significant.[5] Similarly, some prematurity may be the result of HIV infection, but not always or not significantly.[5,13]

The most significant adverse outcome of pregnancy in infants of HIV-positive women is

HIV/AIDS in infants and children

Epidemiology

Globally, the majority of infants and children up to the age of 14 with HIV/AIDS are infants. Most have been infected during pregnancy, and most of the rest by infected blood transfusions. Sexual abuse, early sexual intercourse and unsterilized injection equipment have also contributed to infection in children.

In Africa, because there are many women with HIV, the number of children infected during pregnancy is the highest. In Latin America up to 1989, the overall number of women with AIDS was low. Forty-five per cent of children with AIDS under age 15 were infected during pregnancy, while 24 per cent were infected through blood transfusion. Sixty per cent of paediatric cases reported in children were in Brazil. In Mexico, where blood transfusion has been responsible for most AIDS cases in women, this has also been true in children. Twenty-eight per cent of children were infected during pregnancy to 1989, while 40 per cent were infected through transfusions. In North America to 1989, 64 per cent of children were infected during pregnancy, and 8 per cent through blood transfusions.[2]

As the rate of heterosexual transmission rises, pregnancy-related infection will comprise a larger and larger proportion of cases of new HIV infection in infants.

Manifestations

Some children with HIV have been followed for up to eight years. Of these, some have signs of illness and others do not. If these children follow adult patterns, they may have no signs of infection for ten or more years, if at all. There are few natural history studies in children and adolescents, but increasing numbers in these age groups are living with HIV.[3,4]

Most infants born with HIV infection, or who get HIV through blood transfusion prior to four months of age, show signs of HIV-related illness well before one year of age or in their second year.[5]

Failure to thrive or grow may be the first sign of HIV infection in the first months of a baby's life, and early care should be sought, whether or not either parent is known to be infected.[6] In developing countries, the manifestations of HIV and AIDS are frequently difficult to distinguish from those of other severe and common illnesses of childhood.[7]

Most of the HIV symptoms and diseases that appear in adults also appear in infants and children, except Kaposi's sarcoma, which is rare under the age of 15.[6,8] Infants tend to develop the life-threatening illnesses described in adults more quickly than adults.[6]

The earlier HIV symptoms and disease appear, the more likely an infant is to die at a very young age.[6] This is because its immune system is not fully developed and immunity to many diseases has not yet been acquired – one of the many reasons why breastfeeding is so important.

Many fear that AIDS deaths will erase all the gains made by programmes to reduce infant mortality around the world. In Zimbabwe, where infant mortality has been decreasing for some time, AIDS had become the leading cause of infant deaths in two major hospitals by mid-1988.[9]

By the end of two years of follow-up, 44 per cent of HIV-infected infants in a Zambia study had died, in spite of prompt clinical care. All except two had recurrent episodes of illness, requiring frequent admissions to hospital.[10]

In a Ugandan study, 62 per cent of the babies of HIV-positive women were healthy five years after birth, and 35 pr cent had died. Of the babies of HIV-negative women, 89 per cent were well and 11 per cent had died.[11]

In a hospital serving poor women in Kinshasa, mortality in infants born to HIV-positive women was 22 per cent compared to 3 per cent in infants of HIV-negative women. Of the infants who died, 26 per cent died in the first week of life, 12 per cent within one month, and 62 per cent over one month, with illnesses commonly associated with AIDS.

In contrast, in a Kinshasa hospital serving wealthier women, mortality in the infants of HIV-positive and HIV-negative women (4 per cent and 3 per cent) did not differ significantly. It was similar to mortality observed in the infants of HIV-positive European women.[6]

In the European collaborative study, in most infected babies who have survived to one year of age, disease has progressed more slowly and the babies have remained stable or even improved during their second year of life.[5]

An Italian study found that babies and children who get HIV infection when they are over the age of four months have disease and survival patterns similar to adults.[12]

HIV infection itself. The risk of transmission during pregnancy found in different groups of women has ranged from as low as 6.4 per cent[14] to almost 60 per cent.[15] The majority of studies have found a rate of between 15 and 40 per cent.[5,10,16,17] In other words, 60 to 85 per cent of infants of women with HIV do not become HIV-infected themselves. A lower risk of transmission has been found more often in groups of women in Europe and North America. A higher risk has been found more often in African women. Many factors appear to affect this risk.

When and how does pregnancy-related transmission occur?

It is extremely difficult to determine when and how this form of transmission occurs. It is thought that most infection happens during pregnancy, possibly via HIV in the placenta or if HIV in the mother's blood crosses the placenta.

Evidence of infection has been found as early as 13 weeks of pregnancy in the foetuses of HIV-positive women who had second-trimester abortions, in several studies though not in all of them.[18,19] One study found almost no evidence of infection in foetuses aborted in the first and second trimester of pregnancy.[19] Thus, infection may occur or be detectable only later in pregnancy or at birth.

It is thought, though not proved, that infection may happen during childbirth, possibly during the mixing of maternal and infant blood through the umbilical cord, or through ingestion by the infant of maternal vaginal mucus and/or blood during delivery.

A recent study is widely interpreted as indicating that infection may occur at birth. This study, of 66 pairs of twins of HIV-positive mothers, found that 50 per cent of the first-born twins with vaginal delivery had HIV, and 38 per cent of the first-born twins with caesarean section had HIV, while 19 per cent

of the second-born twins had HIV with both forms of delivery. This difference in the rate of infection in the first- and second-born twins has not been fully explained. It is suggested that if the first-born twins remained longer in the birth canal, they might have ingested more virus-containing fluids, leaving less to affect the second-born. On this theory, it is suggested that some unspecified form of vaginal cleansing prior to delivery might reduce infection.[20] However, this does not explain the difference in the rate of infection in those twins delivered by caesarean. In fact, some or all of these infants may have been infected prior to birth, and any form of vaginal cleansing in childbirth sounds highly problematic.

Seven other studies have compared infection rate with vaginal as opposed to caesarean delivery, to see if that affected the rate of transmission. One found no difference in risk for infants between the two forms of delivery. Six found non-significant lower transmission rates with caesarean than vaginal delivery, including the European collaborative study. Although some European obstetricians seem disposed to carry out caesareans on women with HIV, the data do not support this as a routine or recommended practice. Further studies are needed.[20,21]

Is it possible to know in advance whether an infant will be infected?

No one can predict in advance whether an infant will be born with HIV infection or not, and no antenatal screening test for infants exists. Any invasive test during pregnancy might transmit HIV infection from the mother to the foetus. Even if there were a safe antenatal test, and even if it showed the foetus to be HIV-negative at the time it was done, there would be no guarantee that the baby would remain HIV-negative throughout the pregnancy and birth.

Testing for HIV antibodies in the blood of an infant under 12–18 months does not provide a definitive diagnosis of HIV infection in the infant. This is because the mother's antibodies to HIV may remain in the infant's blood for up to 18 months. Only after 18 months do antibodies to HIV in the infant indicate that it has HIV.[5,7] The lack of certainty this causes for 18 months after a baby is born is one of the most difficult issues for women with HIV to cope with.

What are the risk factors?

The following seem to influence the rate of pregnancy-related transmission of HIV to infants, though these are not predictive for individual women or infants:

- The risk may be greater if the mother becomes infected during pregnancy or near the time that the child is born. This would correspond with the fact that the amount of HIV in the mother would be high in the weeks or months after infection occurs and before enough antibodies are produced to fight it.

  A study underway in Rwanda has preliminary data that link multiple sexual partners in pregnancy to a higher rate of transmission of HIV to infants during pregnancy. Because the researchers had not expected to find this a significant factor, they had only begun to ask women more questions on this subject before reporting their results. They are now asking about frequency of unprotected intercourse and when it took place during pregnancy, to try to determine the actual risk factors.

- The risk may be less in women who are beyond the window period but who have few or no symptoms of HIV-related illness and relatively high T4 cell counts.

- The risk may be greater as HIV-related illness in the mother becomes more advanced, and/or as her immune function decreases.

  This would correspond to the higher presence of HIV in the woman at more advanced stages of infection. Evidence that women are at or progressing to a more advanced stage of infection may not be obvious during pregnancy or at delivery, unless T4 cell counts are done. It may become clear if a woman progresses to AIDS within one to two years after a birth. One or more previous pregnancies combined with poor health and any maternal complications, may contribute to a decline in a woman's health, which may allow HIV to take a greater toll. This could increase the vulnerability of the woman and therefore the infant.

  The European collaborative study found a 6 per cent rate of transmission to infants in women with T4 cell counts above 700 and a rate of 19–22 per cent in women with T4 cell counts below 700.

  Having one infected child may be a sign that the mother's health is declining and/or that an increased risk of transmission exists. On the other hand, the risk may be the same in each pregnancy. Some women who have had one or more infected children have had uninfected children afterwards.

- The risk may be greater if the infant is born before 34–37 weeks of pregnancy, than if born closer to term. Prematurity may be one indication that infection of the infant has occurred. Or, the infant may become infected in the birth canal because prematurity has made it more vulnerable or because it has missed receiving some maternal antibodies later in pregnancy.[10, 13, 14, 17, 21, 23, 24, 25, 26]

Prevention of pregnancy-related transmission

The best way to prevent pregnancy-related transmission of HIV to infants is for women and their partners not to get HIV infection in the first place.

Women and men who are old enough to be having children need to be informed about the risk of pregnancy-related transmission of HIV. For many women, the first indication that they are HIV-positive may come as the result of a test during pregnancy. They will have to come to terms not only with the diagnosis for themselves, but also with the possibility of transmitting infection to the foetus. In this situation, they may or may not want to continue the pregnancy. Adequate counselling is essential to help women make an informed decision about this and any future pregnancies, without pressure or coercion.

Unwanted pregnancy, HIV and other sexually transmitted infection can be avoided through safer sex practices and use of condoms alone or with another effective birth-control method, and with abortion as a back-up. These should be available for all women, regardless of HIV status. However, not all couples use these or use them effectively, and not all couples want to prevent pregnancy, including those at risk of HIV.[27]

Knowledge of HIV status and openness between partners make prevention and risk reduction much easier to achieve. All women/couples who are considering pregnancy should be advised that they can find out their

---

What to tell women and their partners

- Any woman (and her partner) seeking information and advice about HIV and pregnancy should be informed of what is known and unknown about the possible risks to herself, her partner and any infant they might have.
- The information must be accurate and adaptable to the woman's personal situation and stage of disease. Advice to a nulliparous woman in the early stages of infection may be completely different from that given to a woman with many children in the terminal stages of AIDS. The risk for women in the developing world may differ from that in developed countries, as the prognosis for both mothers and infants appears to differ.
- Any assessment of risk must take into account how soon the woman wants to become pregnant, her parity, her health status, and the amount of social and medical support available both for her and any child(ren) in future. The possibility that the children may be orphaned should also be raised.
- Where available, additional tests to assess the prognosis, such as T4 cell counts, should be performed.
- Women should be offered the option of termination of pregnancy, regardless of the stage of disease. In later or terminal stages of illness, termination should be considered even at late stages of pregnancy, in view of the poor prognosis for mother and child if the pregnancy is carried to term.
- Women wishing to continue their pregnancy should be given any additional information they request and referral for support where this is available. Arrangements should be made for antenatal and future care.[17]

HIV status before trying for a pregnancy so that they can make informed decisions in advance.

Women considering pregnancy may have a perceived risk of HIV infection, may have a diagnosed HIV-positive partner, or know that they are HIV-positive themselves. These women, and where possible their partners, should be offered counselling and an HIV test if it is needed/wanted.

However, not everyone may want to know or be able to find out their HIV status at this time.

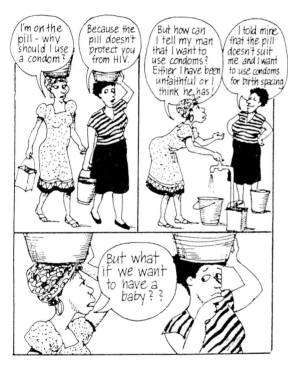

Petra Röhr-Rouendaal

Risk reduction strategies

Practising safer sex and trying to get pregnant are not possible at the same time, at least on fertile days, and it may take many months or years for a woman to complete her family. This simple fact seems to shock many people. They have just never thought about it.

There are a limited number of risk-reduction strategies to prevent sexual transmission of HIV for those trying for a pregnancy. Only a few of them protect the infant as well as one or both partners, and they may not be acceptable to many people.

For all couples

- Practise safer sex except on fertile days.
  A woman can only get pregnant during a few days of each cycle. She and her partner cannot protect each other during those days if they are trying for a pregnancy, but for the rest of the month they can. Doing this requires both knowing when those fertile days are and male cooperation. This is one among many reasons for teaching all women and men the simple techniques of fertility awareness from adolescence on, as part of health and sex education, and in safer-sex workshops.

  Though it will not protect everyone, this technique should reduce risk, since it reduces the frequency of potential exposure to infection. Where both partners have HIV, it will help to reduce the risk of re-infection. Where one partner has HIV, it reduces the risk of them transmitting it to the other partner. And it will be equally valuable for those who do not know their HIV status.

- Good antenatal, childbirth and postpartum care benefits all women and babies, including those with HIV.

- Preventing infection during pregnancy and breastfeeding. It is important for women to protect themselves from infection or re-infection during pregnancy and breast-feeding for the sake of the infant, as well as for themselves, by:
  - abstaining from intercourse or using condoms for intercourse during this period;
  - stopping injection drug use or cleaning any shared or re-used equipment;
  - ensuring that any blood transfusions have been tested for HIV.

If either or both partners has HIV

- Adoption.

  Adoption and techniques developed to overcome infertility are relevant for those willing to consider them. Although these alternatives are rarely discussed or tried in many cultures, they are accepted by more people than even twenty years ago. Even if the initial reactions are of rejection, it is worth getting people to think about them.

  If either or both partners is HIV-positive or think they may be infected, the only way to avoid risk completely is to adopt a child that is HIV-negative.

If a woman has HIV, but her male partner does not

- Surrogate motherhood.

  A way to avoid risk for the male partner and the infant is to find a willing woman who is HIV-negative to have a child for them as a surrogate mother. The surrogate mother can get pregnant by the partner, by intercourse if this is acceptable or by insemination with the partner's semen. In cases of infertility in many traditional societies, a family member is often asked to act as a surrogate, and this practice could be adapted in this instance. The woman would not be the biological mother.

- Insemination by partner.

  A woman can inseminate herself with her partner's semen without sexual intercourse, thus protecting him and making it possible for her to have his child. The chance of infection of the infant during pregnancy is not reduced, however.

If her male partner has HIV and the woman does not

- Insemination by partner.

  Attempts have been made to remove HIV from semen by centrifuge and washing techniques. However, when this was tested with the semen of a man who had HIV in the USA, his wife became infected after three inseminations. More recent attempts to remove sperm from the semen of HIV-positive men in Germany have resulted in three births of uninfected infants.[28] The safety of this procedure remains to be determined.

Self-insemination

Insemination can be done with, but does not require, clinical support.

1. During the woman's fertile days, the man ejaculates his semen into a sterile container.
2. The semen should immediately be siphoned into a clean straw, sterile syringe (without a needle) or similar cannula-like holder.
3. The syringe should be inserted into the vagina and the semen released at the top of the vagina, near the cervix. This is easiest if she is lying down, and can be done by the woman, her partner or another helper.

Inseminations can be done around and during the woman's fertile days, as often as both partners are willing, until she gets pregnant.

- Insemination by donor.

A woman can do inseminations with semen from an HIV-negative male donor or have intercourse with him. This will protect both her and the baby from HIV infection, though her partner would not be the biological father. Again, reference to traditional and modern practice in cases of infertility is relevant.

The technique of insemination by donor is valuable for women with infertile male partners, and lesbians and heterosexual women who do not have male sexual partners, who want to become pregnant. Its use has been increasing steadily in many countries. Now it can also be valuable for women with HIV-positive partners.

It is important that this technique is practised safely, whether through clinics or by a private agreement with a donor known to the woman or arranged by others.

Clinics which do inseminations, usually women's health or infertility clinics, are now required to screen donors for HIV in most developed countries. How well they are doing this is a matter for investigation. Where sperm banks exist, donors are usually anonymous, but policy may differ in each country and women should check this if it makes a difference to them.

If clinics do not have access to a sperm bank, freshly donated semen is the only option. It was the only way inseminations could be done before there were sperm banks, and this may still be the case in many countries. Using fresh semen is not as safe as it was before HIV/AIDS. It is no longer permitted in clinics in Australia.

A donor who provides fresh semen should be asked to have an HIV test though there is a chance he may be in the window period. If a test is refused or not possible, the man's word that he is at low risk would have to be accepted. [29]

Many gay men have been willing to act as semen donors. One counsellor reminds women: 'Not all gay men are infected with HIV. Any man could be infected, regardless of his sexual orientation. Don't assume that gay men are no longer potential donors and/or fathers.' [30] By the same token, not all heterosexual men are HIV-negative, including family members.

Getting pregnant through inseminations takes as long as getting pregnant through intercourse. In countries where HIV tests are not easily available, uncertainty about a donor's status will remain. People need to be convinced in themselves that it is worth the effort.

Donor insemination

- Donors should be volunteers at low risk for HIV infection. A potential donor should be tested for HIV and his semen stored in a sperm bank for at least six months.
- He should be tested again at the end of six months, before his stored semen is used, whether he intends to donate again or not. This is to ensure that he was not in the window period at the time he first donated.
- If he plans to donate semen again, he should be asked to practise safer sex in the interim.
- New donations of semen from the same donor should be used only if he continues to be HIV-negative at six-monthly intervals. [22]

Breastfeeding: the unresolved dilemmas

A very small number of cases of infants who became infected with HIV through breastfeeding by HIV-positive women have been reported. On the other hand, protective effects of breastmilk for infants of HIV-positive women have also been reported. Unresolved dilemmas have arisen.

Breastfeeding is the feeding method of choice

Breastfeeding is enormously beneficial in reducing illness and death in infants. Breastmilk contains all the nutrition a baby needs in the first months of life. A mother's antibodies against many types of infection and disease are passed to a baby through breastmilk, and provide protection that infant formula cannot give. Further, as a widely used method of birth control, breastfeeding contributes to child spacing and supports maternal health.[31]

In contrast, infant formula feeding is a major contributor to the one and a half million infant deaths from diarrhoeal diseases and malnutrition each year. Infant formula may be watered down or the quantity cut down in order to reduce its cost. Malnutrition can result. Lack of clean water is a major problem in many developing countries. If the bottle, teat or water used with infant formula is not clean, increased exposure to illness can occur.[31]

Thus, everything can be said for breastfeeding and nothing against it. Any recommendation to the majority of women with HIV infection not to breastfeed ought to be based on substantial evidence of risk to the infant indeed.

How could HIV infection through breastmilk occur?

In 1985 a Belgian study in three women isolated HIV in their milk, but it was not clear whether it could be infective. In 1988, a study in one woman in Australia indicated that HIV in breastmilk might be infective.[15,32] Whether the quantity or infectivity of HIV in breastmilk is different at different stages of HIV-related illness in the woman and at different stages of breastfeeding is currently being investigated.

Infection via breastmilk would have to occur through tissues in the mouth or gastro-intestinal tract of the infant. Sores or lesions or other infection in the infant's mouth and throat might make this more likely.

Evidence of risk when infection is postpartum

Before 1990, eight cases were identified worldwide in which breastmilk was thought to be the source of infant HIV infection. In six of these cases, the women had been given HIV-infected blood transfusions postpartum or during the breastfeeding period. These women were either known or thought to be sero-negative at the time of the child's birth. In one case, the woman was injecting drugs and sharing equipment. She developed sero-converting illness nine months postpartum. In one case, the woman was a wetnurse who was ill and losing weight. She was found to be seropositive and died when the baby was 17 months old.[32]

On the basis of these reports, most analysts concluded that there is a risk of transmission of HIV through breastmilk if:
– a woman becomes infected around the time of birth or during the period of breastfeeding, or
– she has advanced immune deficiency or AIDS-related illness.[32]

Since these cases were reported, more

evidence has been sought. A further case was reported in Saudi Arabia in 1990 of a woman given an infected postpartum transfusion and infection of the infant during breastfeeding.[33]

A study in Rwanda confirmed these risks. It followed 210 women for almost 17 months after childbirth. All the women had tested HIV-negative at birth. Sixteen of them became HIV-positive during the 17-month follow-up period. All were breastfeeding. Six seroconverted within the first three months postpartum. Five of their babies became HIV-positive, one of whom was already infected at birth. Four of the mothers seroconverted between the fourth and ninth month after birth. Two of their infants became HIV-positive. Six of the mothers seroconverted between the tenth and eighteenth month after birth, and two of their infants became HIV-positive. The study concludes that four cases are attributable to breastfeeding, where seroconversion occurred in the mothers after four months postpartum.[34]

It is possible that only two of these cases, where seroconversion occurred after the tenth month postpartum, were through breast-feeding. It is also possible that all of these women became infected during pregnancy, that the infants were infected at or prior to birth, and that, like their mothers, they remained in the window period for some months. However, it is not possible to rule out breastfeeding as the route of infection either.

Because there have been so few studies and so few cases, the extent of the risk has not and cannot yet be quantified.

Evidence of risk when infection is during pregnancy

What is the risk of HIV-positive women transmitting HIV in breastmilk, but not during pregnancy or birth? The answer to this question affects the great majority of women who have HIV from the start of a pregnancy.

It has been thought that a woman who does not transmit HIV during pregnancy or birth is also unlikely to transmit it in her milk. However, even a small risk of transmission of HIV through breastmilk would increase the numbers of affected infants.[35]

Several studies have compared the prevalence of HIV infection in breastfed versus non-breastfed infants of women infected from before pregnancy, finding little or no significant difference between the two groups. One study found a lower rate of infection in breastfed infants than in non-breastfed infants, implying a possible protective effect of breastmilk.[36]

No distinction was made between babies breastfed for a short or long period of time. Does the length of time a baby is breastfed make a difference to the risk? If breastfeeding has a protective effect against HIV infection, the same question applies. These studies did not address these questions.[32]

Data published in April 1992 from the European collaborative study indicated a significantly higher rate of HIV infection in 36 breastfed infants as compared to 683 bottlefed infants – 31 per cent of breastfed infants compared to 14 per cent of bottlefed infants were found to have HIV. In all cases, the mothers already had HIV during pregnancy.[21]

A number of problems surround this data. First, the small number of breastfed compared to bottlefed infants (36 to 683) weakens the results. Second, data on the time and duration of infection, stage of illness and T4 cell counts in the breastfeeding mothers was not available. Yet these are usually important indicators of relative risk. Third, and probably most importantly, it is not known whether the breastfed babies were already infected at birth.

Lastly, 35 per cent of the 16 infants breastfed for less than four weeks were infected, compared to 26 per cent of the 19 infants breastfed for longer than four weeks.[21] This difference implies either a protective effect with longer breastfeeding or that other factors played a role. Many questions are unanswered.

In spite of these weaknesses, this data is the first evidence of a possible risk to infants from breastfeeding by women already infected from the start of pregnancy. Because the risk is unconfirmed and partly unexplained, there has been a great deal of discussion about what the data indicate. There are worries that breastfeeding may be responsible for many cases of infant infection, and that the higher rate of transmission of HIV to infants in developing countries, as compared to developed countries, may be because more infants are breastfed.

Nothing is proven, and it would appear that it can never be proven, because further studies may never be done. Some consider it unethical to recommend that HIV-positive pregnant women in developed countries breastfeed their infants for the sake of a study, when bottlefeeding is a safe alternative for their babies. And it would be equally unethical to recommend that HIV-positive pregnant women in developing countries bottlefeed their babies, because of the high risk of infant death from causes other than HIV. Control groups, and therefore meaningful studies that might quantify the risk from breastfeeding, would thus be impossible. Others argue that it is so important to find out if there is an increased risk that further studies must be done. From this point of view, it would be unethical not to do further studies.

Maternal antibodies to HIV may protect infants against infection

Possible protective effects of breastfeeding also need to be taken into account.

Maternal antibody to HIV, passed to an infant during pregnancy, may be a source of protection against HIV infection of the infant during and after pregnancy. Maternal antibody to HIV in breastmilk may also confer protection. If a woman becomes HIV-infected around birth or during breastfeeding, the infant would not benefit from her antibodies during pregnancy or part of the breastfeeding period, and could be more susceptible to infection through breastfeeding.[32,37]

Even the extent of the presence of HIV in breastmilk is uncertain. A group in the USA have tried but have been unable to isolate any HIV in breastmilk, though they have found antibodies to HIV. In 1991 this group published evidence that strongly suggests that breastmilk may not be infective if it does contain HIV. They found that certain factors in human milk may prevent HIV from being infective – factors which do not exist in cow's milk. These factors were present at varying levels in the milk of both HIV-positive and HIV-negative mothers, with no differences between the two groups.[37,38]

Protective effect of breastmilk for HIV-positive babies

In 1990, a study in Italy of 100 infants infected with HIV before birth showed that the bottle-fed babies developed AIDS at a median age of 10 months. The breastfed babies developed AIDS more slowly, a median of 19 months. Up to about five years of age, the breastfed babies fared better. This study was retrospective, and again, factors such as the mother's health and period of breastfeeding were not taken into account. However, it is an indication that the health of infants with HIV infection may benefit from breastfeeding.[39]

Thus, there is also evidence of protective effects of breastmilk.

The dilemma for public health policy

How many babies are at risk of HIV infection transmitted through breastfeeding? Unknown. How many babies are protected from HIV infection through breastfeeding? Unknown. How many babies are more at risk from causes unrelated to HIV from infant formula feeding? Millions. The dilemma is that it is not possible to make one recommendation that will protect them all.

It is very difficult to support universal breastfeeding if it might cause HIV infection in infants, even if the risk is unquantified. Where there are safe alternatives to breastfeeding, an unknown number of babies who were not infected during pregnancy will be protected from infection during breastfeeding, without being at serious risk from other causes. Hence, in the late 1980s policymakers in the USA recommended that women who know they are HIV-positive should not breastfeed. The UK went even further and advised in 1988 that women known to have HIV and all women at high risk of infection should be discouraged from breastfeeding.[40]

As an almost immediate reaction, donor milk banks in the UK were closed down because of fear that some of the milk might be infected, even though donor breastmilk can be made safe from infection.[41] Thus, the safest alternative to breastfeeding for the babies of women who cannot or are advised not to breastfeed was removed in the UK.

In 1989, in response to widespread protests at the international ramifications of a no-breastfeeding-with-HIV policy, the UK issued a revised circular. It expressed continuing support for breastfeeding of the majority of infants, acknowledged the hazards of incorrect use of infant formula, even in the UK, stressed that mothers using infant formula needed added support, and stressed the advantages of donor breastmilk over infant formula feeding. But it still said that HIV-positive women should be advised that it is prudent to avoid breastfeeding. It noted that this guidance might be inappropriate for other countries, particularly developing countries, where the balance of risks and benefits might be

different. It said that this guidance was not intended for use outside the UK.[42]

However, the word spread. In November 1990, a national expert on AIDS in the Bahamas said at a conference on women and AIDS that it was Bahamian policy to advise HIV-positive women not to breastfeed.[43] And in Zambia, many mothers began to believe that breastfeeding was dangerous, while health workers made accusations of double standards for developed and developing countries. Surveys in Kitwe and focus group discussions in Lusaka townships found that many mothers were afraid to breastfeed their babies in case they passed on HIV.[44,45] The consequences for infant health from formula feeding are likely to be serious.

Prior to the publication of the European data, two studies had concluded that where the infant mortality rate from all causes is higher in bottlefed babies than breastfed babies, all women should be encouraged to breastfeed to protect uninfected infants. Even if the transmission rate of HIV during breastfeeding were near 100 per cent, which it is not, the more women who did not breastfeed because they were afraid they had HIV, the higher the infant death rate would rise. One found this for New York City, the other for developing countries. These researchers concluded that more infant deaths would occur if fewer infants were breastfed, whether the mothers and infants had HIV or not.[46,47]

World Health Organization recommendations in 1987, reaffirmed in 1991, reflected this awareness. They came down strongly in support of breastfeeding. They said that wherever safe and effective alternatives to breastfeeding were not available, no matter what the mother's HIV status, breastfeeding was the method of choice.[32,48]

In 1992 European data led to qualifications in this policy. Where breastfeeding is the only safe option, babies who are breastfed may be more at risk of HIV infection from breastfeeding than was previously thought – while those babies who are not breastfed are at risk from other causes of infant death. It is not just a double standard, but a no-win situation for the infants of poor women in developing countries.

In May 1992 the WHO convened an expert meeting to discuss the consequences of the European data. In a press release and policy statement, they recommended that:

- Where infectious diseases and malnutrition are the main causes of infant deaths and the infant mortality rate is high, pregnant women, including those who have HIV, should be advised to breastfeed to avoid the risk of infant death from other causes.
- Women in these settings who know they are HIV-infected, for whom alternative feeding might be an appropriate option, should seek advice from their health care providers in making a decision how to feed their infants most safely.
- Where infectious diseases are not the main cause of infant deaths, and infant mortality is low, women who know they have HIV should use a safe alternative to breastfeeding.
- When a baby is to be fed by artificial means, the choice of substitute feeding should not be influenced by commercial pressures. Companies selling infant formula should respect the International Code of Marketing of Breastmilk Substitutes.[31]

These recommendations seem to be the only way to protect the maximum number of infants. But will people understand the complexity of the problem?

To what extent will a policy that advises some women not to breastfeed encourage the existing trend away from breastfeeding in rich and poor countries alike? How many babies will die unnecessarily because they were not breastfed? Will it be more or less than those who may become HIV-infected through breastmilk?

Within days of the WHO press release outlining these recommendations, a Kenyan newspaper headline read: 'HIV transmitted by breastfeeding.' It matters little that the article qualified this headline.[49]

Even before HIV and breastfeeding were linked, it was an uphill battle to encourage breastfeeding around the world. In Zimbabwe, many middle-class women partially breastfeed their babies, but have them bottlefed when they are at work. Poor women often try to emulate the middle class. If a domestic worker is bottlefeeding her employer's baby, she is less likely to fully breastfeed her own. Women's fears that they may have HIV, their refusal to be tested because they do not really want to know, and now the fear of transmitting HIV to their infants will add immeasurably to this tendency.[50]

It is more than unfortunate that so few studies and incomplete data have had to be used to determine such major policy. It is a painful lesson that studies of infant health which do not look at maternal health, and those that look at AIDS issues without looking at other health issues, are inadequate. More harm than good may result.

It is hard to see how this uncertainty can be resolved unless more is learned about the actual extent of risk to infants of infection through breastfeeding by HIV-positive mothers. It is difficult to accept that any further research on the subject would be unethical when so much is at stake.

Safe alternatives when breastfeeding is not possible

- Pasteurization of mother's breastmilk.
  Breastmilk can be pasteurized at 56 degrees centigrade for 30 minutes, with gradual heating and cooling conditions, in either Vickers or Axicare pasteurizers. HIV that was added to breastmilk was no longer detectable when the milk had been heated to this temperature.

  A higher temperature of 62.5 degrees centigrade is recommended in UK guidelines. The lower temperature of 56 degrees may be better as it preserves more of the immunological and nutritional properties of breastmilk, which may be partially destroyed by the higher temperature.[41]

- Donated breastmilk.
  Breastfeeding women can be asked to donate breastmilk and could be given nutritional supplements to help with milk production. To ensure their milk is safe:
  – they can be tested for HIV antibodies and asked not to donate if they think they have been at risk of infection in the six months prior to donation.
  – their milk can be pasteurized, as above.
  Or both procedures can be used for extra insurance. The milk can be stored in a milk bank.

  The advantages of pasteurization are that milk can be pooled and stored, and donors need not be tested. The advantage of screening and testing donors is that milk need not be pasteurized. But the technical resources for HIV testing, pasteurization and storage of milk are costly.

  Where there are no refrigerators, breastmilk can be stored in a cool place for up to six hours in an earthenware pot that has been soaked in cold water. This is how water and cow's milk are kept cool, and breastmilk contains less bacteria than cow's milk when kept in this way.[50]

  There are other disadvantages. Donors and recipients have to go to the hospital or clinic regularly. This may not be feasible for many women. In developing countries it may be more realistic in small, organized communities. Cultural taboos and stigma may also be prohibitive. In parts of North Africa, for example, women traditionally do not go out for 40 days following childbirth.

  More research and development of appropriate and affordable technology for donor milk banking in developing countries is needed.

- Wetnursing by women known to be HIV-negative.
  Where milk donation is not possible, wetnursing – breastfeeding by another woman – may be a viable alternative. It is still widely practised in many cultures, and there is good reason to suggest bringing it back elsewhere.

  Women willing to wetnurse can be tested for HIV antibodies and asked not to volunteer if they think they have been at risk of infection in the six months prior.

  Again, there are disadvantages. Women in many parts of Africa will not use a wetnurse unless she is a relative, for fear of witchcraft. No matter who does the wetnursing, the wetnurse may be blamed if the baby becomes ill. Such issues require discussion with and among women.

- Artificial feeding.
  This should only be suggested if:
  – the mother's milk cannot be pasteurized;
  – breastmilk from a donor or wetnurse is not available;
  – the mother is given or is able to afford adequate supplies of infant formula, has access to clean water, is taught how to measure and mix formula and to clean bottles or containers used, and can be supported in feeding the baby.

  In many rural areas in developing countries, there may not be enough water or fuel to boil water to sterilize bottles and teats. Teats can harbour harmful bacteria even more easily than bottles. A feeding cup or cup and spoon can be recommended instead of bottle and teat. Cleansing these requires less water and is easier, especially for older children looking after younger ones while mothers are working.

The dilemma for women

'What would you do if you had HIV and it was your baby? Would you breastfeed?' The bottom line is that every woman will have to make her own decision, and health care providers will have to advise women on the basis of the women's own personal circumstances.

But how many health care providers are advising women with balanced and full information, to counter media headlines such as the Kenyan one? How many governments are prioritizing public education for women and providers on this issue?

How much support will be given to women who decide to use an alternative to breast-feeding because they are afraid to breastfeed? In their 1992 policy statement, the WHO failed to mention the alternatives of donor breastmilk or wetnursing for women who cannot breastfeed, though they had suggested both as being preferable to infant formula in 1987.[32]

How many women will use infant formula because there is no alternative? Will govern-ments make the water supply clean where it is not? Will they provide infant formula free to women who cannot afford to buy it? Will the companies give it away?

Surveys of how clinicians are advising women are needed, and monitoring of what women are doing and how this is affecting infants should be extensive. Will it be?

It is worth repeating that women need to be advised before and during pregnancy and after birth that if they themselves have HIV in pregnancy there is a well-studied risk to the foetus of infection, and an unquantified risk to their infants of transmission through breastmilk, particularly if they become infected perinatally or post-partum, or are at advanced stages of illness.

These risks underscore the importance of safer sex, safe blood supplies, and the importance of drug treatment programmes and education for women users. It cannot be said often enough that preventing infection in infants means preventing infection in women. The transmission chain that infects infants is a public health problem, not just a woman's problem.

Strategies for prevention of pregnancy-related transmission

by Janet L. Mitchell

Prevention of perinatal transmission of HIV can be looked at in terms of primary and secondary prevention. Primary prevention can be viewed as:

- preventing pregnancy in the HIV-infected women,
- identifying which woman is most likely to transmit the virus to her foetus, or
- identifying early in pregnancy which foetus is likely to be infected or become infected.

We have the technology to do the first – the use of an effective contraceptive method. However, technology and society have not kept up pace. Many of the women who are HIV infected or at high risk of infection are not consumers of our contraceptive technology. The reasons vary from country to country, and from woman to woman, but are closely related to the perceived role or function of women in that society or culture.

Therefore, the appropriate application of contraception must be linked to an understanding of the various cultures and may involve extensive re-education of an entire society. If a society defines the primary function of a woman as bearing children, not bearing children makes that woman a dysfunctional part of that society. To change that focus on childbearing entails a re-education of every member of that society.

Since 70 per cent of children born to women who are HIV infected may not themselves be infected, a more acceptable approach for many women may be to identify those who are at highest risk of transmitting the virus to their unborn children, or identifying those foetuses who are at highest risk of developing infection. If available prior to pregnancy, this information may persuade a woman to delay or postpone pregnancy. Or, if the information is available early enough in pregnancy, it may give the woman the option of terminating the pregnancy – if her society or culture allows this and if she so chooses. Definitive information given to a woman and her family about her own, individual risk for that particular pregnancy may make it more likely that she will not pursue or continue the pregnancy. When given information about the risk for the general population only, many of us would like to feel we will be the exception. The need for self-worth and self-esteem from a baby make our odds appear even better.

Secondary prevention can be defined as preventing or interrupting transmission of the virus to the foetus or newborn. It is this strategy that may be the most promising. Presently, two approaches are being explored.

The role of anti-virals in preventing or interrupting transmission in utero or at delivery is being aggressively pursued. This approach has challenged us to re-examine the exclusion of pregnant women from most research, which has a sound basis in protection of the foetus. In HIV disease, however, the question must be asked: 'How is the foetus best protected?'

It is critical that this issue be resolved in a timely fashion, because pregnant women are the ideal candidates for an alternative approach to secondary prevention – the development of an effective vaccine. An effective vaccine that would block perinatal transmission of the virus would allow HIV-positive women to again be able to exercise their rights to all reproductive choices within the confines of their individual societies and cultures.

Safe motherhood and HIV/AIDS: the issues for women

Women found to have HIV are marked out as different from other women by health professionals, no matter whether they decide to continue or terminate a pregnancy, or seek infertility treatment. While concern for the welfare of the woman and her infant is partly the reason fear, disapproval and rejection may also play a major role.

Deciding to continue pregnancy

Many countries are failing to prevent maternal and infant mortality and morbidity from causes that are more easily preventable and treatable than AIDS. Because AIDS has been seen as a unique threat, rather than as a new cause of these deaths, HIV-positive women's decisions to have children have called down the disapproval of certain professionals.

This disapproval has been expressed in public policy and professional advice to women with HIV not to have children. Like the American College of Obstetrics and Gynecology (ACOG) in 1987, they have recommended that 'infected women should be encouraged not to become pregnant and should be provided with appropriate family planning assistance',[1] sometimes including the option of abortion.

Despair is often expressed when women with HIV say they intend to continue a pregnancy. As a result, women have often been compelled, not only by the reality of the virus but also by their doctors and counsellors, to confront their own and their children's possible early mortality in a direct and sometimes brutal fashion.[2]

Is this ethical? The status of a woman depends on her ability to have children. In many parts of the world, a woman is still a girl until she has her first or second child, and her reproductive capacity is often seen as the possession of her husband or of his family. Even where women's status has begun to move beyond these narrow confines, women with no children are often pitied or considered incomplete.[3] Having children is central to women's identity, whether married or single.

Counselling for those with HIV, as with all chronic illness, encourages living positively, believing in the ability to stay well and carrying on with life. Women with HIV are having children because they are women, regardless of colour, culture or class.[3,4,5] They are choosing to live until they die. Having children is one of the most concrete expressions of positive living that women can make.

Professionals have begun to recognize that their focus has been too narrow. In trying to reduce the numbers of infants with HIV, they had forgotten to take women's lives into account. By 1990, the ACOG had changed their recommendation to say: 'An individual woman's reproductive choices should be respected regardless of her HIV status.'[1] This acknowledges not only that women with HIV are having children, but that it is their right to do so, and that informed choice is the only ethical basis on which to counsel them.

Women do think about the situation and ask many questions about the risks to themselves and an infant before making a decision.[6,7] They can even forget themselves in their concern for the infant.[8]

Women often look at the risk of infection during pregnancy from the positive side. They see that 60–85 per cent of children will not become infected, and hope theirs will be among them.[9] Counsellors may be afraid that providing this information will encourage women to get pregnant who might otherwise have decided against it. But this assumes an importance of counselling over and above women's life experience and hopes. Those giving counselling to women need to examine their own feelings about HIV and AIDS, as well as about pregnancy, having children, abortion and death.[4] The demands of women's lives and the desire to have children override many other considerations.

'Several times, women I am seeing have got pregnant immediately after their HIV test, even between the pre- and post-counselling period of two to six weeks. Sometimes testing positive for HIV seems to accelerate their desire to get pregnant. The reality of a baby's suffering and dying from AIDS may be an unknown quantity to a young, first-time mother.

In the beginning I was astounded when this happened, and was concerned that I was not being an effective counsellor. Then I began to talk it through with the nursing staff and some of the women themselves. It became clear that not having children was not an option for these women. They felt that as long as they were healthy, they would go ahead and take their chances.'[3]

HIV can also create compelling reasons for having children. For women with HIV who have experienced AIDS deaths in their families, having children is a chance to leave survivors behind and to leave someone for their families to care for in the future. One woman, whose husband, two brothers-in-law and one sister-in-law have died of AIDS, reasoned that: 'For every single infected child averted to limit the transmission of AIDS, two healthy children would be eliminated. I ponder what the reality of such a proposal will be . . . applied to me and my family, where an entire generation of men have ceased to exist'.[10]

Some women with HIV have expressed the determination to have even more children than they might otherwise have done, in order to ensure that some survive.[11] This is far from unusual in communities used to a 10–30 per cent infant mortality rate. The greater the perception of threatened infant mortality, the more a woman may feel she has to take her chances.[4] There is a Rwandan proverb that says: 'In order for a child to die it must be born.'[2]

'We do not agree that there is an absolute standard by which the birth of an HIV-infected baby is morally unacceptable. There is no intent to create harm. In fact, the intent is just the opposite – to bring good into the world. There is no certainty that harm will be done. The majority of babies born to HIV-infected mothers will not be infected. HIV-infected women have the same moral obligation as men to refrain from behaviours that put their sexual or needle-sharing partners at risk. Although there are alternatives to unsafe sex and sharing needles, there is no safe alternative for an HIV-positive woman who wants to give birth to a baby.

Although the birth of HIV-infected babies

Grace

'Grace is 32 years old. She arrived in the UK last year. Her partner was keen for them to start a family because they had been together for several years and he was 35 years old. After three to four months, Grace fell pregnant. Both she and her partner were delighted. She booked in at a relatively large London maternity hospital where, on booking, she was tested for HIV without consent or knowledge of what she was being tested for.

Four weeks later, Grace returned to the antenatal clinic for a routine check-up. She was told very briefly by the doctor that she had been tested for HIV and was found to be seropositive. He said not to worry, he would refer her to an excellent physician at a nearby hospital, where she could be counselled and told what she should and shouldn't do.

During the time since Grace was diagnosed, her partner left her, she became homeless and was financially ruined. Not only did she have to come to terms with the fact that she was HIV-positive, but she was now in a country where she didn't really know anybody. She was desperate.

Through great strength of mind and determination, she managed to get part-time work in a hotel and accommodation. I suggested that she might benefit from going along to a support organization, which she did. They have been extremely helpful and supportive and, it is hoped, will continue to be so in the future.

She is keen to know as much as possible about HIV and AIDS, and has expressed a desire to become active in a supportive role for other women who might be in a similar situation to herself. She appears to have accepted her condition at the moment and wants to work and focus hard on making a future for herself and her child.'[6]

Elise

'Elise was very happily married, was in a good job with responsibilities and was very pleased to be pregnant. She decided to take out life insurance when she was 20 weeks pregnant. To her surprise, she received a letter from the company, informing her that she was HIV-positive.

She had gone to the antenatal clinic and told the obstetrician/midwife about her diagnosis. She felt that on that and subsequent visits the staff's attitude towards her had become cold and non-communicative. She felt so isolated and rejected that she went and told her doctor, who referred her care to us. We arranged antenatal check-ups on a regular basis, liaising with a paediatrician, health visitor and obstetrician. Elise delivered a beautiful baby girl and has since gone home. She is asymptomatic.

Her partner confessed later how very guilty he felt about the whole situation. He had known his previous girlfriend was HIV-positive, and she had died of AIDS about five years before. He had always thought he might be positive, but was never tested. It was almost as though he wanted that part of his life to be shelved and forgotten. Unfortunately, in the stark reality of it all, this was not possible.'[6]

has clearly desirable consequences from the point of view of mothers, public health officials, medical professionals, and society, it is in our view the tragic but inevitable price we must pay for previous and current neglect of their mothers.'[10]

Fear of telling partners

Although the majority of partners might be supportive if they learn that women have HIV during a pregnancy, many women do not tell their partners of their HIV infection. In a large study in Zaïre, more than 97 per cent of pregnant women were unwilling to inform their partners because of fear of divorce, physical harm or public scorn.[12]

Men also do not always tell their women partners of their own risk of infection.

Conflicting feelings

HIV can make uncertainties about pregnancy more problematic. Most women do not know when they became infected. Because the risk to both the woman and the infant may be higher or lower at different points after infection, there is pressure to choose the right time to become pregnant, if at all. If already pregnant, whatever decision she makes, a woman will fear it was the wrong one. There will be guilt if the child proves to be HIV-positive, and uncertainty over whether it was infected if abortion is chosen.[4]

In the USA, one woman was so angry and depressed about her own and her child's HIV infection that she was unable to make an active decision, and carried her next pregnancy to term. She then became pregnant again, had an abortion, and planned to be sterilized. Another woman had decided to continue her pregnancy but miscarried. She got pregnant twice more. She had an abortion with the first of these pregnancies and continued the next one.[13]

It is no wonder that many women prefer not to know their HIV status during or just after a pregnancy. The conflicting feelings may become too great to resolve or cope with all at once. The more difficult a woman's circumstances generally, the more likely this is to be true.

Deciding to terminate pregnancy

Not all HIV-positive women continue their pregnancies if they learn they have HIV.

In a group of women in Scotland, knowledge of positive HIV status did not influence the rate of abortion and the HIV-positive women's reasons for abortion were only sometimes different. Forty-four women knew they were positive before they became pregnant, and 21 had a termination. HIV infection was the main or only reason given for termination by nine of the women, including two who had AIDS and two who had HIV-related illness. Of 25 women who learned they were positive during pregnancy, nine had requested a termination before their test result was known, and one asked for a termination after receiving her result.[9]

In New York City, four out of 18 women who learned they had HIV during pregnancy decided for abortion, on the grounds of risk to themselves and the infant of HIV infection. Among 11 seropositive women who had learned their HIV status during a previous pregnancy and had become pregnant again one or more times, one woman decided for abortion.[13]

Women's circumstances may make it impossible to consider or carry out the decision to have an abortion. In New York City, among women with a history of injection drug use, one woman made attempts to get an abortion but could not find an outpatient clinic that would take a methadone patient at her dosage. She refused inpatient procedures because she did not want her family to know.

One said abortion was unacceptable to her.

Another overtly denied her infection. Another with mental health problems and learning disabilities had a limited understanding of HIV infection and an aversion to abortion.

Two others made attempts to get an abortion. One was too incapacitated by chronic drug use to follow through. The other had problems arranging inpatient services because she needed childcare. Her partner was against abortion and would not assist her. When he learned of her arrangements, he assaulted her and broke her jaw. She may have become pregnant again later.[13]

In addition to individual problems, all of the existing legal and political restrictions on women's access to safe abortion in every country in the world affect HIV-positive women too. For example, an HIV-positive woman might have to tell an abortion provider her HIV status in order to have grounds for abortion, though this would violate her right to confidentiality.

Access to abortion after 12 weeks of pregnancy is restricted in many countries. Many women do not find out they are HIV-positive until they are pregnant, and often only in the second trimester or later, when they first attend for antenatal care. If women are to have a real choice of whether to continue their pregnancies, early and later abortion services need to be accessible to them.

For poor women with HIV, abortion may be too expensive to consider.

The illegality and consequent risks of abortion in many countries create additional hurdles. No published study has asked how many HIV-positive women seek or get terminations in countries where abortion is illegal, nor whether these abortions are safely provided.

During HIV counselling, if abortion is raised with women or if women bring it up themselves, there may be limited or no help that can be offered. There is anecdotal evidence that some doctors are providing safe abortions for women with HIV in Africa, but practice is likely to be inconsistent. Everyone knows that women will risk their health and lives to have clandestine abortions. If women with HIV are seeking clandestine abortions, abortion mortality could increase because of HIV/AIDS.

Some countries were considering changing their abortion laws in the late 1980s specifically to allow abortion on grounds of HIV infection. French Polynesia did so,[14] but in Mexico, although it was discussed by health officials, no changes have been made.[15]

An awareness of these issues, let alone changes in law and policy, have not been raised publicly or at policy-making level. In fact, the subject of access to safe abortion rarely if ever comes up in relation to HIV/AIDS.

Women from countries where abortion is illegal have said that campaigning for legal abortions for HIV-positive women may be a socially acceptable way to start raising the whole issue of abortion publicly.[16] This seems sensible, especially if all other routes are closed.

The issue of confidentiality should not be forgotten, however. It would be better to say that HIV is a reason for women's access to safe abortion, rather than arguing that HIV should be made a legal grounds for abortion.

Discrimination against pregnant women with HIV

The following are examples of how health care providers have discriminated against pregnant women with HIV in ways that threaten their health and lives.

Consequences of coercion

The logical endpoint of controlling the pregnancy decisions of HIV-positive women would be mandatory and repeated HIV testing of all women of reproductive age, forced abortion, criminalized childbirth and compulsory contraception or sterilization.[17]

Even without these, there are reports of women who have been pressured or coerced to have an abortion or be sterilized because they are HIV-positive. Racism and prejudice might contribute to a climate in which overt pressure and coercion are seen to be more tolerable.[17]

In Scotland, six HIV-positive women reported in 1988 that they had been told they could not continue their pregnancies and were forced to have abortions. They had all become pregnant again afterwards. One doctor found that some HIV-positive women were waiting to seek antenatal care until they were 26 weeks pregnant, in case they were told that the pregnancy had to be terminated.[18] Similar cases have been reported in London and in New York.[6,13] In Australia, HIV-positive women have been told by doctors that the rate of transmission to infants during pregnancy is 80-100 per cent, in order to convince them to have abortions.[19]

In Scotland an informal follow-up of 80 HIV-positive women, two years after they had been pregnant, found that six were dead. Only two had died of AIDS. The other four had died from drug overdoses, three of them following termination of pregnancy.[20]

In the USA, where there is a long history of sterilization abuse of poor and disadvantaged women, there are fears that the hard-won protection against such abuses will start to disappear. Involuntary sterilizations were again being reported in New York City's hospitals in

---

One woman's experience of coercion

A 38-year-old Haitian woman in New York City learned that she was HIV-positive during her antenatal care in a hospital with an excellent record for high-risk pregnancy care. She was advised not to tell anyone of her HIV status, that her chances of having a baby with AIDS were extremely high and that she should abort the foetus. She was also told to go home and write her will, because she was going to die. She was asymptomatic.

She chose to continue her pregnancy. When she went for her next routine check-up, she was taken to another building for a meeting with several high-ranking medical personnel. They told her that having a child with AIDS was worse than having a child with spina bifida, which her older daughter has. They said such a child would be a burden to society, and that she would be wrong not to abort. She insisted that she wanted to have the baby and pleaded that they continue her care. They refused, stating that the hospital was not equipped to treat her.

She was referred to another hospital for a second-trimester abortion. This was performed without counselling or obtaining her signed consent. She was placed in a room marked 'Isolation' during her induced labour and was left alone screaming for help for 15 minutes after the foetus was expelled. When she haemorrhaged because the abortion was incomplete, she was made to walk down the hall to the operating room. In both hospitals, as soon as they knew she was HIV-positive, she felt they wanted to get rid of her.

The Center for Constitutional Rights in New York filed a case against both hospitals for discrimination, inflicting emotional distress, negligence and failure to obtain consent for abortion in the second hospital.[21]

1990. There are fears that these may have been related to HIV.[17]

Refusal of infertility treatment

The most invisible of the many reproductive health issues related to HIV is infertility. In 1991, the *British Medical Journal* featured a debate on whether doctors should provide treatment to an HIV-positive couple to help them achieve a pregnancy.

The case involved a married couple who had sought infertility investigation and treatment at two clinics. Both had had children with previous partners. They had had unprotected intercourse for two years without conception. At the first clinic, the woman's treatment was discontinued when she was found to be HIV-positive. At the second clinic they told the staff of their seropositivity. After counselling, they continued to want treatment. The doctors decided the couple had a right to know the cause of their infertility, but refused to treat them. They felt that they would share the responsibility for the birth of an infant with HIV and for the child's likely future status as an orphan, even if not infected. They said they had also taken into consideration the risk of HIV transmission to staff during any procedures, though they admitted this was slight. They told the couple they could go elsewhere for treatment, knowing that the couple might decide not to reveal their HIV seropositivity at a third clinic.

Ironically, this same clinic had previously helped another couple where the woman alone was seropositive. Here, the only cause of infertility was that the couple had been practising safer sex. The clinic taught them how to do inseminations at home using the husband's semen, so that he would be protected from infection. This, they said, removed them from active management. They did not justify why they felt less responsible in the one case than the other, when the risk of infection for any infant was the same in both. They helped the seronegative man to protect himself from infection, yet were inadvertently encouraging the other couple, who went away still wanting a child, to have unprotected sex. These contradictions were not mentioned by the other professionals who commented on the case.

The lawyers discussed whether an infected child could hold the doctors or parents legally responsible for negligence, and concluded that it could not. The director of a private infertility clinic believed that refusing to treat a healthy HIV-positive couple was the same as refusing to treat anyone with a severe life-threatening disease, e.g. a woman with unstable diabetes or severe hypertension.

Two other doctors felt there was no positive duty to treat an infertile couple wlth HIV. They believed doctors must make moral decisions about what is in the best interests of patients and any child. A medical ethicist in turn questioned this view. If doctors believe they must be concerned with the welfare of children resulting from treatment, they are forced to impose a personal judgement on potential clients. He believed in treating all people who might benefit clinically, unless scarcity of resources was a limiting factor.[22]

Only one letter was later published from two doctors in London who directly supported the desire of women with HIV to have children. They felt there was no distinction between the fertile and the infertile in the need or right to have children, if they so desire.[23]

The space-suit approach to childbirth

Fear of HIV infection during childbirth is a common reaction among inexperienced professionals, and reactions can be extreme.

In 1990 a woman in Chile was tested for HIV in her third month of pregnancy, when she donated blood. She was only told she was HIV-positive in her eighth month of pregnancy, and the medical and paramedical personnel of the maternity and neonatal departments of the hospital were also told. Reactions were varied. On the one hand, staff expressed insecurity and even panic about the possibility of infection. On the other hand, everyone concerned, including the doctors, admitted their ignorance about HIV/AIDS and any precautions they might need to take.

A hospital resident offered to research the measures to be taken to prevent any risk to the staff during childbirth. Information sessions were organized. More than 150 people were shown a video that gave a concise explanation of HIV/AIDS and safety measures. A detailed plan was drawn up for handling her birth, including treatment and emotional support, and designating the labour, delivery and recovery rooms she would use. Norms were established requiring double gloves, caps, masks, boots and robes, and communicated to everyone who would be in direct contact with her. There was a contingency plan in case of caesarean birth.

The birth took place without problems, but the paediatrician, who was herself pregnant, was nervous and pricked her finger with the needle when taking a sample of the baby's blood. She panicked, but was not later found to have HIV.[24]

The recommendation to use double gloves, caps, masks, boots, robes, and isolation of the woman during labour, delivery and recovery are common responses of inexperienced health professionals. While some precautions need to be taken, these are overreactions and serve to make women feel more anxious during childbirth than necessary.[6]

Further, up to 150 health care workers may have been informed that this woman was HIV-positive, a gross and unnecessary breach of confidentiality. Not surprisingly, she was initially unwilling to tell her story to anyone else.

Abandonment in childbirth

It is universally agreed that pregnant women need good antenatal care and continuing care for themselves and their babies following birth. This assumes that such care is available, when for many women it is not.

With or without HIV, pregnancy, childbirth and abortion are often not a safe experience for women. Half a million women die each year, most in developing countries, from lack of or negligent care. International campaigns have led to some improvement in services, but they are far from reaching their goals. In the midst of global economic recession, services are in decline or ongoing crisis. Maternity care is still a privilege, not a right.[25]

Fear of HIV and AIDS is endangering the lives of pregnant women and their children in new ways. In 1989 a bitter public debate in the Dominican Republic began when doctors in the public health care system refused to attend the births of women with HIV. The assistant director of the country's only specialist obstetric hospital justified this stance, saying that doctors face a high risk of contracting HIV from patients and have a right to be afraid.[26]

At a press luncheon on AIDS in the Philippines one woman recounted that all the doctors in a hospital in her province had taken leave of absence when she was about to give birth. Only one of her relatives, who was a nurse and who could not bear to leave her alone, attended her birth. Afterwards, a sign was posted on the door of her room which said 'Isolated AIDS Patient: Keep Out'.[27]

The same year, the Egyptian public were said to be horrified by media reports that no one would assist an HIV-positive mother at birth. According to the press, the Deputy Minister of Health backed down on his offer to deliver the child and eventually supervised the birth through a window. A midwife finally volunteered to deliver the baby. Although the press heralded her as a heroine, she was subsequently ostracized by colleagues.[28]

In 1990, the Family Welfare Training and Research Centre in Bombay reported that an HIV-positive sex worker was abandoned by health care personnel at the time of her delivery and afterwards. Her birth was attended by her friends and her brothel keeper in the hospital where she had been admitted. The Centre decided to train some of the sex workers in first aid and home nursing as a result.[29]

In another case in Sri Lanka in 1990, doctors from the National AIDS Committee came forward to handle the delivery. Plans for national education on AIDS were probably implemented sooner following from this incident.[30]

The same year, among more than 900 community midwives in the UK, who do home visits after a woman has left hospital with her baby, 64 per cent were afraid of HIV infection from patients. Forty per cent believed they should have the right to refuse to provide care or did not know if they could refuse care for women known to have AIDS or HIV infection. Ninety-seven per cent thought they had a right to be informed of a patient's HIV status, and 77 per cent of these thought this could be without patient consent. Confidentiality was seen as a lesser concern than their own protection.

A major concern was lack of experience in dealing with infected patients. Two-thirds were worried about the resources available for this purpose. Many questioned the reliability of the information they were receiving, as this information was changing all the time.[31]

Refusal of abortion services

There is evidence from the USA that abortion providers are refusing their services to women who are HIV-positive. In 1989 an investigator for the New York City Commission on Human Rights phoned 30 abortion clinics to book an abortion. After making the booking, she would tell them she had HIV. Twenty of the clinics refused to keep the appointment. Twelve said they had inadequate infection control precautions.[32]

The following are examples of what the abortion providers said to her:

– Private doctor: the secretary said she did not know what HIV was. A nurse came on and told her they could not perform the procedure. When asked why, the nurse put the phone down and yelled, 'What do I tell her now?' The nurse came back and said the doctor would be on holiday for the next few weeks, and hung up. A call some days later ascertained that the doctor was not away.
– Clinic: the man on the phone said, 'We don't handle that type of patient. Please don't call for that,' and hung up.
– Clinic: the doctor told her that he would not perform the abortion because his staff would refuse to touch any person infected with HIV, and that he would not force them to do so. He advised her not to tell any other doctors that she was seropositive, and that she should go to a hospital for her abortion.
– Clinic: she was told that the clinic did not have the necessary 'special sterilization procedures'. When the investigator said they must have done abortions for HIV-positive women before, she was told that this was not the case. The clinic tested all clients for HIV without their knowledge.[32]

In a government information pamphlet about AIDS for women in Zaïre, there is one question and answer about abortion, which strongly discourages women from pursuing this option by giving medically false information:

Is abortion a solution for a seropositive woman who is already pregnant?

The ideal would be for an HIV-positive woman to avoid becoming pregnant. But where pregnancy has occurred, it is best for her to be under medical care. Abortion does not seem advisable with the current state of knowledge. It would even seem that abortion carries an increased risk of precipitating the start of disease. In the end, it is the doctor who must decide, taking into account not only the woman's history but legal considerations and each specific case, since in medicine, each patient's situation is unique. [33]

Overcoming discrimination by health professionals

If medical professionals are not well informed, are exposed to conflicting information, do not trust the information they receive, have seen relatively few women with HIV and have little of their own experience, fear and self-protective action can adversely affect the care they provide.

Identifying HIV-positive women will not keep health workers safe from HIV infection. There is no justification for routine HIV testing of women needing any reproductive health service. Service providers cannot possibly know whether every women they see has HIV or not, nor should they presume or expect that women who know their HIV status will reveal it, especially when confidentiality cannot be or is not assured. Nor should routine testing be the main priority of services with already scarce resources.

Fear is a human issue, however, not a technological one. Initial feelings of fear and anxiety can be turned into supportive and engaged care through education, training and informal discussions about the experiences of working with HIV-positive patients, where staff have the chance to talk freely about their own feelings. [7] And the need for supportive health care does not end when women with HIV become mothers.

Mothers living with HIV/AIDS

Women face many hurdles as they enter motherhood with HIV. Frequent clinical check-ups for the woman, and after delivery, for the child, are constant reminders of HIV infection. [7]

Waiting for up to 18 months to find out if the child is infected, and coping with illness in an infant and not knowing whether it is HIV-related, are stressful. [34] Uncertainty is present all the time and continuing support is needed. If the child is infected, it is a hard blow. Health care staff and support organizations are very important at this time.

A woman might fear that if the child was not infected during pregnancy, it can become infected later. Women need reassurance that holding and showing love to a baby and giving normal care cannot pass on HIV. [34]

People's fears of infection make it difficult for an HIV-positive woman to tell others that she has HIV and that her child may also. Many women keep this knowledge to themselves, though they are always aware of their own child's situation and what it is doing. Women say they try to guide the child's behaviour so that it cannot possibly harm other children, and this can be very isolating. [7]

Children very quickly become aware that the close monitoring they are undergoing is something out of the ordinary, and they look for reassurance from their mother. This places even more pressure on the woman, who is probably already stressed because of her own HIV infection. [35]

In 1989, a group in Scotland tried to find out what support women drew upon, to see if it could be improved in any way. They asked 28 HIV-positive mothers whom they felt able to talk to about HIV. Eighty-two per cent of the women said a health professional, including doctors, nurses, social workers, researchers or voluntary sector workers. Sixty-eight per cent said a parent or sibling, 64 per cent said their partner, and 46 per cent said a friend. Seven per cent said they could not talk to anyone.

Eighty-two per cent of the women knew other HIV-positive mothers, and 29 per cent discussed HIV with other mothers. Of those who did, 88 per cent found this useful. When asked if they would like to meet other parents who were HIV-positive, 32 per cent said yes. Several said 'not at this time, perhaps later'. The rest said no.

The main conclusions were that:

- HIV remains a closely guarded secret and women are selective about where they draw their support from.
- Most of the women preferred not to meet others for support.
- The type of support offered needs to be tailored to each family's needs if it is to be of any value. Some women will require practical and financial help, others will require emotional support because of relationship complications or their own psychological difficulty in coping with HIV infection.[35]

The women frequently asked: 'What can I say to my child about what is happening?' There is no single, simple answer to this, but honest information at a level that the child can understand is the most reassuring, rather than denial or half-truths which may have to be retracted at a later date.[35] There are a number of books for children, and in a few countries, support services and training exist to help parents to teach children, not only about HIV and AIDS but about their bodies, health care, sexuality and reproduction.[36]

Drug use is not necessarily incompatible with adequate child care and no woman should ever have her child removed from her care solely on the grounds that she is using drugs, though child care may be compromised when drug use results in a chaotic lifestyle.[37]

Partners may become ill and die of AIDS, leaving women to cope on their own.

Psychologists in Mexico have found that women have a great deal of difficulty leaving a child or partner with HIV or AIDS, but instead will care for them, even at the cost of

their own health. In contrast, men more frequently abandon their families if the woman has HIV.[38]

Often, mothers with HIV are single parents. Some may not be able to turn to their families for help, or may live far from their families.[2] Others may be unwilling to involve their families because they do not want to reveal that they have HIV or do sex work, or they may have become alienated from their families through their own or their partner's drug use.[4]

Failing health will make women less and less capable of being sole caretakers.[39] Women should not have to take on alone the burdens of the larger society.[3] Again, social services, self-help groups and support from voluntary organizations make a tremendous difference if women become ill.

Families affected by HIV/AIDS

Women whose children have got HIV other than through pregnancy may not have HIV themselves. They will see these children through a varying number of years, healthy and ill, and possibly dying.

> 'The extent to which families have had to suffer the loss of beloved children, and have had to do even their grieving in secret, for fear of discrimination or perceived disgrace, is a real blemish on our society.'[39]

With or without children or partners with HIV/AIDS, and whether or not they are infected themselves, women may have adult children, other family members or friends who have HIV or AIDS. They may be involved as caregivers during illness and death, and may take responsibility for any children left behind if the people they are caring for are no longer able to cope.

Children of all ages are affected by deaths

of one or both of their parents from AIDS, and are doubly affected if they have HIV infection or AIDS themselves. These children are a community responsibility. No one wants orphans institutionalized, but in many cases that means that they must be cared for by the extended family.[3] Not all children can live full-time with other members of their families or friends/neighbours of their parents.

Babies and children who test positive for HIV are being left in hospitals for many reasons:

- Mothers have just left them there.
- Mothers are too sick to care for them.
- Mothers may have died from AIDS.
- Fathers are nowhere to be found.
- Fathers might not be aware of what has happened.
- Family members, through fear, anger or limited resources, are not in a position to help.[40]

In developed countries the standard alternative is to children them with foster families, in the hope that the families will eventually adopt them.

In Germany, under the auspices of the 'AIDS and Children' programme, supportive services are offered early to those affected. The goal of the programme is to keep families intact, despite obstacles, and to make it possible for them to remain together as long as they can. Some children have had to be moved into foster homes because of their need for care when parents are ill. One of the most difficult problems has been the placement of a child in the absence of parents, due to an AIDS-related death or prolonged hospital stay.[41] Families able and willing to cope with these children are hard to find because the children may have special needs and because of the stigma of AIDS. Training and support are needed.

A chilling anecdote

'There is a chilling anecdote that was told to me by a social worker in New York City. She was trying to help a young woman with AIDS whose two children were also infected. The woman was able to continue working and paying an outrageous rent in a crummy flat because her mother was paying for the AZT.

Relations between the mother and daughter had been strained at one time, since the initial infection came from the injection drug use of the daughter's deceased spouse. The fact that the injection drug use was the mode by which her daughter had become infected caused the mother to have an especially virulent hatred for illicit drugs.

So they were struggling and coping, until one day the daughter called the social worker hysterically. She said that the ceiling had just fallen into the meal she was cooking. That she was too sick and too tired after a day's work to go downstairs for more food, and besides, she did not have the money. The social worker said, "Come, come now! You have survived much worse than that. What is really the matter?" After a pause, the woman said, "You're right. There is something else. You know that crack raid last night that was in the papers? My mother was caught in the sweep. She had been selling crack (cocaine) to pay for my AZT."

So that is what an awful tangle we are in right now, and women are in the middle of the mess in a dozen poignant and dreadful ways: as people at risk, as parents of small children and adolescents who are not yet adequately warned; and as mothers of adult children, who need love, solicitude and help, as they always did, but now more than ever.'[39]

Some developing countries, where the numbers of orphans is high and increasing, are also turning to foster care as a solution. Often, community-based groups or non-governmental organizations arrange placements, since no formal government-run social services of this kind exist.

Other solutions are being sought. In Uganda, where the number of orphans is among the highest, many children whose parents have died of AIDS are living on their own, as no one has come forward to take care of them. This has worked best when the eldest child is a girl and takes over the mothering role.[42]

Zambia is considering a solution that involves help from extended families and communities, using kibbutz-style homes. In Israel, where the kibbutz model originates, responsibility for children is shared by the parents and the community. Children live in children's houses staffed by houseparents, and spend certain times each day and week with their parents.[43]

To get ideas for how to adapt this model in Zambia, both orphaned children and adult members of their extended families have been interviewed and proposals drawn up. Members of the extended family, who are willing to help but cannot take full responsibility, would act as parents do on the kibbutz. All the siblings from one family or more would live together in group houses, depending on their ages. These would be sited near the helping family members, with whom they would spend an agreed amount of time each week.

The children would attend school and recreational facilities in the community with other children, and might be moved to the group house gradually. For example, when one parent has died and the other is still alive, they might begin to take meals or attend a play group after school at the group house. Community leaders and extended families would be involved in planning and supervision. Church groups and women's clubs and organizations have said they are very willing to be involved in such programmes.[43]

Children who have lost their parents to AIDS are not only small children but also teenagers. Because of the association of AIDS with immoral sexual behaviour, these children may think their parents were immoral and may themselves carry the shame and stigma. Often it seems that the stigma carried within a person is much greater than that placed by society, and these children are unnecessarily carrying this burden.[3]

'I sometimes try to insist that we could always talk about AIDS as a family disease, for it has had an extraordinary impact on families, and sometimes it really is the disease of a dying family. In Africa this dynamic is very obvious now, but also in the United States there have been stories – growing more frequent all the time – of older children who have been left standing, like sole surviving trees in a burned-out forest, after their mother, father, and younger siblings have died around them. In one such poignant anecdote, a 13-year-old was quoted as saying how happy she was to be pregnant, because at last she would have someone she could keep.'[39]

A London midwife's experience and recommendations for infection control policy for all pregnant women delivering in hospital

by Sandra Dick

The quality and type of services for HIV testing in pregnancy vary enormously from one antenatal clinic to another. At St Mary's, where I work, we send women leaflets with information about HIV with their booking letter, before they come for their first visit to the antenatal clinic. One is called *HIV Testing: Your Questions and Answers*. The other explains that we carry out anonymous screening for HIV with all pregnant women coming to the clinic unless they tell us they do not want it.

This procedure has the advantage of raising awareness of HIV prior to the woman's booking visit. The disadvantage of raising the issue of HIV testing at the first visit is that women already have too much information to take in. They may feel more obliged to accept an HIV test. They may feel more vulnerable, they may consider it offensive or threatening, and levels of anxiety may be raised unacceptably.

Midwives are encouraged here to raise the issue of HIV at the first visit, usually by asking the woman if she received the leaflets. I feel it is important to explain to all women how HIV is transmitted and how it is not transmitted, before the woman makes a decision about whether she would like to see a counsellor, and/or have an HIV test. There is a counsellor available one day per week to see any women who request this.

Relationships between a woman and her midwife are usually based on mutual trust and respect. Breaches of confidentiality can be extremely damaging for the woman and her infant. In some circumstances, the woman's partner and family may not be aware of her HIV status and relationships with those people in her life may be placed at risk.

Should confidentiality be breached? I have known of a woman who delivered herself at home for fear of breach of confidentiality. Here at St Mary's, consent must be sought from the woman before discussing her case with members of other services.

Obviously a crucial time for the woman is when she receives an HIV-positive test result. My own experience is that most women wish to carry on with the pregnancy regardless. There is a very low uptake of termination of pregnancy. There is now a feeling that in the past there was over-enthusiasm about termination of pregnancy.

Some women have claimed that terminations were carried out after they were placed under enormous pressure to accept. I have spoken to several HIV-positive women who, in the past, had abortions on the grounds of possible foetal transmission, congenital malformation and HIV disease progression. They have subsequently fallen pregnant again and elected to carry on with the pregnancy. The inability to diagnose accurately whether the foetus was infected was given as the most common reason for their wishing to continue their pregnancies.

Infection control policy

At present I am trying to streamline our infection control policy, so that the health care workers do try to adopt a single-tier system for all women. In the past, dating back to 1985–6, we have focused on elaborate infection control measures which have probably done more harm than good. These have ranged from exaggerated visors to wellington boots to almost space-suit type clothing. Restricting our focus to issues of infection control, we may be distracted from other important issues, e.g. the psychosocial and physical impact of HIV on the woman herself.

The new policy is based on an assumption of HIV seropositivity and hepatitis B infection in all women, to avoid discrimination. This means a change for most health care workers and new ground rules for everyone.

Ground rules for normal childbirth and post-natal care in hospital

With all deliveries

- Staff to cover abrasions and, if extensive, skin lesions. This means wearing gloves when in clinical areas until lesions are healed.
- No re-sheathing of needles or sharps.
- Disposal of sharps in approved rigid containers.
- Minimizing of blood taking.
- Avoidance of exposure to blood, amniotic fluid and vaginal secretions.
- Glasses to be worn at delivery.
- Eyewash bottles to be available in case of splashes.
- Alerting staff to deal with splashes or injury from sharps immediately – good washing with soap and water.

- After delivery of the infant, mouth mucous extractors for aspiration of infants to be used only in emergencies. Otherwise, wall suction or mechanical suction to be used at all times, if possible.
- The bathing of the baby is important. It must be done before transfer from the labour ward to the post-natal ward, to ensure that all blood is removed (as long as temperature and overall condition of the baby allow this).
- The correct disposal of soiled linen in the appropriate bag.
- Disposal of soiled sanitary towels.
- Instructions to staff about spillages of blood.
- Good housekeeping practices, i.e. cleaning of surfaces, stethoscopes, laryngoscopes.
- Universal precautions apply with blood and other body fluids that contain visible blood. They also apply to semen and vaginal fluids, though these are not implicated in transmission from client to health worker.
- Universal precautions do not apply to sweat, tears, saliva, urine, faeces, or breastmilk (unless working in a milk bank). Urine and faeces should be dealt with in the usual manner, with gloves and careful handling. No extra precautions need be taken.

Additional precautions if a woman is known to be HIV-positive

- The membranes should remain intact as long as possible, when in labour.
- Invasive procedures such as use of foetal scalp electrodes and foetal blood sampling should be avoided, to reduce risk of transmission of HIV from mother to baby in labour.
- Midwives and others caring for women with HIV need not wear any protective clothing unless performing a procedure which may involve contact with blood or amniotic fluid. The main procedure where this is necessary is artificial rupture of membranes. when a plastic apron, gloves and eyewear should be used.

Post-natal care

After giving birth is the period when most HIV-positive women may experience stressful situations. In the past, they have been isolated in separate rooms and made to feel like outcasts.

It is not necessary to isolate the woman in a single room, nor is it necessary to provide her with separate toilet facilities. She need only be reminded that blood spillage should be dealt with promptly.

The emphasis in the care of all women during the post-natal period should be on self-care as far as possible.

If the midwife needs to touch the perineal area, discharge or caesarean section wound, then gloves should be worn – as with all women.

The infant goes to the post-natal ward with the mother unless there is a problem and the infant goes to the special care baby unit. The mother is taught how to care for the baby by the midwife. e.g., cord care, nappy changing, bathing. It is not necessary to wear gloves for nappy changing unless visible blood is seen.

Most of the women I've cared for have all been fully aware of the care taken with regard to spillages of blood, disposal of sanitary pads, etc. I usually go through the precautions that are taken by staff, and this should be done with all women.

Post-partum counselling of HIV infected women and their subsequent reproductive behaviour

by M. Temmerman, S. Moses, D. Kiragu, S. Fusallah, I. Amola and P. Piot

A study investigating the impact of maternal HIV infection on pregnancy outcome was conducted in 1988 at Pumwani Maternity Hospital, a large referral hospital serving 12 smaller health centre maternity units in Nairobi, Kenya. Women with an adverse pregnancy outcome (low birth weight or stillbirth) were recruited into the study along with women delivering normal birth weight infants. Out of a total of 1,507 women, 94 HIV-infected mothers were identified.

All were invited to a follow-up clinic 7–14 days post-partum, where they were to be informed and counselled as to their HIV status by a trained counsellor. Sixty-one of the 94 women returned for the follow-up visit.

HIV-positive women were more likely to be single, younger at age of first sexual intercourse and to have more sexual partners than the HIV-negative group. Twenty-three per cent of HIV-positive women had a history of perinatal death as compared to 10 per cent in the HIV-negative group. Positive syphilis serology was also associated with HIV infection.

Of the 61 women, 36 reacted calmly or indifferently to their diagnosis, while the remaining 25 expressed anxiety or shock.

For the HIV-positive women, information was provided on the transmission of HIV, how to prevent further transmission, and how to recognize the symptoms and signs of HIV-related illness. Emphasis was placed on informing the women of the potential effect of future pregnancies on their health, the risks of pregnancy-related transmission and the high mortality risk in infected children. The use of condoms and other appropriate methods of family planning was encouraged. The women were advised to inform their spouses of their diagnosis and to return with them to the clinic in two weeks' time for further counselling. A free supply of condoms was also offered to the women. Children born to HIV-positive mothers were referred to a paediatric follow-up clinic.

Only two seropositive women returned with their partners to the clinic for further counselling.

One year post-partum, the HIV-positive women who could be contacted (51 of 94) were asked to return to the clinic; 24 returned. Use of oral contraceptives and condoms was low among them, as it was among the HIV-negative women who were followed up. Only nine of the 24 HIV-positive women had informed their partners of their diagnosis. Two of the 18 married women in the HIV-positive group had been divorced by their husbands (one who had informed her husband and one who had not), as compared to two divorces among 26 married HIV-negative women. Only two of the 24 HIV-positive women considered their lives to have changed because of the HIV test. One was regularly using condoms with her husband and the other one was divorced. Fifteen of the 24 HIV-positive women expressed the desire to have many more children to ensure that some were healthy. Only one of the women had progressed from being asymptomatic to having symptomatic disease.

Although in our population legal abortion is not an option (and the majority of pregnant women do not attend antenatal clinics before the sixth month of pregnancy), we had hoped that our counselling sessions would encourage women to make more use of condoms, or failing that, to limit their family size through the use of other methods of contraception. However, the majority of women, when confronted with the notion of a high risk for child mortality, expressed the desire to have even more babies to increase the number of uninfected children. On being informed that the risk of pregnancy-related transmission may be 30 per cent or more, many women drew attention to the 70 per cent chance of having an uninfected child.

The low rate of partner notification found is also worrying. Among this population, coming home with information regarding an STD (called a woman's disease) generally puts the blame on the woman, and there is danger of being abandoned by the husband or replaced by another woman. The majority of these mothers therefore preferred to keep the information to themselves. Most of them were in good health and not prepared to worry unduly about future eventualities.

More intensive counselling than what we were able to provide might have yielded more positive results, and we are currently planning new studies to evaluate the impact of more intensive counselling on modifying behaviour. However, in the busy maternity and antenatal clinics found in most African countries, providing more counselling sessions and more time than what we had offered is probably not a realistic proposition.

Reproductive concerns of women at risk for HIV infection

by Ann B. Williams

As part of a wider study, I interviewed 15 women at risk for HIV infection through their own injection drug use and 6 who were at risk through drug use by their male sexual partners. Five of the six used non-injection drugs themselves. Twelve of the women were white, seven were African-American, and two were Puerto Rican.

Five of the women knew that they were HIV-positive. Three of these women had clinical symptoms of HIV; the other two were asymptomatic. Eight women had been tested for antibody to HIV and knew that they were HIV-negative. The others either had not been tested or did not share that information with me. Two women were married to men who were seriously ill with AIDS, and two women had HIV-positive children. Women with and without HIV infection were included in the sample to provide a fuller range of perspectives, not for the purposes of comparison.

The sample included non-high-school graduates and high-school graduates. Only two of the women were employed full time: one was a nurse and the other was a drug rehabilitation counsellor. The remaining 19 were homemakers and mothers. Ten women were married or in an exclusive relationship with a male partner, and 11 were single. All were heterosexual. All the women were in some way associated with a drug treatment programme.

The concern expressed by the women about the effect of AIDS on their families and communities was impressive. Many of the women said they wanted to do what they could to help fight AIDS.

Children were central to the lives of the women. Often estranged from other family members as a result of drug use, relationships with children were the most important connections they described. In the face of fear and hopelessness, their children gave them strength. All but one of the women interviewed had children or was pregnant at the time of the interview. Most were deeply involved with their children. Sometimes their children were the only people they spent significant time with.

Being a good mother was important. Being a good mother included not using drugs during pregnancy. Several women who had been addicted to heroin for more than 15 years described how they had stopped drug use when they were pregnant. Children were the greatest, sometimes the only source of strength in the women's lives. One said she used to think that if she had AIDS she would kill herself, but now she knows she would struggle to live for her baby. Others said that their children were what had helped them stop drug use. A woman with AIDS tearfully explained: 'You know what keeps me strong? My daughter. If I wouldn't have her, I think I'd be cracked up.'

The women worried what would happen to their children if they (the mothers) got AIDS. One woman, whose husband died of AIDS, refused to be tested because she did not want to tell her children that they might lose both parents. For the HIV-positive women, this was the most painful issue they faced: 'Cause once you're gone, ain't nobody going to love them like you. That's all I really care about, her and leaving her behind. I don't care about anything else.'

Although all but one of the women in the study believed that abortion was the right decision for an HIV-positive pregnant woman, no one had had an abortion for this reason. Three women had been pregnant in the past year, and one was pregnant at the time of interview. Each had had different experiences, but the theme of guilt and fear was common to all.

The first woman had been distressed during her pregnancy by pressure from her care providers and her husband to be tested for HIV. She was afraid that she would discover that she was positive and did not want to be tested. Looking back, she accuses herself of selfishness.

The second woman was also afraid of her HIV test results. Four months pregnant at the time of the interview, she had been tested but had repeatedly missed appointments to be given the test results. Although she said that if she were HIV-positive she would have an abortion, the time for abortion had passed. She also used the word selfish to describe her actions.

The third woman knew that she was HIV-positive before she became pregnant. She discovered her infection during a hospitalization for a spinal abscess. She was immobilized by fear, first, by fear of returning to the hospital for a tubal ligation and then,

after she became pregnant, by fear of how an abortion would affect her. This is her second HIV-positive child, and she talks about guilt if anything happens to the child because she chose not to have an abortion.

The fourth woman discovered her pregnancy and her HIV infection at the same time. She had always wanted a baby and felt this was her last chance. She sought information from nurses, physicians, and social workers about how likely it was that her baby would have AIDS. She took a positive view of the risks explained to her and interpreted the professionals' willingness to let her make her own decision as a sign that it was safe to continue the pregnancy.

Because we cannot predict which children will acquire infection in pregnancy, she based her decision on how she felt. 'I felt that if I felt well, the baby must be well. And I really needed her, for myself. In a lot of ways my decisions were selfish. They definitely were.'

If clinicians and public health officials concerned with preventing pregnancy-related AIDS focus solely on the prevention of pregnancy among women at risk for HIV, their programmes are likely to conflict with the desire of the women to become mothers and raise issues of the reproductive rights of minority and disenfranchised women.

For every infant with HIV acquired in pregnancy, there is also a woman with HIV infection. Mother and child are a unit whose best interests are served by preventing HIV infection in women to begin with, and by developing comprehensive clinical and supportive services for women who are already infected.

Reflections on the AIDS orphans problem in Uganda

by Christine Obbo

Rakai district has suffered most from the AIDS scourge and for some communities there the problem of AIDS orphans is a grave one. It takes time to raise the consciousness of patients with a fatal disease to continue leading economically productive and socially meaningful lives. It takes determination and commitment to focus their attention upon the survivors, and both rich and poor need reminding to plan for them.

The Save the Children Fund estimated in 1989 that there were 24,524 orphans in Rakai, almost 13 per cent of all children under 18 years old in the district. Of those, 48 per cent had lost their fathers only, 12 per cent had lost their mothers only, 30 per cent had lost both parents, and for 10 per cent there were no details. Officials would prefer to regard as orphans only children who have lost both parents. But the local communities define as orphans children who have lost a father or both parents. Because women have been outliving their husbands by six months to two years only, fatherless children are perceived as potential orphans. The number of AIDS orphans increases daily in Uganda, and the situation is going to be worse in districts where the rehabilitation of war orphans has not been completed.

The limitations of poverty

It is a widely held view that according to African tradition the extended family will absorb the orphans. The reality of the situation is that the problem is so enormous that the extended families cannot cope as they used to.

The problem of orphans cannot be regarded in isolation from the social and economic changes that have taken place in Uganda. The AIDS epidemic followed a decade and a half in which the Ugandan economy deteriorated so much that poverty became a reality and a threat to many families. Thus, with regard to the orphans, the extended families are doing all they can, but poverty limits what they can do. And in some families, individualism, wealth, and personal dispositions have inhibited closeness and sharing.

The majority of Ugandan women rarely control valuable resources such as land and livestock, and often have little claim or entitlement to the labour of others except their small children. As a consequence, widowhood represents impoverishment in general. In the case of AIDS widows, they may even have to pay off the debts incurred during the prolonged nursing of their husbands.

The lucky orphans

The lucky orphans are those taken by the extended families, but some families offer more potential for the future than others. Families of paternal and maternal aunts and uncles as well as grandparents below 60 years of age do not seem to suffer visible disruptions in their lives. These families are usually still in the child-raising cycle in their lives. Orphans do not constitute an assumption of new family burdens, as happens in the case of aged grandparents. Lucky orphans are also rescued by family friends. All these arrangements are traditional. In fact, children are usually exchanged between families and raised in the above situation even when their parents are alive.

Mention must be made of a category not usually regarded as extended family – divorced stepmothers. They have been rescuing orphans when both parents are dead and there is no one to take them. In some cases, they may have had no children in that particular family and may have a new family. Again, the children in these families appear happy. Hitherto it was not regarded as desirable to entrust parenting to grandparents or stepmothers because the former were indulgent and the latter spiteful.

Children-alone families

An increasing number of orphans are left on their own. Certain factors seem to favour the viability of children-alone families left on a plot of land and in a house. The most viable families have at least one girl, as the eldest child. Based on their early training in work, they manage to cook, grow food, and even make mats to generate income for basic subsistence needs and even school fees. Families with boys only or boys as elder children tend to resort to begging once the neighbours reduce the amount of help they can offer.

Viable children-only families also need to be near relatives who, although they may not provide labour or other economic support, nonetheless offer social and psychological support by including the children in social celebrations. In families that are not coping well, the children typically show physical signs of lowered nutritional status. This affects their school attendance as they succumb to frequent colds and fevers.

One of the main problems faced by community leaders is providing food and medication for these children. In some active communities, day care centres have been organized in the homes of widows, or in abandoned homes. Food is provided and volunteers feed and wash the children.

In two instances, individuals had solicited supplies of food, clothing and medicine as well as cash and had set up informal orphanages. Officials were unaware of these until a researcher pointed out dangers observed in these houses. There was overcrowding and many children were sharing a few eating and drinking utensils and toilet outlets. Many children had running stomachs, sore eyes and rashes on their bodies. They ate only small meals most days, except on days when members of assisting foreign NGOs were known to be coming. In both cases, the individuals lacked the experience to set up good orphanages. Because the officials did not have the resources to re-allocate the orphans, some of whom had come from outside the district, the homes continue to operate but with increased support from the international NGOs.

Orphans who are homeless need suitable home arrangements, security for themselves and their property, bodily comfort and shelter, growth through skills training and good health. Above all, their social, cultural and religious needs must be fostered.

The local chapter of the Uganda Women's Efforts to Save Orphans, together with interested Resistance Council members, try to arrange for food, day care and school fees for the orphans, but the few volunteers are always overworked, so their impact is limited. In response to the government's declared desire to reach the orphans through a community-based system, a Resistance Council member has proposed the formation of an Orphans Community-Based Organization in Rakai, which will coordinate locally the support and relief assistance programmes of the international NGOs. It will register the orphans and identify well-intended volunteers to be responsible for the orphans and to be answerable to the local Resistance Committees.

Prototype leaflets for women

The following are examples of leaflets about HIV, pregnancy, birth and children which can be used or adapted locally.

I. HIV/AIDS and Pregnancy: Information for You and Your Partner

ARE YOU PREGNANT?
ARE YOU THINKING OF GETTING PREGNANT?

THEN YOU NEED TO KNOW ABOUT HIV AND AIDS . . .

Having HIV, the virus that can cause AIDS, is not the same as having AIDS. It means the virus is in your body, and you could infect someone else. You or your partner could be infected and still feel fine for many years.

Being infected also means that you might become sick in the future. If you have HIV, no one can tell you if or when you might get AIDS.

If your partner has HIV, he could pass it to you:
- during sexual intercourse – including while you're trying to get pregnant or when you are already pregnant.

If you have HIV, you could pass it to the baby:
- during pregnancy and possibly during childbirth.

WHAT ARE THE RISKS FOR YOUR BABY?

The chances of your baby being infected during pregnancy can be as low as one in six, or as high as one in three.

The amount of HIV in your body is highest in the first months after you are infected, and again if you have HIV-related illnesses or AIDS. At those times, your baby may be more likely to become infected. If you are not well because of HIV or AIDS, pregnancy may affect your health too.

If you feel well and have minor or no symptoms, the chances are probably better that your baby won't be infected and that your health won't be affected by pregnancy either. No one can tell you for sure how great the risk is with any pregnancy.

There is no test you can have during pregnancy to find out if the baby is infected. At the moment, it may take up to 18 months for doctors to know if your baby is infected, unless the baby becomes ill before that from HIV-related causes.

Infants with HIV have about a one in four chance of becoming ill with AIDS in the first year after they are born. Some of these babies don't survive more than a few months or a year. If a baby doesn't become ill in the first months, it may live and be well many years with HIV. It may or may not need more medical care than other babies.

This is the chance you have to take with HIV and pregnancy.

WHAT SHOULD YOU DO?

If you think there is a chance that you or your partner has HIV, you first need to decide whether to have a blood test to find out for sure. If you're pregnant, you can still take the test.

If your partner agrees, it is always better for both of you to have the test at the same time. Then you can decide what to do together.

Not everyone wants to have an HIV test. If you're not sure, you should talk it over with your partner if you can, and with a health worker or an AIDS counsellor or information centre. You can do this together or alone.

If you are going to have the test, it's always better to do it before you become pregnant. But not everyone thinks about it until they are pregnant. Maybe you didn't know you could be tested. Maybe you didn't think about your risk. Or maybe you preferred not to know.

There is still time when you are pregnant, but again, if you want to be tested, it's better to be tested early in pregnancy.

If you or your partner have HIV and you decide not to be tested, you may learn of your infection if the baby becomes ill or is found to be infected after it is born.

Only you can decide.

IF YOU THINK YOU ARE AT RISK AND YOU DECIDE TO BE TESTED AND . . .

. . . THE TEST IS NEGATIVE
If both you and your partner test negative for HIV, you can get pregnant with no worries about HIV. But you need to make sure you don't get the virus between the time you are tested and the time you have your baby – or afterwards!

. . . THE TEST IS POSITIVE
If one or both of you tests positive for HIV, and you decide to try for pregnancy, you should practise safer sex with your partner except around the days you are fertile, the only days you can get pregnant.

If you want a child, but you don't want to risk infecting a baby, you could consider:

- adopting a child, or
- asking an uninfected woman to have a baby for you (if you are infected and your partner isn't)
- getting pregnant by an uninfected man (if your partner is infected and you aren't)

You can do this by one of you having sex with the other person or by inseminations with uninfected semen. An infertility clinic can advise you if you want to try inseminations in this way or use an anonymous male donor.

IF YOU'RE THINKING OF GETTING PREGNANT . . .

Take your time and decide what you think is best for you and your partner.

There's no need to rush into a decision or to get pregnant immediately. Practise safer sex and use contraception until you've made a decision.

IF YOU ARE ALREADY PREGNANT, YOU CAN . . .

. . . CONTINUE WITH THE PREGNANCY
Many women and couples make this decision, because they really want to have a baby.

In this case, it is important for you to have good care during your pregnancy and birth, and for you and your baby to get good care after it is born.

Always practise safer sex during pregnancy, for your own sake and for protection of the baby.

. . . DECIDE TO HAVE AN ABORTION
Many women who didn't want to be pregnant or weren't sure make this decision.

Some decide on abortion because they just don't want to take the risk.

Only you (and your partner) can make the decision for yourselves.

You and your partner still need to protect yourselves and each other afterwards:

- Use an effective contraceptive against pregnancy – go to a family planning clinic or your doctor for advice.
- Practise safer sex – use condoms during intercourse or avoid intercourse. Condoms may be your contraceptive choice too, or can be used in addition to another contraceptive.
- If you and your partner use injection drugs, don't share needles or always clean your needles and syringes with bleach before re-using them.

YOU CAN GET HELP MAKING YOUR DECISIONS

A midwife, a family planning clinic, your doctor, a social worker, an AIDS counsellor or information centre, or a women's health organization can help you think about what you want to do or refer you for the help you need.

You don't have to decide all alone!

II. HIV/AIDS, pregnancy, birth, breastfeeding and post-natal care

If you have HIV or AIDS and you are pregnant, it is very important that you have antenatal care for yourself and the baby that is coming.

PREGNANCY

- Seek antenatal care as soon as you know you are pregnant.
- It will help both you and your midwife if she knows that you have HIV. But you may not want anyone else to know. You need to find a midwife you can trust. You have a right to ask her to keep your HIV status private and to ask for your consent before she tells anyone else.
- Your antenatal care during pregnancy should be the same whether you have HIV or not, but you should also be checked for HIV-related problems. Some pregnant women experience nausea, shortness of breath, etc. Keep an eye on these problems, as they may also be HIV-related.
- It is important to practise safer sex with your partner throughout your pregnancy and after you have given birth. This will help to protect both of you and your baby.
- If you use injection drugs, pregnancy is a good time to try to give up – both for your own sake and for the sake of your baby. Professionals used to think there was a risk to the baby if a woman stopped using drugs during pregnancy, but that has changed now. Try to find an agency who can help you.

BIRTH

Every woman should be treated the same – before, during and after birth. Unfortunately, this is not always the case. Until attitudes change, women who are HIV-positive will always encounter a certain amount of ignorance. Extra precautions are sometimes taken when a woman has been honest enough to reveal her HIV status.

- Giving birth to your baby normally does not put your baby more or less at risk of HIV infection. There is no reason why you should have a caesarean section because you have HIV.
- There are precautions that health professionals should take with every woman and baby during and after birth – these should be explained to you. For example, everyone who will assist the birth should wear simple protective gloves and glasses to avoid skin and eye contact with your waters when they break and with the blood and fluids that are present with all births.
- There is no reason why you or your baby should be isolated in any way after your baby is born. Again, simple precautions like cleaning up any blood spillage apply with all women. These should also be explained to you.

BREASTFEEDING

Almost all babies who have HIV infection became infected during pregnancy or childbirth. There is a possible risk of infection through breastmilk, though only a few cases have been identified worldwide.

Your baby might be at greater risk from breastfeeding if you were infected with HIV late in pregnancy or in the months after you gave birth. You need to protect yourself from HIV at these times.

Breastmilk will also help to protect your baby, whether or not it has HIV. Breastmilk protects babies against many childhood illnesses and infections, while infant formula does not. For many babies, the risk of other infections and malnutrition with infant formula feeding is much greater than the possible risk of HIV infection from breastmilk.

It is important to get advice from a health worker about whether to breastfeed your baby. The health worker will help you to choose the feeding method that is safest for your baby.

One safe alternative would be to express your milk and have it pasteurized in a clinic, so that you can feed it to the baby. This would make it safe from HIV infection.

There are several other options for feeding your baby:

- arrange to feed your baby with breast-milk from a milk bank which tests donors for HIV or pasteurizes their milk.
- find a wetnurse who is not HIV-positive.
- get support from a health worker in using infant formula safely.

POST-NATAL CARE FOR YOU AND YOUR BABY

Both you and your baby deserve good post-natal care, whether or not you have HIV. Again, this care should be the same for all women and babies.

Because your baby may have HIV infection, doctors and midwives will want to keep an extra careful eye on you and your baby's health. This may mean more visits from the community midwife or to the clinic than you might otherwise have had.

Your baby should be immunized against the same childhood diseases as other babies, and vaccinated against polio and whooping cough using an inactivated vaccine. Only the live vaccine BCG is not recommended, and even this advice is changing, so ask a health worker.

III. HIV/AIDS: you and your children

Your child cannot be taken from you just because you, your partner, or the child has HIV infection or AIDS.

Social workers and everyone helping people with HIV will try to support you, your partner and your children so that you can remain together for as long as you are able to look after your children.

If you or your partner have AIDS or HIV-related illness, you may need support. There may be help you can get – don't be afraid to ask for these.

CHILDREN WHO ARE HIV-POSITIVE

Like adults, children can be infected with HIV and remain completely well.

Children who are HIV-positive may suffer from ordinary childhood conditions such as diarrhoea, running nose, sore throat or ears, skin rashes, and fevers. More serious difficulties include: failure to thrive, lung disorders (pneumonia or tuberculosis), lack of coordination or seizures.

If your child is or may be HIV-positive and shows any signs of these infections, seek medical help and prompt treatment. The condition may or may not be HIV-related. It is often difficult to tell the difference.

If your child comes into contact with chickenpox or measles, even if they have been immunized, you should contact your doctor within 5 to 7 days. They may need a shot of immunoglobulin in case they have not developed enough antibodies to cope with these infections.

It is important to allow your children to play freely with other children. There are no known cases of children infecting each other through everyday activities.

Day nurseries and childcare facilities should always accept a child with HIV infection.

CHILDREN WHO ARE HIV-NEGATIVE

Many HIV-positive women have said they are afraid to have a loving relationship with their children who are HIV-negative. There is no need to worry. It is impossible to infect a child through normal loving and affectionate behaviour.

Make sure you carry out standard hygienic procedures. Cover any open sores, cuts or grazes with a plaster. Mop up any split blood yourself, using bleach in the water. Wash any clothes or bedclothes containing blood, urine or faeces in the hot cycle of a washing machine or with a disinfectant in the water.

SCHOOLS

There is no record of children infecting each other in school. Children with HIV should receive a normal education and have access to the full range of school activities. Parents whose children are HIV-positive need not tell the school authorities. You may find it preferable to inform the head of the school, to make sure your child gets full support. Ask the head to give you an assurance that the staff and teachers will not write or talk about it, as confidentiality is important.

LIVING IN THE COMMUNITY

If you want to tell your neighbours, friends or others in the community that you or your child have HIV infection, think about it carefully first.

A lot of people are still ill informed. If you feel you have to tell them, talk about HIV infection in a general sense first and see how they react. If they seem not to know very much, or have a negative reaction, slowly try to educate them yourself. Then you may decide to go ahead and tell them about you or your child.

You'll want to keep your life as free of stress as possible. If telling people is going to cause you any problems, don't say a word. If you have to tell them, get someone who knows about HIV to be present to support you.

SAFEGUARDING YOUR CHILDREN'S FUTURE IF YOU HAVE HIV/AIDS

If you or your partner have HIV infection or AIDS, think about and plan for what will happen to you and your child(ren) if you fall ill.

The obvious thing to do is to arrange support from your family or close friends. If you don't have any family or friends who are willing or able to help, social services departments or AIDS support agencies can help you to ensure that the child(ren) get community care, foster care or are adopted if need be.

For your own peace of mind, make a will that says exactly who is going to care for your child(ren). A lawyer can help you, or you can write it yourself. You will need to get two other people to sign it as witnesses. Give a copy to someone you trust in case something happens to you.

HAVING SOMEONE TO TALK TO

Even if you want to keep silent about your situation with most people, everyone needs someone to confide in and talk to. If there is no one in your family, your community or among your friends who you think you can trust, look for a specialist AIDS agency and find someone you can talk to through them.

Many women have joined support groups where everyone has HIV infection and they have felt much better for it. They feel safe in talking about all the worries and problems on their minds. If you can't find such a group, you might want to start one yourself.

7

Sexual transmission of HIV

How sexual transmission of HIV can occur

Unprotected vaginal and anal intercourse

Nearly all sexual transmission of HIV occurs through unprotected vaginal or anal intercourse between a man and a woman, or through anal intercourse between men, if one partner has HIV. Vaginal and anal intercourse are the most common and frequent sexual practices in most, if not all, cultures.

A number of studies have shown that heterosexual couples have anal intercourse as often as gay men.[1] One study in the USA found that bisexual men have more anal intercourse with both male and female partners than exclusively gay men do together, and that they use condoms even less with their women partners than with other men.[2]

In different studies in the USA, between 6 and 61 per cent of women report having had anal sex. Of sexually active girls attending an adolescent inner-city health centre in New York in 1987, 25 per cent had had both vaginal and anal intercourse, and the practice of anal intercourse increased with age. These young women were less likely to use condoms during anal sex than vaginal sex.[3] They may have been

less aware of the risks or considered anal sex part of foreplay, and not intercourse. It may have been more difficult to ask for condoms to be used. Or condoms may have been seen as unnecessary, since anal intercourse is often used as a form of contraception. In some cultures, anal intercourse is a common way of preserving virginity before marriage and when infibulation prevents vaginal intercourse.

Studies among college students, sex workers, clients of sex workers and partners of injection drug users have found anal intercourse to be a common sexual practice between men and women in Nigeria, Zaïre, the Dominican Republic and Puerto Rico. In a large survey in Brazil, 40–50 per cent of those questioned considered anal intercourse between men and women to be normal sexual practice. In a focus group discussion in Malawi, people were asked how sex would take place with a seropositive partner if abstinence was not possible. Anal sex was seen as a more likely option than condoms.[4]

Thus most women who are in a sexual relationship with a man experience one or both forms of unprotected intercourse as part of normal sexual practice.

HIV can live in the semen and sperm in men, in the lining and mucus of the cervix and vagina in women, and in the lining of the rectum in both. During unprotected inter-course, semen is deposited in the vagina or rectum, and the penis comes into contact with vaginal or rectal mucus. If HIV is present in either partner, it can penetrate the lining of the vagina and cervix, the glans and the opening and the tip of the penis, or the rectum, and enter the bloodstream of the other partner.

Unprotected oral sex

Only very few cases of HIV infection have been reported where oral sex was the only risk-related sexual contact between two men or two women. Oral sex is very common, but it appears rare for male-female couples to have oral sex only and never sexual intercourse.

Semen, vaginal and rectal mucus and possibly menstrual blood in the mouth or swallowed could cause HIV infection. This form of transmission could occur when a man or woman sucks or licks a partner's genitals or anus. Transmission risk may be higher if the mouth, gums or throat are irritated, inflamed and/or have open sores, lesions or bleeding, if reproductive tract infection is present,[5] or as immune deficiency increases in the partner. Oral sex is probably less safe if semen or menstrual blood is frequently involved but it is still much safer than unprotected intercourse.

Sexual practices involving other body fluids

Practices that cause bleeding during inter-course are highly risky. Inserting fingers or a fist in the vagina or rectum may cause damage, e.g. from fingernails or rough insertion. Rough penetrative sex may also bruise tissue. Damage to tissue in the rectum may occur easily because the lining is thin and dry, which may make the rectum very vulnerable to infection.[6]

Faeces and urine may carry HIV in small quantities. If sexual practices involve vaginal, anal or oral contact with these, they are considered unsafe, though no cases of HIV transmission have been reported from them.

Kissing and deep kissing have never been found to transmit HIV. Although tiny quantities of HIV have sometimes been found in saliva, it is not enough to cause infection.

Woman-to-woman transmission of HIV

Women rarely seem to transmit HIV sexually to other women, but it does happen. Only a few cases have been recorded internationally, so sexual practices between women are assumed to be safer than those that involve men, not least by many lesbians. Lesbian activists in many countries are challenging this assumption.[7,8]

Sex between women is safer because inter-course is not involved. But lesbians get reproductive tract infections, and sex between women may involve oral or other exposure to vaginal and rectal mucus and menstrual blood, shared use of sexual aids for vaginal and anal penetration, and practices that cause irritation or damage to tissue or bleeding. And lesbians sometimes use drugs and have sex with men.[8]

Intercourse is the major route of HIV transmission sexually. The following are the more important factors that increase the risk.

Risk factors

It takes only one partner with HIV to put their other partner(s) at risk. Having more than one partner is not, in itself, a risk. But people cannot always know whether they or their sexual partners have HIV or have had other partners with HIV. Hence, the more partners, the more unknown risks involved. This has been shown to be true for getting other sexually transmitted diseases as well.

Unprotected intercourse would not be a problem in itself, if everyone were in lifelong, mutually monogamous relationships. However, having more than one lifetime partner, in relationships and liaisons of many kinds, is widespread among people of all ages and all sexual preferences – single and married, men and women.

HIV is less efficiently transmitted through intercourse than hepatitis B, gonorrhoea or syphilis.[6] Studies of heterosexual HIV transmission reveal marked differences in the rates of infection among previously uninfected partners of people with HIV. One review of typical studies found that the rate of HIV infection among female partners of HIV-positive men ranged from 9 per cent to 54 per cent. Similar differences have been observed in female-to-male transmission rates.[9,10]

People with advanced HIV-related illness are more likely to pass on infection to their partners than those who are still well or have only minor symptoms of infection. This implies that the risk of infection is related to the stage of immune deficiency or illness.[11] It is more likely that one infected partner will infect the other the more frequently they have unprotected intercourse. This variation can also be explained by the presence or absence of other risk factors.

Do women become infected more easily than men?

Some studies have found that, other factors being equal, men with HIV are two times more likely to transmit it to their women partners than vice versa.[12] There are several reasons for this. First, there may be much more HIV in semen than in vaginal mucus and therefore more HIV to transmit.[13] Second, the lining of a woman's vagina and rectum are more vulnerable to infection than the penis, because the mucus membrane surface can more easily be penetrated by virus. Third, semen remains longer at body temperature in the vagina and rectum than vaginal/rectal mucus does on the penis, so there is more time for exposure to occur.

There is also evidence that the partner who is penetrated during intercourse (the receptive partner) is more at risk of infection than his/her (insertive) partner. Women are always the receptive partner in both anal and vaginal intercourse.[12]

However, some studies have shown that female-to-male transmission rates are similar to male-to-female ones. Other factors are not always equal and can make the risk for men as great as that for women.[14] A man may have more partners, more frequent intercourse, and other co-factors that affect risk.

Co-factors that affect risk

Reproductive tract infections are the most thoroughly studied co-factor in sexual transmission of HIV. But there are other conditions and practices that may make internal and genital tissue more vulnerable to HIV infection.

Reproductive tract infections (RTIs)

RTIs involve open sores or lesions, ulcers or localized irritation or inflammation of some kind, which allow HIV to penetrate tissue and enter the bloodstream much more easily.[15]

RTIs also cause the activated immune system to send certain infection-fighting cells to the lining of the reproductive tract. HIV can live on these cells and may be able to replicate in their presence. This can increase the amount of HIV present in the reproductive tract, which increases the risk of transmission to a partner. If the partner also has an RTI, the risk is increased even more.

Many women are not aware that they have RTIs or do not get or have access to treatment. Many more have little or no choice about having sex even if they and/or their partner has an RTI.

Menstrual blood

A few studies have reported some increased

risk of HIV infection related to intercourse during menstruation,[16] but other factors were also involved. People are very unlikely to have sex only during menstruation, so the extent of risk is difficult to determine.

Traditionally, many cultures forbid sexual relations during menstruation, but this taboo has been disappearing in many places.

Effects of the menstrual cycle

Formation of the tissue that protects a woman's vagina and cervix against infection may depend on hormonal changes that initiate menstruation. The lining of the female genital tract does not go through certain changes until well after ovulation is established, up to some months after the first menstrual period. Without that protection, girls who have not passed menarche may be particularly vulnerable to HIV infection. Gonorrhoea has been found to cause severe lower tract infection in girls because of the immaturity of this tissue, and coital injury in child brides can be very severe.[17]

Among more than 2,000 Ethiopian women, it was found that half had had sexual intercourse before onset of menstruation and had much higher rates of STD and pelvic inflammatory disease, especially if sexual activity started at age 12 or less. The rate of cervical cancer was also higher.[17]

Hormonal changes during the menstrual cycle may make women more vulnerable to infection at certain times in the cycle. Some women with recurrent genital herpes report outbreaks with their periods, for example.[18]

Cervical ectopy, a normal condition, occurs when certain cells from the interior of the cervix move towards its surface and form a thin, reddish layer. These patches change with normal hormonal fluctuations during the course of each menstrual cycle, during normal pregnancy, and in association with taking oestrogen, e.g. in oral contraceptives. They can

bleed easily if irritated. They occur more commonly in adolescent and young women in their 20s and in women taking oral contraceptives containing oestrogen.[6]

Menopause can change the lining of the vagina, making it dry and more easily irritated during intercourse if a lubricant is not used.

Certain contraceptives

Two contraceptive methods, spermicides and IUDs, may increase the risk of HIV transmission.

Spermicides

Spermicides were shown to be safe as vaginal contraceptives by 1980, though they are far less than 100 per cent effective against pregnancy if used alone. For this reason, contraceptive advice has always been to use spermicides in combination with a diaphragm, cap or condoms if possible. Contraceptive sponges which contain spermicide are not the same as using spermicide with another barrier method, as the sponge itself is not a barrier, but only a vehicle for the spermicide.

It is widely believed that spermicides also protect against reproductive tract infections. In fact, few good studies before 1990 substantiate the extent of protection, if any, with each form of barrier method, alone or in combination, for many RTIs. Whether spermicides reduce risk or are safe for anal use is also unknown.

Papers since 1990 have attempted to re-evaluate previous studies and to assess the level of protection against RTIs more thoroughly. No protective effect of spermicide has been shown for any of the viral RTIs and there is conflicting evidence in the case of thrush.[19]

Among a group of Thai sex workers there was an increased risk of thrush with frequent contraceptive sponge use, compared to a control group.[20] In contrast, among a large group of women attending an STD clinic in the USA, there was no increased risk with the sponge. Diaphragm users did have a significantly higher rate of thrush; it was assumed that they were also using spermicide. Those using the contraceptive sponge, diaphragm or condoms had significantly lower rates of gonorrhoea and trichomoniasis and somewhat lower rates of chlamydia than in a control group. Previous studies have confirmed these findings, to varying degrees, though there is more information about gonorrhoea than chlamydia and trichomoniasis. There are few studies on bacterial vaginosis. This study found no protective effect against bacterial vaginosis among users of spermicides, sponges, diaphragms or condoms.[20] It should be noted that most studies have only looked at effects over a short period of time, e.g. one to three months or only one or two clinic visits.

Among another group of Thai sex workers at high risk for RTIs, most of whom had two or three partners daily, use of nonoxynol-9 spermicide with condoms provided significantly better protection against gonorrhoea and chlamydia than use of condoms alone. No increased risk of thrush or genital ulcers was found in either group. Protection from condoms used alone was considerable. Irritation from nonoxynol-9 was also considerable, though mostly not severe. These data confirm that nonoxynol-9 can decrease the rate of cervical infection and should be used with condoms or alone if condoms cannot be used, for this purpose. However, these researchers conclude that spermicide should not be the only protection used against all sexually transmitted infection, since it does not protect all possible sites and the amount of protection is less than that conferred by condoms.[21]

Most studies in the past 20 years have indicated that nonoxynol-9 and other substances in spermicides can irritate vaginal and anal/rectal tissues in women and men, especially with frequent use.[6,19] Further, a reproductive tract infection or other existing problem could be an initial cause of irritation, which spermicide could exacerbate.

Sex workers in Canada reported in a recent study that they experienced not only vaginal irritation and, to a lesser extent vaginal thrush, numbness and burning from condoms lubricated with a nonoxynol-9 spermicide, but also soreness, numbness and burning of the lips from oral sex using these condoms.[22]

Forty-two per cent of nonoxynol-9 spermicide users in another small Thai study experienced disruption of the cervical lining and/or bleeding with frequent use, compared to no abnormal findings in a control group. All symptoms disappeared within a week of stopping use.[23] In a large, controlled study that lasted nine weeks in Bangkok, use of a nonoxynol-9 spermicide up to 22 times a week was associated with higher rates of irritation and a higher drop-out rate from the study.[24]

This level of frequency of use would, in general, apply more to sex workers and others having frequent intercourse. For contraceptive purposes and with less frequent use, which applies to the majority of people, these effects are less important. Most people experiencing irritation can usually find a brand that does not bother them, and irritation has been shown to disappear with a short period of non-use. However, it is not known whether even minor irritation may increase the risk of HIV transmission.[19]

Tests in 1985 showed that nonoxynol-9 and a number of other spermicides destroy HIV rapidly in vitro, that is, in laboratory conditions.[25] However, it is unknown whether consistent use of nonoxynol-9 spermicide will reduce the risk of HIV infection,[21] particularly over longer periods of time.

The only longer-term study in women before 1990 was among a group of sex workers with a high rate of reproductive tract infections attending an HIV research clinic in Nairobi. By 1987, over 85 per cent of women tested in this clinic had HIV. All the women who were HIV-negative were invited to participate in the study. They had a mean number of 34 sex partners per week. The women were randomly assigned to use either placebos in the form of vaginal pessaries or contraceptive sponges with nonoxynol-9. All the women were strongly encouraged to use condoms at all times. Reported compliance in using the spermicide and the placebo (81 per cent and 90 per cent) was somewhat better than in using condoms (58 per cent and 63 per cent). However, condom use increased during the study.

Follow-up was for a mean period of 14 months for the sponge users and 17 months for the placebo group. This study was terminated in 1990 when it became clear that no protective effect of nonoxynol-9 could be shown, as hoped, against HIV infection. Almost half the nonoxynol-9 users developed vulvitis, burning sensation or ulcers on the vulva, and it was feared that this might have increased their risk of HIV infection. After two years, 56 per cent of nonoxynol-9 users and 41 per cent of controls had become HIV-positive. Only the rate of gonorrhoea was reduced by nonoxynol-9 use. [26]

Condom use at all times by subjects and controls and careful attention to potential adverse effects was and is recommended for any future studies of this kind. [19,26]

Spermicides containing nonoxynol-9 have been widely recommended for use with or as an alternative to condoms, where condom use is considered impossible, to protect against sexual transmission of HIV and other STDs. Women have been told in some safer sex workshops and leaflets that although condoms are safest, if men refuse to use condoms, a nonoxynol-9 spermicide is better than nothing for protection.

This may well prove to be true for some women, and new studies are under way to attempt to find out. It may prove to be more true for women who have intercourse only a few times a week or less with one or few regular partners. Using a spermicide will certainly make women feel they are doing something, rather than nothing, to protect themselves if their partners will not use condoms. And no one seems willing to say that it is better to use nothing for protection against HIV than to use spermicide alone.

On the other hand, recommending spermicides alone may reduce women's motivation to continue to fight for condom use. The current lack of a proven alternative to condoms is a dilemma that must be faced by and with women, and more discussion among women is needed. [27] Any woman who decides to use spermicide in the absence of condoms requires continuing support to try to use condoms with her male partner(s).

Many condom brands are now lubricated with spermicide, and condoms without spermicide may be more difficult to find. Some condoms popularly used for anal intercourse also now contain spermicide, in the absence of sufficient tests on anal safety or efficacy for purposes of prevention of HIV infection. Further, condoms with spermicides are extremely unpleasant tasting, in addition to the adverse effects reported, and the spermicide may discourage their use for oral sex.

Until further work on spermicides, RTIs and HIV is done, users need to be aware that:
- spermicides have not been shown to be effective in preventing HIV transmission with frequent use in high-risk situations;
- spermicides may provide some protection with infrequent use, but no studies have yet shown this to be true;
- there is a risk of oral, vaginal and genital irritation from spermicides, particularly with frequent use;
- irritation to tissue, particularly with frequent use or in the presence of RTIs, may increase the risk of infection;
- use of spermicides anally and orally cannot be recommended for women or men. [19,22,26]

Condom manufacturers should continue to make non-spermicidal condoms at least as available as those with spermicide, and brands advertised as safe for oral and anal use should not be permitted to contain spermicide until tests show that this is safe.

Intra-uterine devices

Intra-uterine devices (IUDs) can cause minor inflammation in the uterus and the cervix. If infection enters the upper reproductive tract during insertion, pelvic inflammatory disease and infertility may result. This may occur either because of pre-existing lower tract infection or unsterile insertion practices.[28]

In the UK, IUDs are currently recommended only for women in mutually faithful relationships and not for women with a history of pelvic inflammatory disease, because of the risk of infection.

Men sometimes complain that the IUD tail in the vagina irritates the penis.[29] IUDs are also associated with an increase in certain cells in the vagina that can harbour HIV and may increase both a woman's and her partner's risk of infection. Because HIV affects the immune system, reproductive tract infection may be more likely to occur in HIV-positive women in the presence of an IUD.[30]

A few studies indicate that there is an increased risk of infection for women who use an IUD with an HIV-positive partner. A European-wide study among 153 women partners of HIV-positive men found that 40 per cent of those using IUDs became HIV-positive, the highest rate of infection associated with any one factor in that group.[31] An Italian study found that women with IUDs who had seropositive partners were three to four times more likely to be HIV-positive than women using condoms or oral contraceptives.[32]

In 1991, the International Planned Parenthood Federation (IPPF) Medical Advisory Panel recommended that women who are known to be HIV-positive should not use an IUD. They advise that if a woman with an IUD in place becomes HIV-positive, she should have the IUD removed, both for her own sake and for the sake of her partner. They also advise that testing for HIV infection should not be a prerequisite for women who wish to use an IUD.[30]

If a woman and her partner are willing to use condoms with the IUD all the time, these risks are greatly reduced. Hence, the use of an IUD should not simply be dismissed, especially if a woman prefers it for contraception.[33]

Other contraceptives

As regards what is known about other contraceptives, studies in Rwanda, the USA, Zambia and Zaïre have found that oral contraceptives (OCs) do not affect the risk of HIV transmission. An early study found a possible increased risk with OC use and a more recent one found a protective effect, but neither has been confirmed.[34]

Neither the diaphragm nor the cervical cap used alone have been shown to be protective against HIV infection, though they do protect against cervical and upper reproductive tract infection.[14]

Some clinicians have suggested that HIV-positive men have vasectomies, in order to reduce the number of white blood cells in semen, which can carry HIV. But one study found that HIV can enter semen through other routes in vasectomized men,[35] so this cannot be recommended.

Only the use of condoms would allow women and their partners who may be at risk of HIV infection to use the contraceptive of their choice to prevent pregnancy without concern about the possible negative effects it might have for HIV infection.

Lack of male circumcision

It has been found in both developed and developing countries that uncircumcised boys and men have more infections on the penis and in the urinary tract than circumcised men, and that uncircumcised men are more at risk of penile cancer, a leading cause of cancer deaths in men in some countries. This may put women at increased risk of reproductive tract infection and possibly of cervical cancer through intercourse.

It needs slightly more effort to clean the penis well when there is a foreskin. The warm, moist environment under the foreskin can harbour infections, possibly including HIV.[36,37] Studies in Africa in 1988 and 1989 found that lack of male circumcision was a risk factor for HIV infection in the men,[38] though it was not necessarily the only factor.

Male circumcision done safely carries very low risks in newborn boys.[39] After circumcision, the glans of the penis develops a cell covering similar to external skin, which may help to protect against infection, irritation and injuries. Some medical researchers have suggested that universal male circumcision could help to prevent HIV and other infection in both men and women.[36] However, in many cultures male circumcision is not practised or accepted. Campaigns that stress good hygiene or encourage male circumcision health reasons may be effective in changing prevailing practices.

Female circumcision

Depending on the cultural practice of the ethnic group or region, female circumcision may be done at a girl's birth, at first menstruation, just before marriage, or during pregnancy.[40] Unlike male circumcision, female circumcision has no protective value for women's health. On the contrary, it carries many health risks, some of which may be life-threatening.

Infibulation (the stitching together of the two sides of the vulva, leaving a small hole to permit the flow of urine and menstrual blood) may result in later complications, including:

– Accumulation of menstrual blood for many months.
– Recurrent urinary tract infection.
– Chronic vulval infection.
– Difficulty in penetration during intercourse. If penetration is forced and scar tissue does not yield, tears in tissue and bleeding may occur, and a false vagina may be opened. If penetration is not possible, anal intercourse may be used as a substitute for vaginal intercourse.
– Problems during childbirth if labour is obstructed and there is perineal tearing and laceration. These may have implications when intercourse is resumed.[41,42]

If HIV becomes prevalent in areas where female circumcision is commonly practised, circumcised women may be at increased risk.

Pregnancy, childbirth and abortion complications

Women can suffer damage to tissue from complications of pregnancy, childbirth and unsafe abortion. Examples are tears in external and internal tissues that may not heal properly even with repair, and may be re-torn during intercourse. Women from lower socio-economic groups in developing countries suffer disproportionately from maternal morbidity, as do young women who have had children before they themselves are fully grown.

Prolapsed uterus, common in older women and those who have had many pregnancies, makes women more prone to reproductive tract infection.

Vaginal agents and sexual aids

Many herbal and chemical preparations are used by women in the vagina and on the genitals for sexual, medicinal, contraceptive and cleansing purposes. Some of these can irritate tissue and may increase the risk of HIV infection. Studies on the types of preparations used and the extent of risk are still in their infancy.

Agents for drying and tightening the vagina appear to be widely used. A study among 50 sex workers in Zaïre found that they often used agents for tightening the vagina for sexual purposes. Those who did had visible inflammatory lesions on the walls of the vagina.[43] A study among sex workers in the Dominican Republic found that 14 per cent reported drying the vagina for intercourse.[44]

In Zimbabwe, 60–70 per cent of women surveyed at a family planning clinic in Harare were concerned about vaginal secretions during intercourse and used a variety of substances to try to control these. Eighty per cent of sex workers interviewed in Harare reported using herbal agents to enhance male sexual arousal during intercourse. And 50 per cent of women with cervical cancer attending a hospital clinic in Harare reported using herbs vaginally.[45]

Another small study in Zimbabwe found that 93 per cent of women attending urban clinics and 80 per cent of nurses used a variety of agents before intercourse. Thirteen different herbs were named. Forty per cent of clinic attenders and 75 per cent of nurses also reported using non-herbal agents. These included cold water most commonly, but Dettol in water, tissue paper, dry cloth, salt in water, Betadine antiseptic solution, pessaries, and gauze were also reported.

The main reasons the women gave for using these agents were either to contract the vagina, reduce the amount of vaginal secretion, or increase the warmth of the vagina. Specific agents were used for specific effects, for example, to make the woman 'like a virgin' or change the quality of intercourse. Most of the women used them before every act of intercourse. Certain agents were inserted several hours in advance and removed before making love.

The main outcomes hoped for were sexual gratification for the husband, joint gratification, maintaining the husband's fidelity, and an increase in sexual compatibility. Many of the women knew the agents might have adverse effects, and a small number said they had experienced pain with intercourse using them.

Most of the women started using agents after the birth of their first child. Most had been taught to use them by an aunt, grandmother, friends or peers. Over half the women said their husbands were unaware that they used them. Almost all the clinic attenders and half the nurses said they would advise their daughters or nieces to use the agents, and that they themselves would continue to use them as long as they remained sexually active.[45]

In Malawi a study among almost 4,000 pregnant women found that over a three-year period, 35 per cent reported using one or more agents to treat discharges, and these brought a small increased risk of HIV transmission when other factors had been controlled for. Another 12 per cent had used something as a tightening agent for sexual purposes. Agents used included herbs, aluminium hydroxide powder, silica gel, pumice-like stones, and cloth. An increased risk of HIV infection was found with stones used as tightening agents.[46]

Some tribal women in India use half a partly scraped-out lemon in the vagina as a contraceptive. The juice probably acts as a spermicide, while the lemon skin is intended to cover the cervix as a barrier. The men believe that if a woman has any reproductive tract infection, she will not be able to tolerate the lemon inside her. They consider this a form of protection against infection for themselves and a means of keeping women faithful.

The women also use pieces of cloth soaked in various solutions for contraception before intercourse. Solutions are also used as vaginal douches for post-coital contraception and cleansing purposes, including diluted vinegar, alum solution, diluted lime juice, herbal solutions and medicines from traditional practitioners.[47]

Vaginal deodorants, available in some developed countries, have not been studied. Healthy vaginal discharge does not have an unpleasant smell. An unusual or unpleasant smell from the vagina is a sign of infection, whch should be treated. Regular washing of the genitals with water and mild soap is good hygienic practice and will reduce smells from menstrual blood and after intercourse. The use of tampons during menstruation and of condoms for intercourse works as well.

Sixty-nine per cent of adolescent girls visiting a family planning clinic in Houston, USA, in 1986 said they douched. Most learned to do so from their mothers and most began when they started having sexual intercourse.[48] It has been estimated that half of women in the USA douche occasionally.[45] Many women sex workers in the Philippines believe douching after sex helps to prevent STDs and HIV.[49]

Douching does not clean the vagina or prevent conception. The vagina makes mucus in order to clean and protect itself. Douching reduces protective mucus, and can make the vagina more susceptible to infection until mucus naturally replaces itself. Douching may also help to push sperm and any existing infection into the upper reproductive tract through the cervix.

A wide range of sexual aids exist, which may or may not be a risk factor for HIV, depending on what they are made of and how they are used. Objects used for penetration of the vagina or anally and then shared could possibly transmit infection, though no cases have been reported. Bananas are also reported to be used for this purpose. If the banana skin contains pesticides, this may act as an irritant.

Men in the Philippines use a range of chemicals and substances on the penis, to prolong erection. Their safety has not been evaluated.[49]

Rings of many kinds are often used on the penis to increase stimulation. In the Philippines, rings with hair were popular until recently, and now a growing number of men are using 'bolitas', small balls made of metal, fiberglass or semi-precious stones, which are sewn under the skin of the penis, usually under the loose fold beneath the glans. Irritation and infection of the penis, vaginal irritation, and painful anal intercourse have all been reported anecdotally. Bolitas could damage a condom or make it difficult to use one as well.[49]

There is no need for people to stop using all vaginal agents or sexual aids, and their psychological value in relation to sexual needs must not be undervalued or dismissed. There is a need to find out which agents are safe, and for those found to be unsafe, substitute something safer. Sex education courses, safer sex workshops, and antenatal clinics are all places to take this up with women and much research is needed.

Any adverse effects that most of these agents might have on condoms is unknown. Whether the use of some of these agents would make women and men less likely to want to use condoms is also unknown.[45]

Although lubricants may help to protect against trauma to tissue during penetration, oil-based lubricants damage condoms, and the types of lubricants people use also need to be investigated.

Sexual assault, rape and sexual abuse

Although the number of documented cases is small, both children and adults can get HIV infection through sexual abuse or rape.

In the UK, 23–30 per cent of rapes involve two or more assailants. Assault involves oral or anal penetration and ejaculation in up to 35 per cent of reported cases. Prevalence rates of STDs among victims range from 3.9 to 43 per cent. Whether these result from the attack or were already present, they increase the risk of

HIV transmission. Physical violence also regularly involves damage to oral, genital, vaginal and rectal tissue, though this has not been studied in relation to infection. Major vaginal and genital lacerations were reported in 6.8 per cent of women in one study, and that did not include more frequent, less serious injuries in this area.[50]

Several preventive treatments against STD/HIV infection have been suggested for rape victims. These include the immediate use of zidovudine (AZT), vaginal douching with vinegar and use of a nonoxynol-9 spermicide. However, there is no evidence that any of these help and some chance that they may even be harmful. Until they are evaluated, they cannot be recommended.[51]

Following rape or sexual assault, women should be encouraged to attend a clinic for preventive treatment for oral and reproductive tract infection, for postcoital contraception to prevent unwanted pregnancy, or referral for abortion if pregnancy has occurred. Counselling about HIV infection should be given and testing for HIV can be done at a follow-up visit in three to six months' time.[50] There should be no pressure to report the assault to the police. Women counsellors and clinicians should be available.

If the assailant is known to the woman, as is often the case, she may know whether he was at risk of HIV. The fact that possible exposure to HIV was once only should give some reassurance to women that there is a good chance they were not infected.

Women whose children have experienced incest or been sexually abused, especially by a family member or friend, may find it very difficult to take the child to a clinic because the abuser is likely to be known to them. These situations are beyond the bounds of biological solutions. They are the subject of legal, social and political action.

Few countries provide adequate or good quality services for women and children who have been assaulted. Abuse and rape should be the subject of sex education from an early age, to teach young girls and boys how to protect themselves, and to teach young men how devastating forced sex is for girls and women. Self-defence should be part of physical education classes for young women. Rape crisis phone lines and centres provide support, referrals for care, and campaign against these forms of violence. But as long as rape and abuse continue, all the services in the world are only palliatives, and the risk of HIV infection will only add to the fears and emotional trauma they engender.

Improving reproductive health education and services

Increased risk is multi-factored. In a large group of men and women attending an STD clinic in Kampala, Uganda, almost half of whom had HIV infection, genital bleeding or bruising during sex and/or sex during menstruation was reported by 64 per cent of the men and 58 per cent of the women. These increased the risk of HIV infection only somewhat more than a history of genital discharge or lack of male circumcision.[16]

Reproductive health is important for prevention of HIV infection. Given the extent and range of causes of reproductive tract infection and trauma in women, much needs to be done.[52]

Women and their families need to know to seek medical help early when complications occur with pregnancy, childbirth and abortion, with female circumcision and after sexual abuse, assault and rape.

Genital hygiene needs to be taught more widely. Women may not be aware that the vagina cleans itself, and men may not be aware that the foreskin can harbour infection. Women may perceive normal, healthy discharge as a sign of infection, and need only simple instruction on how to tell the difference.

More research is needed on the safety and effectiveness of herbal and chemical agents used vaginally, and on self-prescribed drugs for the same purpose. In many developing countries, resistance to low-cost drugs for RTIs has developed partly due to inadequate and inappropriate use.[53]

Women and men need to know how to recognize signs of infection so that they can seek treatment for themselves and their partners. People may currently know more about HIV than other RTIs because there have been so many educational messages about HIV. In contrast, few messages exist about RTIs, let alone other causes of vaginal and genital trauma.[54]

The industrialized world realized during both world wars that sexually transmitted diseases had economic repercussions. Measures such as wide distribution of condoms, walk-in clinics where no referral or appointment are needed, anonymity, and free services helped to reduce the spread of infection. Tracing of people's sexual contacts, voluntarily as in the UK or compulsorily as in the USA, has also made a major difference.

Services for RTIs and HIV/AIDS can benefit from being linked. For over three years the European Community has supported the planning and implementation of combined programmes in more than 20 developing countries. They have found that this approach has advantages but does not work well enough for women.[55]

Where such programmes are integrated into primary health care, they are mainly seeing men who have symptoms. RTIs are more likely to be diagnosed and treated in pregnant women during antenatal care, if at all. Non-pregnant women are neglected unless they ask to be treated, which few do because of the stigma. Where it is mistakenly thought that sex workers are the only women who have sexually transmitted diseases, programmes may target only these women. Even then, only a minority of sex workers may be reached. Contact tracing is often not feasible or is poorly done. Women who have no symptoms or do not recognize symptoms are not seen.[53]

The existing structures, planning and implementation, management strategies and available diagnostics and therapeutics are limited. New approaches are needed.[53,55]

Because women may be culturally or socially constrained from using these services, it is important to consider combining investigation and treatment with other consultations, especially those requiring an internal examination.[52] This makes even more sense when cervical disease in women is taken into account.

Women could be offered this care as a 'well-woman' service at antenatal, maternal and child health and family planning clinics. But from women's viewpoint, comprehensive reproductive health education and services that are open to all women, and not dependent on needing care in pregnancy or to prevent pregnancy, would be the most effective.

AIDS and sexually transmitted diseases: an important connection

by Mary T. Bassett and Marvellous Mhloyi

The changing nature of marital and sexual relationships in Zimbabwe has profoundly influenced patterns of transmission of not only AIDS, but other STDs as well.

In 1990, over 900,000 cases of STDs were treated nationwide, which averages out to nearly one quarter of the adult population. Popular ideas about STDs suggest that little stigma is attached to male infection. Having an STD is almost a rite of passage into manhood, proof of sexual activity: 'A bull is not a bull without his scars.' Consistent with both data and belief, a study on HIV infection among male factory workers found that a history of prior STD was common among both seropositive and seronegative men: 100 and 75 per cent respectively. Other risk factors, now documented in numerous studies of AIDS in Africa, were also more common in the HIV-positive group, e.g. multiple partners, a history of payment for sex. What was unexpected was the high prevalence of high-risk activities among the seronegative men: 40 per cent reported an STD in the previous year, and 67 per cent had paid money for sex. Seropositive men were more likely than seronegative men to report a history of genital ulcer. In the light of these data, one can hardly characterize the seronegative comparison group as 'low risk'.

The focus on genital ulcers as an important co-factor for HIV transmission has both positive and negative features. While it offers new approaches for intervention programmes, it also shifts emphasis from the broader social context of STD occurrence to more narrow medical concerns. Certainly any intervention that results in reduced rates of STDs, such as increasing public awareness about the availability of treatment for STDs, will also mean a diminution of HIV transmission. It is said that some women now inspect men for signs of genital ulcer before agreeing to have sex, a strategy that may be particularly useful for women engaged in commercial sex. The focus on genital ulcer is also appealing because it seems to eliminate all of the value-laden issues that accompany interpretation of other risk factors, such as multiple partners and prostitute contact. Zimbabwe's Ministry of Health has generated protocols for STD treatment, and the nation's independence made access to medical care effectively universal. None the less, the number of cases of STDs in Zimbabwe increases yearly. To reduce the problem of HIV transmission to the problem of controlling genital ulcer is to search for a 'technological fix' that fails to address the social factors that jointly underlie both problems.

Safer sex

Confronting sexual risk

Many AIDS educators find that when they talk about sexual transmission of HIV, a lot of questions are asked about kissing and rare forms of sexual transmission. One Philippine doctor reassures people that it takes 32 litres of saliva to accumulate enough HIV for kissing to be a risk.[1] Such reassurances are important, but behind these questions may lie unwillingness, embarrassment and fear of confronting the real risk factors for HIV infection.

People may immediately react: 'Then I can't have sex any more.' Or, 'My partner is OK. I don't need to worry about him/her.' Before discussions about safer sex begin, reactions like these must be confronted and overcome.

Neither the amount of information people have been given about sexual risks nor the level of their own risk are always a measure of whether they will change their behaviour. Some people have changed to safe practices some or all of the time. Some have changed only when they find out that a partner has HIV. Some do not change even then, whether out of a feeling of duty to share their partner's fate or because at some deep level they still do not believe they will become infected. Many

would like to make changes, but are simply not in control of the sexual situations they are in. Many have not known or believed they were at risk until they themselves became infected.

Public education messages have offered a limited number of sexual strategies for protection from HIV/AIDS. But these urge people to act as individuals in an individual way. A decade of the AIDS epidemic has proved that this is not enough. Sexual practices are part of social norms, and individuals cannot alter these on their own or overnight. More account must be taken of the differing realities of women's lives and the need for social acceptance of change.

While it seems to be agreed that behaviour change is the goal, we must ask: Behaviour change to what? For what? For how long? And for whose sake? Dictated by whose values and needs? And with what power and resources for women to achieve it?

Should the goal be to let HIV dictate sexual practice as a short-term expedient? Or is there a longer-term aim, for women to be able to express their sexuality in a self-determined way and at the same time be safe? What about the future? Is it not also important to give young people the chance to grow up into a safer and more satisfying sexuality from the start?

Such a focus may be thought idealistic or

impractical when people are at risk of a virus. Everyone needs information and the means to protect themselves here and now, but HIV/AIDS have created an opportunity that cannot be ignored to talk about and act for the long term.

Analysis of safer sex strategies

The following are the most common safer sex strategies that public education messages offer, with comments on the value and limitations of each.

• **Be faithful to one partner.**
This strategy works as long as neither partner has HIV, is not at risk from other sources of infection, and as long as both partners are alive, together, and faithful to one another all the time.

Many women with HIV have had only one lifetime sexual partner, and many others only two or three partners, one at a time, over many years. Being faithful has not protected them when their partners were not faithful in return or already had HIV when the relationship began.

• **Say NO to sex.**
This message has been widely directed at young people of both sexes, particularly young women. If young people delay starting a sexual relationship until they are ready to marry and are then faithful to each other, they greatly reduce their risk of infection.

However, the traditional age at marriage used to be much lower than it is now, and fewer young people are waiting to get married before having sex. Adolescence is often a period of experimentation with both sex and relationships. Young and older men often pressure young women to have sex with them. Some young women would rather refuse, and can find this strategy supportive. It will help

them for a time, but not indefinitely, and the problem becomes one of anticipating when they will need other advice. Others definitely want to have sex, and will. For them, this strategy is not appropriate. Ironically, the advertising media have made use of sex to sell products all over the world, creating a very sex-aware culture from an early age.

One AIDS educator tells parents, 'Don't teach your kids to say no. Half of them have already said yes!' When she meets a mother who tells her daughter to say no, but does not want to tell her daughter about AIDS, she warns the mother that she is putting her future grandchildren at risk.[2]

Being able to say no to sex is something women of all ages would like to do when their experience of sex is negative or demeaning. Not all can. Negative experiences and social and economic dependency on men can disempower women, making this difficult or impossible. Many women would like to refuse when they know their partner is having sex with others. Some find the courage and social support to do so; others do not. Women whose partners have HIV may be able to say no or insist on safer sex only if their partner becomes ill.[3] Saying no to sex is also being suggested to those who have lost their partners to AIDS, in case they have HIV themselves. But this does not take into account their own emotional, social and economic needs, let alone sexual needs.

Refusing to have sex has been one strategy people have used to protect their partners, without having to reveal their HIV status or how they became infected. A story circulating in Brazil tells of a bisexual man with HIV who decided not to have sexual relations with his wife any longer. Although he stayed with her until he died, she felt totally rejected by him. After his death, she learned he had had AIDS, and only then realized he had meant to protect her.

Desertion of partners with HIV/AIDS is not

uncommon. This strategy, one form of saying no, is being used by some women and even more men. It is a drastic step for many women, but a last resort where there are no apparent alternatives. Losing her partner can be disastrous for a woman. She may be unable to support herself and her children, and in the absence of social support may well turn to selling sex.[3] Deserted and deserting men are likely to turn to other women for sex.

Overall, saying no may appear the most effective strategy, on the grounds that 'what you don't do can't hurt you'. In practice, it may be problematic. Yet it is the strategy most often promoted, partly because, in addition to mutual faithfulness, it is the only strategy many religious leaders will condone.

• **Reduce the number of your sexual partners – or avoid having multiple sexual partners.**

For those with more than one partner, reducing the number of partners is a practical, if imprecise, approach to lessening the chances of infection.[4] But there are many definitions of 'multiple partners'.

For women who exchange sexual services for money, food or housing, multiple partners are a source of survival. This strategy would reduce their income and conflict with basic needs. Women who charge money for sexual services could raise their prices in order to gain the same income from fewer clients. This would only succeed if all the women working in the same premises or area agreed to do this together, and even then, some men might stop visiting them or might visit them less often.

For others, multiple partners means having 'one-night stands', where there is no emotional involvement, and is a euphemism for promiscuity. But being promiscuous also means different things to different people. Does one new partner a year constitute multiple sexual partners? What about three or four?[5]

Some women and men seek sexual contacts for their own sake, and perhaps with great frequency; for them this advice is useful. For most, however, sexual contact is not a goal in itself but occurs in the context of relationships, which may not be prolific nor easily found. To suggest that someone not begin a relationship because of a need to cut down on the number of partners will not work.[3]

Women often form relationships with a number of men before finding a long-term or marriage partner. Some women face a sex-ratio imbalance, especially women who are not young and for whom eligible partners may be scarce. Should the warning to avoid multiple partners be a reason for women to accept or remain in a safe but unsatisfying relationship?

Women who consider sex a form of commitment to a partner may not view having serially monogamous relationships as multiple partners. For many, a safe relationship may be one that lasts more than a few months and where there is simply the intention that it will continue.[5]

• **Ask your partner his/her sexual history – or, select a partner carefully, excluding people at high risk.**

This strategy falsely assumes that people with a history of high-risk behaviour or experience are infected with HIV while others are not. It also assumes that no one should have a relationship with anyone at risk of HIV. These are invalid and stigmatizing assumptions. Most people who are asking for information about a potential partner, let alone being asked, do not know if they have HIV.

Many people do not easily discuss sexual matters. The vast majority engage in sexual relationships without investigating the lifestyle and history of potential partners extensively. They are left unprotected by this strategy.[4]

Even taking it at face value, this strategy entails finding out the actual or probable HIV status of a potential partner before having sex with them, by asking the person to have an HIV test and sharing the result, or asking them to give details of their sexual history and risk-related behaviour and weighing up the risk.

Although one person's sexual history can in principle be elicited, their previous partners' sexual histories, and those of their previous partners' previous partners, cannot. This completely negates the value of the exercise.[6]

Further, at what point should someone ask a sexual history or start being selective? The nearer two people are to starting a sexual relationship or actually making love, the less likely they are to ask or feel able to walk away or stop.

Women have tried to reassure themselves that unprotected sex is safe with a new partner by bringing up the topic of AIDS and asking if he has had an HIV test. The partner may falsely reassure her that he has and that the result was negative. But 'stories' such as this have joined the many common pretences when two people meet. Believing such stories, also common, may now be more risky than it used to be.[5]

A group of US college students were asked how much they thought men and women would lie when asked about their risk factors for AIDS. Both men and women thought that men would lie significantly more than women. When asked if they had ever lied to someone in order to have sex, 35 per cent of the men admitted to having told a lie compared to 10 per cent of the women. When asked about their experience of being lied to by partners, they reported that partner dishonesty was quite prevalent. When they were given several hypothetical scenarios in which honesty threatened the opportunity to have sex or to maintain a desired relationship, a sizable percentage of both sexes indicated that they would not be honest, with the men less willing to be honest than the women. This study demonstrates very clearly that the strategy of asking one's partner about HIV risk factors is itself a risky technique, particularly for

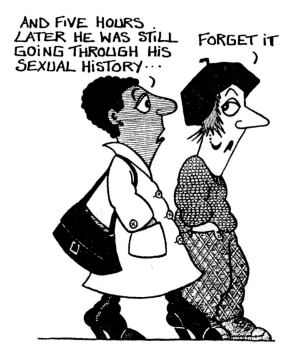

AND FIVE HOURS LATER HE WAS STILL GOING THROUGH HIS SEXUAL HISTORY...

FORGET IT

Cath Jackson

women. Yet this strategy is increasingly being used by women.[7]

Obviously, in preventive interventions it is important to distinguish between the goal of increasing communication between partners to facilitate safer sex practices, and using information gained during this process to circumvent the consistent practice of safer sex.[7]

• **Use condoms.**

This is the only effective strategy for safer intercourse if either partner has had, is having or will have intercourse with others.

Intercourse with condoms is much safer than unprotected intercourse. The more often condoms are used, the lower the frequency of exposure. Very low and even nil rates of HIV transmission are reported with consistent and correct condom use. Even sometime-use is reported to be protective.[8]

Using a condom with every partner and every act of intercourse is, in practice, not easy to achieve. While no one wants to encourage only sometime-use, people may think that if they do not use condoms all the time, they might as well not bother at all, and this is not the case.

In fact, many people use condoms some of the time but not always, or with some partners but not others. Many men and women are more willing to use condoms with casual partners than with their spouses or regular partner. Thus, spouses and regular partners may be most at risk with each other through an unwillingness to question or threaten love or trust. This is as true for sex workers as for others. In addition, many women fear violence and/or desertion if they ask for condoms to be used.

Yet condoms are not always used with casual or one-time partners either. Sex workers who do not operate a condom-always policy can find it extremely dispiriting to convince every client individually, especially when it is economically difficult to turn anyone away.

Some men with HIV are not using condoms because they do not want their partners to ask if they are infected. Fear of rejection can also lead them to prefer one-night stands if they feel that such fleeting relationships do not commit them to using condoms or telling their partners that they have HIV.[9]

And this is only a partial list of reasons why many people do not use condoms when they or their partners may be at risk.

No matter what the level of risk or the type of relationship involved, people often reject condoms as a symbol of mistrust and because they are seen to interfere with sexual pleasure. This image needs to be challenged and turned on its head.

Emphasizing only the resistance to condoms is self-defeating and can help to sustain an undeserved negative image. Trust and sexual pleasure do go together with condoms for the many people who use them.

Few experienced and satisfied condom users have been asked why they use and like condoms, even though their positive reasons could form the backbone of condom-promotion campaigns. These reasons include but are much broader than contraceptive/prophylactic protection. For example, many women dislike it when semen seeps out of the vagina for hours after sex, wets the bed and leaves a bad vaginal odour. Men may be able to maintain an erection longer with condoms, and condoms can be used as sex toys.

Instead of giving in to short-term defeatism, condom-promotion campaigns need to be broadened and intensified.

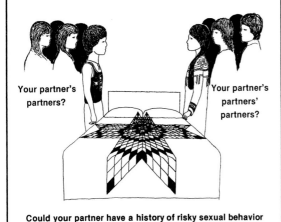

How well do you know your partner?

Your partner's partners?

Your partner's partners' partners?

Could your partner have a history of risky sexual behavior in the last ten years that you do not know about?

Because you might not know everything about your partner, talk about the risk of AIDS. It is up to you to protect yourself.

NATIVE AMERICAN WOMEN'S HEALTH EDUCATION RESOURCE CENTER

P.O. BOX 572 • LAKE ANDES, SOUTH DAKOTA 57356 • 605-487-7072

Native American Women's Health Education Resource Center, USA

• Alternatives to intercourse.

The strategies described so far assume that sex equals intercourse and that safer sex equals safer intercourse. For relationships between men and women, not having intercourse has rarely been encouraged as a way to have safer sex, and the fact that all other forms of sexual practice are much safer than intercourse is not widely publicized.

Finding safe alternatives to intercourse does not mean stopping sex. It means replacing intercourse with other pleasurable practices – all of the time to be very safe, or some of the time to reduce risk. Reduction, not just elimination, of risk is better than nothing.

Most religious leaders would not encourage alternative sexual practices, because all religions preach that sex is for procreation. In the dominant male-centred point of view, intercourse is considered essential to male sexual pleasure. Implicitly, intercourse continues to be legitimized as the definition of sex, and most heterosexual men and women have not questioned this norm.

Yet people enjoy and seek other modes of sexual expression. Many men go to sex workers specifically for oral and other kinds of sex because they are unwilling or afraid to ask their partners for them. And women often say that intercourse does not always give as much pleasure as other forms of stimulation.

Other forms of sex may be seen as immature, unnatural, perverted, abnormal or dirty. For example, in Africa, oral sex is considered a strictly Western practice[10] and is frowned upon by many women. People may be afraid of condemnation if they admit to, let alone ask for, such practices.

When asked to recall their first sexual experience, people often identify the time they first had intercourse. In reality, many people stimulate themselves and each other sexually long before puberty, and many experience orgasm this way before having intercourse with another person. Adolescents discover various forms of sexual expression, such as petting and mutual masturbation, without 'going all the way'. People masturbate when they have no partner, when they do not get enough pleasure with partners, or just because they like it. Most people have sexual fantasies and become excited by them.

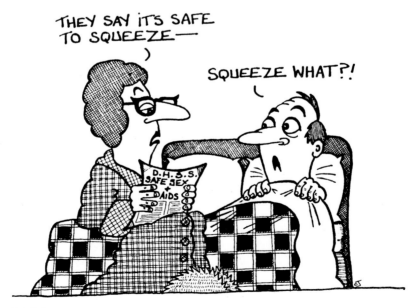

Cath Jackson

None of this is viewed as 'real sex'. Hence, once people start having intercourse they may abandon these practices as childish or immature, or devalue them by calling them foreplay or a substitute for the real thing.

AIDS poses a challenge to intercourse-centred views of sex. While it may sound unrealistic, the best way to reduce the transmission of HIV sexually would be to call a global moratorium on intercourse, even for a day or a week, as a consciousness-raising tool.

The desire for intercourse is a powerful one and will not disappear but it need not be a part of every sexual encounter. It could be saved for starting a pregnancy or for special occasions. Penetration can be achieved through oral sex, for example, or the use of non-abrasive sexual aids, fingers, and some imagination. The imagination does not have to stretch very far to find new ways to achieve pleasure.

The problem is that people find it difficult to talk about sexual needs and desires and to try something that is not socially condoned. No one can be expected to take these steps if they fear they will be ridiculed, appear inexperienced or inept, or be condemned as immoral.

Somehow, this circle must be broken. Alternatives to intercourse should be a major part of the agenda on sexuality for the future. Not only, as some feminists argued in the past, because women do not want it, but because other forms of sexual expression are equally pleasurable and legitimate and much safer.

Women's movement groups and sex workers' organizations have good reason to work together on public sex education. As Nana, the owner of a brothel in Uruguay has said, sex workers know best what people want and how to give it:

Interviewer: Do you see your experience in the brothel as something good and positive?
Nana: Yes, it is positive. You learn a lot about men and about what men want. Everyone knows how much I know about that. Women call me to find out how they can get their husbands back and what they should be doing in bed.[11]

Women religious leaders who advocate a women-centred religious ethic are taking new stances on the subject of what is moral and could become a positive force for change in religious views on sexuality as well. Eventually, public education and health officials may feel safe to follow such leads.

Translating strategies into practice

In practice, strategies for preventing sexual transmission of HIV are the same for everyone, whether people know they have HIV or not. The more strategies there are, the more people will be able to use one or a combination, in ways that fit their personal situations and relationships.

Women will try a number of strategies until they find one that works. In one San Francisco study of women at risk, some women stayed with partners who were at high risk but tried to have safer sex. Some women with more than one partner stopped seeing men they considered unsafe, rather than change their own sexual behaviour. Many women attempted to practice safer sex but met resistance from partners, especially to condom use. More women reported changing to partners they thought had lower risks than to low-risk practices.[12]

The same researchers found that among a group of HIV-positive women 35 per cent abstained from sex for a period of six months after learning they were HIV-positive, and eight per cent were still abstaining after a year. Most of the women changed to low-risk practices when they resumed sexual activity. Only a third were having vaginal intercourse without condoms, compared to 75 per cent before they knew they had HIV. Of 11 women still exposing partners to vaginal mucus after a year, five practised only oral sex and three had partners who refused to use condoms. A big question was whether a relationship would break up if the women told their partners they had HIV. Often it did, but the women usually found new partners who knew their HIV status and were willing to practise safer sex. [13]

Who needs safer sex?

Should everyone having intercourse be advised to practise safer sex, or only people most at risk of HIV/AIDS?

Of 17,655 women attending family planning clinics in the Philadelphia area in the USA from mid-1988 to mid-1989, 14 per cent were at high risk of HIV infection, 31 per cent at moderate risk and 55 per cent at low risk. Risk was measured according to the number of STDs acquired in the previous five years, number of sexual partners in the previous year and sex with an injection drug user. [14] Even on this relatively crude measure, at least half the women would have benefited from counselling about HIV/AIDS and safer sex.

Identifying those at higher risk and concentrating on them may appear to make sense in the short term. However, determination of risk is not foolproof. It is not always possible to recognize who is at risk. Many mistakenly believe married women not to be at risk. Women themselves may not believe or realize they are at risk. And women who are at high or low risk today do not necessarily remain that way indefinitely.

A major disadvantage of encouraging safer sex and condom use only among those with identified risk behaviour is that everyone else is helped to believe they are not vulnerable. [15] This can contribute to double standards of 'good' and 'bad' sex and discrimination against people with identified risk. It also encourages many people not to question their sexual practices or assess their risks at all.

A combined goal of reducing the incidence of unwanted pregnancies, cervical cancer, infertility, treatable STDs and HIV suggests a policy that applies to everyone, not just those at perceived risk of HIV. This may be more obvious in areas of high HIV prevalence, but it is true everywhere.

Most importantly, in the long run, it may be the only effective way for safer sex to become the social norm at a global level.

Safer sex practices for women

The point of safer sex is not to give up pleasure. The point is to find ways of pleasuring yourself and your partner that put both of you at less or no risk of unwanted pregnancy or reproductive tract infections of all kinds, including HIV.

Safe practices

- Massage
- Masturbating yourself
- Masturbating each other, at the same time or separately
- Licking, kissing, nibbling each other

- Touching yourself and each other everywhere
- Hugging and cuddling
- Body-to-body rubbing
- Acting out fantasies, dancing, sexy movements
- Using a vibrator, sex toy or aid (not shared)
- Contact with semen, anal and vaginal mucus on unbroken skin.

Possibly risky practices

- Oral sex on a man – lips, mouth and tongue on penis (riskier if semen is taken into the mouth and in the presence of reproductive tract infection)
- Oral sex on a woman – lips, mouth and tongue on genitals (riskier if menstrual blood is taken into the mouth and in the presence of reproductive tract infection)
- Oral-anal sex on either partner
- Urinating into the partner's mouth or eyes
- Sharing sexual aids used in the vagina or rectum.

High-risk practices

- Unprotected vaginal or anal intercourse
- Any practice that causes bleeding or trauma to tissue, e.g. hand or fist or rough object on the penis or in the vagina or anus, during or followed by unprotected intercourse.

Risk reduction

- Genital hygiene – the genital area should be cleaned daily, and before and after having sex. Men should take particular care to clean under the foreskin. Use mild soap and clean water. Urinating after sex helps to prevent urinary tract infection. Do not use douches; the vagina cleans itself.
- Seek treatment for all reproductive tract infections. Abdominal or lower-back pain, sores, warts, itching, burning, swelling, redness or irritation in the vagina or genitals, an unusual discharge or bad smell, or pain during intercourse or urination are all signs of possible infection.
- For intercourse, use condoms alone for protection against RTIs/HIV and pregnancy, or condoms with another effective contraceptive. Use a male condom on the penis for all vaginal or anal intercourse. Or use a female condom for vaginal intercourse if available. Do not use the same condom anally and then vaginally.
- Do not have intercourse or have it less often and substitute other pleasurable practices.
- During menstrual periods avoid intercourse and oral sex on a woman. Or, use a diaphragm or cap to catch menstrual blood. Or, use a tampon and do not have intercourse.
- For oral sex – use a latex square or cut a condom down the side as a barrier on the anal area and the woman's genitals. Use a condom as a barrier on the penis. Some sources consider this necessary for all oral sex. Others think this is an overreaction, considering the few documented cases from this route. Use of one of these barriers at least during ejaculation, menstruation and in the presence of an RTI is sometimes recommended.
- For inserting fingers or hand into vagina or anus, if hands have cuts, wear thin latex gloves or finger-cots like the kind used in medical and dental care.
- Avoid substances, sex toys and practices that can cause trauma to the genitals, vaginal and anal/rectal tissue.[16]

Ways to present safer sex messages

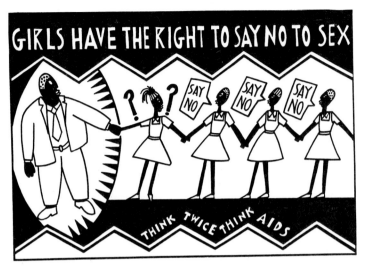

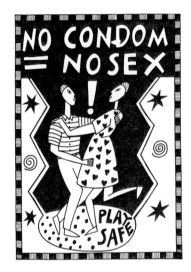

AIDS Counselling Trust, Zimbabwe

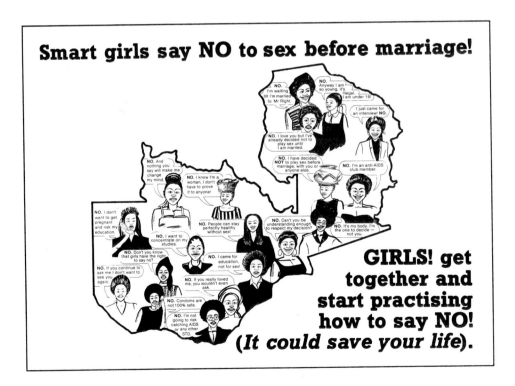

Anti-Aids Project/Copperbelt Health Education Project, Zambia

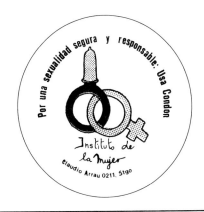

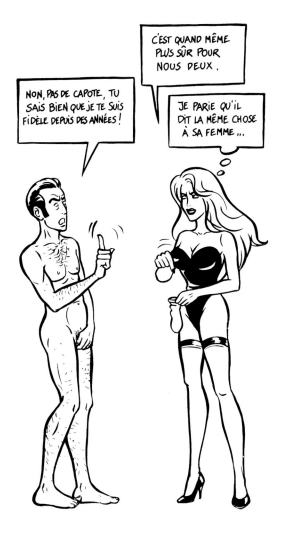

Swiss Aids Foundation

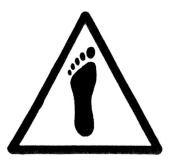

Comite de Lutte contra le SIDA, Zaire

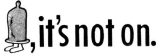

Pacific AIDS Alert Bulletin

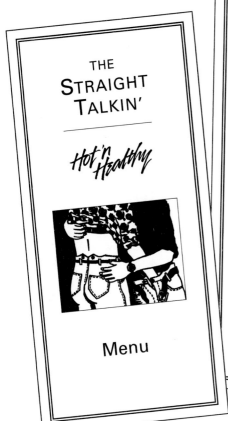

THE STRAIGHT TALKIN'

Hot 'n Healthy

Menu

Hors d'Oeuvres

DISCUSSING HOW HUNGRY YOU ARE. EAR NIBBLING, KISSING, CUDDLING. TICKLING, STROKING, TEASING NIPPLES. SHARING FANTASIES, DRESSING UP. UNDRESSING EACH OTHER SLOWLY. WATCHING YOUR LOVER UNDRESS. SHOWERING AND BATHING TOGETHER, SOAPING, WASHING AND DRYING EACH OTHER. GENTLY RUBBING OIL ON ALL OVER. MASSAGING FEET AND BACK

Are you ready for the main course.... why not have some more starters?

Plat du Jour

ROLLING AROUND, GETTING HOTn'STICKY KISSING AND LICKING ALL OVER. SUCKING, BITING AND TUGGING. TALKING-SEX AND TEASING. TIBBLING HIS BALLS*. KISSING HER FANNY. FINGERING AND RUBBING. SUCKING HIS PRICK. LICKING HER CLITORIS. WANKING EACH OTHER.

REMEMBER

Safe Sex is about what you can do, not what you can't!

* We thought Tibbling was a spelling mistake, then we tried it!

Don't forget to leave room for pudding

THE DISHES BELOW ARE SERVED WITH CONDOMS ONLY

PUTTING IT ON FOR HIM. WATCHING HIM PUT IT ON. LUBRICATING IT (WITH WATER BASED LUBRICANT **) PULLING HIM INSIDE YOU SLOWLY. ENTERING HER IN A TEASING WAY SLIDE INSIDE, TAKE YOUR TIME. MOVING IN AND OUT SLOWLY. WAIT A WHILE, APPRECIATING YOUR LOVER. START AGAIN ANYWHERE ON THE MENU.

Why not skip the rest ..... Pudding might just be best!

Pudding

LICKING WHIPPED CREAM OFF EACH OTHER. THE SAME WITH YOGHURT OR MAYONNAISE. HOLDING EACH OTHER AND TALKING. CUDDLING UP AND SLEEPING TOGETHER. HAVING BREAKFAST OR A LATE NIGHT FEAST. A LONG LAZY BATH TOGETHER.

STARTING OVER !

** Any Petroleum Based lubes such as vaseline or oils can damage the condom and weaken it.

Leeds AIDS Advice, England

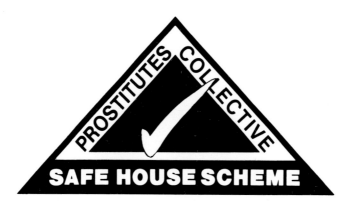

Prostitutes Collective of Victoria, Australia

Activity: using sexual language

by John Hubley

Communicating with others about AIDS inevitably means that we have to discuss sex. If we want to be helpful to people, we must be very frank about specific sexual practices and not hide behind general terms like 'sexual relations'. Using polite or medical terms rather than everyday words in some situations can build a barrier between ourselves and our audience. In other situations, using local equivalents of words such as 'screw' or 'fuck' can cause offence. We have to be sensitive to when it is appropriate to use everyday language or polite words.

Preparation:

On each of eight large sheets of paper, write one of the following at the top in capital letters:

- Male genital organ
- Semen
- Vaginal secretion
- Female genital organs
- Vaginal intercourse
- Anal intercourse
- Oral sex
- Masturbation

With the group:

Start by explaining the importance of feeling at ease with using sexual terms in our work and the need to be specific about details of sexual practices.

Split the participants into eight smaller groups. Give each group one of the sheets.

Give them ten minutes to brainstorm and write down on the sheet all the medical, polite, rude, and everyday/street words that they know for that item.

Ask each group to pass their sheet to another group and add to the list on that sheet any other words that they know. Do this until each group has had a chance to add words to all eight sheets.

Put all the sheets up on the wall where everyone can read them. With each, discuss with the group (or get people to work in pairs) their feelings about all the words, and what these words tell us about sexuality and how we view our bodies as men and women.

Ask them which words they would use and which would be unacceptable in different situations related to their work.

Condom etiquette

Adapted from Girls Night Out, *Chicago Women's AIDS Project*

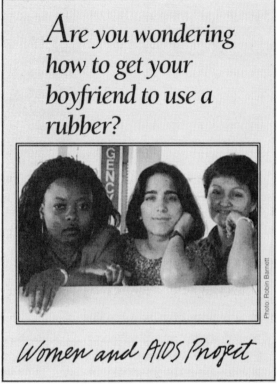

Women and AIDS Project - AIDS Vancouver, Canada

The following are some suggestions on how to raise the subject of condoms with a male partner and could be used for role-play practice. When working with groups, participants could also be asked to brainstorm a list of reasons why people refuse to use condoms, and create role plays around those.

When and where
• Bring the subject up at a party or over drinks with friends, for general discussion first.
• Bring it up when you are alone together, feeling comfortable and free of tension.
• Wait to bring it up when you start making love, but only if you are sure you can stay in control enough to manage it.

What to say
- This is awkward for me, but I've been thinking it would be a good idea to use condoms. What do you think?
- Have you ever used a condom? No? I haven't either. Let's try them.
- Have you ever used a condom? Yes? Oh, good, then you can show me. Here, someone gave me one today and I wasn't sure how to use it.
- I'd love to make love with you. Have I told you that I always use condoms?
- I'd love to go to bed with you. And don't worry, I have some condoms with me.
- I always use condoms. I always have. It just makes sense with all the things you can catch.
- I thought you said you didn't want to be a father . . . Come on, then, prove it.
- I was at the family planning clinic today and they gave me these to try. Have you ever used them?
- I was in the pharmacy this morning and saw a condom display they just put up. It made me start thinking about how things are changing. Look, I bought a packet. Shall we try them?
- Have you seen/heard the TV/radio advertisement for condoms? I never thought I'd see/hear something like that, but it did make me think.
- Listen, what do you think about using condoms?
- I was talking to some friends the other day and they're all using condoms now just to be

careful. I think it makes a lot of sense. What do you think?

- Have I ever showed you my condom collection?
- I'm not using any birth-control method, so we're going to have to use condoms. Do you think I should use something else as well?
- But condoms *are* for birth control. That's what I use.
- Look what I bought for us to try today!
- This whole AIDS thing has got me nervous. I decided I wasn't going to give up sex, so I use condoms every time.
- Listen, if we're going any further, let's get a condom.
- (Don't say anything. Have one nearby and when it starts to get hot, reach out and pick it up and wave it in the air. Then smile at him and start opening the packet. Either hand it to him or put it on yourself.)
- You know, we could have completely safe sex, but I feel like taking chances. Let's just use a condom.
- (As you approach the bed with condom packet in hand, wave it in the air and say:) Honey, can you help me think of something we might possibly do with one of these?
- I want you inside me . . . (as you say this, put a condom on him yourself.)

If he resists

Don't give in. He'll probably come round. Promise him a reward he can't resist. Or maybe it's time for a long talk, not for lovemaking. Your own self-esteem and commitment to using condoms will help you overcome the obstacles he throws in your path. Sex will still be an option when you both understand each other better.

And at the worst

Show him the door. If a man refuses to wear a condom when you are offering him intimacy, sex, a part of yourself . . . after you have patiently told him why you think it is best, after you have tried to accommodate him in every way, then let's face it: you're no worse off without him. You're lucky you found out so soon.

Perhaps he will call you or come round later and apologize and be ready to talk about it. Next time you see him, have a gift-wrapped box of condoms ready to give him as a present.

If not, good riddance! You deserve to be protected.

Women talking about safer sex

from Women, HIV and AIDS: Speaking Out in the UK

The following comments are from a group of women brought together to talk about their feelings about sex and HIV:
'Most people think you've not had a proper sexual relationship if you don't have intercourse. You can do whatever you like – oral sex, masturbation, etc. – but that's just petting as far as they're concerned. And when you work up to an orgasm, the main way you should wish to, is by penetration, actual intercourse. But it's quite interesting, because I think you can have orgasms in lots of different ways.'

'That's right, as far as men are concerned there is a proper way to have an orgasm. I've had girls coming to me and saying, "I can't orgasm the proper way, what should I do?" When I say to them, "Well, you tell me what the proper way is," they say: "My boyfriend says I should come when he's inside me." I say, "Well, isn't that his problem?" '

'Men think of different kinds of sex as having a repertoire of different positions for intercourse.'

'They just want regular sex, basically.'

'I think if men were allowed to get away with it, what they'd like is sex without commitment, even within a marriage, so it's just a function, and I think women have to coach them and tell them it's more than this quick physical gratification, you know, there's more to it than that, you actually want to be loved.'

'Often women are working to fixed times, especially if they're going out to work . . . most women don't value themselves. They think, "I've got to cook the dinner, look after the children, go shopping . . ." As a woman you've got to say, "I need some time for myself and what I want to do is make love." A lot of women make time for everything else but themselves.'

'I use condoms as a method of contraception . . . I feel more in control using barrier contraceptives because I decide when I use a diaphragm and condoms, so we decide when we want to use one or the other and make a partnership of it. It doesn't matter if you drop the condom or whatever, that's part of it. If you're so embarrassed with your partner that you can't put a condom on his penis, how can you talk about sex or have sex with him effectively or enjoy it properly?'

'I've started using condoms. I got militant and decided I wasn't going to take drugs any more, so I stopped taking the pill and started using condoms five or ten years ago. At that time they did feel quite thick and clumsy but I think now they're so thin, they've made them much more sophisticated. I don't think you can tell the difference. I think HIV and AIDS have given condoms a better name but I don't think it's changed people's attitudes because they still think it's not going to happen to them.'

'It's great when you're using a condom. It can be great fun, we call our condom Willy, like a friend. I flick it about, I think it's lovely, and I like how you can use it as part of sex.'

'There are some women who feel well, OK, they will carry condoms around with them, and there are some who think it's still degrading and they're going to be seen as whores. I think at least you've got control and you can then take control in terms of deciding whether you want to have sex, how you want to have sex.'

'But this emphasis on the condom as a way of coping with HIV and AIDS puts the pressure back on penetrative sex and that reduces your freedom as a woman . . . The pressure is on women not to demand different types of sex, not to express their different pleasure areas, like orgasms without penetration . . . You put the condom on and he can carry on in the same old way.'

'It's difficult for young people, particularly girls, to be assertive because you've got to be very comfortable with your own sexuality to be assertive. When you're growing up you're not taught that sex is something that you give to someone else, basically.'

'If I was going out with a guy who was HIV-positive, well, penetrative sex would be out, full stop, because there's no condom in the world that can say you're having safe sex with this guy.'

'You don't know how much you can trust the other person. It's something very personal to say you're HIV-positive. How will he take that information? What will he do with it? Will he still love me or can he not love me? Maybe he would shut down and maybe you're just not willing to risk that.'

Over the dam

by Susie Bright

. . . There were about 100 people gathered in the lecture hall. About half were AIDS care-givers, and the others were HIV-positive women and their lovers. A significant group of lesbians attended. But the part that got me, the stupid obvious thing I didn't expect, was that most of the affected women were so young. I met a couple of middle-aged seropositive women, but the rest were in their 20s. The care-givers in the crowd were the ones who looked like they needed nutrition and exercise. It was the HIV-positive women who sparkled, the kind of girl you would notice walking down the street.

Of course, this was an unusual group; these are the women who take the most activist, pressing role in their diagnosis and treatment. I met the women who knew that a panel like this existed, and they must be in the minority.

I began my talk by explaining I could learn much more from them than they could from me. The mainstream has no information about HIV-positive women's sexuality, so we can only start at the ground floor and share each other's experience. I wasn't about to give a condom-on-banana talk to a group of people who are dealing with the idea that their very body is poisonous. The crucial identity point for women with AIDS is that, like all women, they were raised to be fearful and ignorant of sexual desire, to be estranged from their bodies. To then be infected with the stigma of AIDS must feel like the ultimate denial of anything good, enriching and female about sexual experience.

A woman struggling with AIDS-phobia and her own positive diagnosis is confronted with the dilemma of loving and healing her sexuality in a way she has likely never prepared for before. Of course, many women won't deal with it, ever. They will become celibate, unsexual, anti-erotic.

I asked the audience to jot down on a slip of paper some quick thoughts on a series of questions I had.

I wanted to know, since their HIV-positive diagnosis, did they:

- have more or less sex with a partner,
- masturbate more or less,
- give up a sexual practice they really loved and what it was, and
- start up a new sexual practice they loved, and what it was.

I asked the partners of the infected women to answer for themselves, and for all others who are not HIV-positive to answer the questions as if they were seropositive and had to make such decisions. I madly counted up the replies during the rest of the panel. The biggest surprise was the difference between the people who have HIV and the people who don't. I would say the non-infected respondents were more pessimistic – the attitude that if we were diagnosed positive tomorrow, we'd just crawl into a casket and wait to be carted away.

The majority, in every case, said they had less sex with a partner since their diagnosis. But 32 per cent of the HIV-positive women said they had either the same or more sexual relations with their lover, which I think is a sizeable minority. These women are staying close to their sexual lives.

Fifty-seven per cent also said they masturbated as much or more than usual. It was the large minority, the 43 per cent who masturbate less, that made me sad. There is zero risk in making love to oneself, and yet when sexual self-esteem goes out the window, masturbation seems to be one of the most potent experiences that gets cut.

Seventy-nine per cent of the HIV-positive women, and 90 per cent of their partners, said they have given up something very important to them: unprotected oral sex.

Fifty per cent of the audience said they had incorporated new sexual behaviour that they would never want to give up. The most common was vibrators and fantasy scenes.

The big difference between infected versus non-infected responses was that the people who are not seropositive imagined that they would turn to more gentle, sensuous foreplay type activities if they were practising exclusive safe sex. The seropositive group, however, immediately understood the orgasmic intent of my question and told me what they needed and wanted to get off.

Two HIV-positive heterosexual women said they now enjoyed 'gentleness' and 'more sensitive communication'. One heterosexual woman said how she now loved getting finger-fucked, and all I could think of was: 'You had to wait for this?'

Something puzzled me about the furore over oral sex. On one hand, all the women who spoke up about it seemed convinced that mouth to genital contact was no risk if the woman wasn't bleeding or suffering any infections, etc. Certainly the absence of blood or semen is an argument for no-holds-barred oral sex.

I asked them, 'If you're not worried about oral sex, why have so many of you given it up?' One woman burst out, 'Because if you tell anyone where you're at, they don't want to touch you down there, let alone do it orally!'

That about sums it up. We can talk about safe sex techniques from dusk until dawn, but it's a lot of precise talk about plastic and positions. The real dilemma of women's sexuality and AIDS is fear, stigma, humiliation, estrangement. The goal is to feel close, sexy, passionate and turn on and dig yourself.

The techniques of safer sex can distract us from the bare bones. For example, one girl asked me, 'I was with a lover for six years who had AIDS. I've been alone for a year and I'm just about ready to go out again so I want to know how to use rubber dams.'

That was the moment I was waiting for. I handed her a couple of mint-flavoured squares and said, 'I can tell you how to use a barrier in two minutes, but it seems that's the least of your dilemma. How do you feel about having sex again? Do you fantasize about oral sex, do you long for it, are you afraid of it?'

These questions could be applied to any woman. In this forum, with these women, the basic sexual choices are simply illuminated by the fact that it is now a matter of life and death.

At the end of my presentation, a few people thanked me for showing off my sex toys. One woman said, 'I like that you said that the vibrator was yours, not just saying, "it has been known to be effective".'

'Oh, yes, all these toys and books are my own. I brought them not because I thought it would be so new to any of you, but because I wanted to demonstrate how making the first change in your sexual behaviour is the hardest. The next changes come much more sweetly. I started with a vibrator, but then that opened me up to so much more – not just things to buy and consume, but an understanding of my capacity, a hook into my imagination. My sexuality developed more in the past seven years than in all the 23 preceding.'

There was so much more to say. We had 15 minutes to talk about sex and we needed a good 15 hours. Yet it was the most powerful 15-minute sexual discussion I have ever been a part of.

Contraceptives and condoms

Becoming pregnant requires unprotected intercourse on fertile days. Not becoming pregnant the rest of the time is equally important. In many parts of the world, women are having one or two children at most and can need protection against pregnancy for more than 40 years. Even to have five or six children, most women will want to avoid becoming pregnant for 30–35 years.

The past three decades have seen a phenomenal amount of research to improve and increase the number of safe and effective contraceptive and abortion methods and the clinical services to make these available worldwide. Confronted with women's calls for the right to pleasure in sexual relationships and the right to decide the number and spacing of children, along with the pressure of the growth rate of world population, researchers have sought birth control methods that are both highly effective and do not interfere with intercourse.

Most people are not currently protecting themselves during intercourse from reproductive tract infections, including HIV. Worries about these faded with the discovery of antibiotics, and campaigns initiated by women to encourage condom use against syphilis and gonorrhoea were mostly forgotten after the Second World War. Then barrier methods were abandoned when the contraceptive pill appeared in the 1960s.

Now a potentially fatal sexually transmitted disease is again widespread. Even if a drug or vaccine against HIV is found, other sexually transmitted diseases may appear in future. To find a way forward is a matter of great urgency. Convenience has had its price. Modern contraceptives and antibiotics have influenced the expectations and sexual behaviour of two to three generations around the world.

The responsible thing to do

Using contraception is considered the only responsible thing to do when pregnancy is not wanted. It has taken the whole of the twentieth century, many challenges to traditional religious views, and much concerted work on the part of activists, service providers and policymakers to gain social acceptance for this 'norm'. In many areas, much remains to be achieved.

Effective contraception has supported increased sexual freedom in many parts of the world, but this has often benefited men more than women. For sexual freedom to be of value for women, the welfare of both women and any children must also be taken into account.

Practising safer sex is considered the only responsible thing to do to prevent sexually transmitted infection. Because of AIDS, a new ethic has been born – based for some on a return to monogamy and for others on a form of sexual freedom that protects lives and health. There are many parallels.

About 50 per cent of couples of childbearing age worldwide are using some form of birth control method to prevent pregnancy. This reaches 70 per cent in the more developed regions, and 15–75 per cent, with an average of about 45 per cent, in the less developed regions.[1] On present trends, the demand for contraception will increase by over 60 per cent by the end of the twentieth century, from about 505 million to almost 795 million couples.[2]

In contrast, condom use has been extremely limited in the past few decades. In the late 1980s in most countries, less than 16 per cent of couples were using condoms for contraceptive purposes, and in most countries the figure was 1–5 per cent. The only exceptions were Scandinavia, Hong Kong, Singapore, the UK and Japan, where figures were higher than 16 per cent.[3,4] Data about use of condoms prior to 1990 for protection against reproductive tract infections were rarely collected.

For safer sex, that is, to avoid HIV/RTIs and prevent pregnancy, women need both an effective contraceptive and condoms together, or condoms on their own for both purposes.

Condoms prevent infection

Some women do not currently need or use contraception but may need protection from HIV/RTIs, including:

- pregnant women
- breastfeeding women
  Breastfeeding is effective for contraceptive purposes for up to six months if it is done exclusively and on demand. Condoms used during breastfeeding would increase both contraceptive effectiveness and prevent HIV risks to the woman and infant.
- couples where one or both partners is infertile

DOES YOUR BIRTH CONTROL PROTECT YOU AGAINST AIDS?

YES	NO	
☐	☐	BIRTH CONTROL PILL
☐	☐	IUD
☐	☐	STERILIZATION (having your tubes tied or vasectomy)
☐	☐	RHYTHM or WITHDRAWAL (or no method at all)
☐	☐	DIAPHRAGM or CERVICAL CAP (barrier methods)
☐	☐	TODAY SPONGE (barrier method)
☐	☐	FOAM

Please open up for answers.

ANSWER: NONE OF THE ABOVE. ONLY CONDOMS.

Women and AIDS Project - AIDS Vancouver, Canada

- women past the menopause
- women who have been sterilized or have a partner who has had a vasectomy
  Sterilization has been the most widely used method of birth control internationally since the mid-1980s
- women who see contraception or sterilization as something to use when they want to stop childbearing, but not before.
  Focus group discussions with rural women in Kenya, in 1987, found that they were very knowledgeable about contraception and wanted to use it later, but did not consider it necessary for birth spacing purposes.[5] Many women in India intend to be sterilized when they finish childbearing, but do not use contraception in the meantime.

The use of condoms can be crucial in these situations, but women are rarely encouraged to use them in public education campaigns or by the clinics that see them for health care.

Condoms are also contraceptives

Many people see condoms as a method for preventing sexually transmitted infection, or as a contraceptive method, but not both. This split in thinking probably originated with the attitudes of service providers in family planning, STD and, more recently, AIDS services.

In Haiti, for example, there used to be two delivery systems for condoms: one through the AIDS programme and one through the family planning programme. Some family planning programmes have found that they can get 'AIDS condoms' free, but have to use their own resources to obtain 'family planning condoms'. Any such differentiation is clearly absurd and counterproductive from the users' point of view.[6] Condoms serve both purposes.

The need for protection against HIV changes the definition of 'safe and effective' as this applies to contraception. Before AIDS, 'safe

and effective' was only about the prevention of unwanted pregnancy. Now 'safe and effective' has taken on new meaning. Where the risk of HIV infection is high or even moderate, being safe may mean taking a higher risk of unwanted pregnancy by using condoms, rather than risking HIV infection by not using them.

Using condoms alone depends on how the woman/couple would feel about an accidental pregnancy, and whether or not they would be willing and able to get post-coital contraception or an abortion in case of condom failure. An increase in the rate of abortion may result and would need to be accommodated through increased services. This challenges the prevailing view that fewer abortions are always preferable.

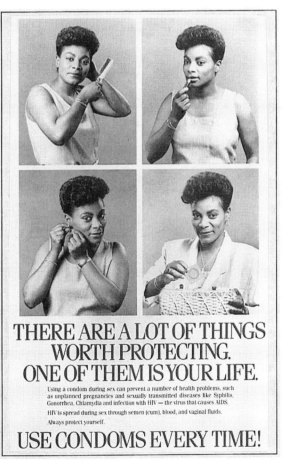

THERE ARE A LOT OF THINGS WORTH PROTECTING. ONE OF THEM IS YOUR LIFE.

Using a condom during sex can prevent a number of health problems, such as unplanned pregnancies and sexually transmitted diseases like Syphilis, Gonorrhea, Chlamydia and infection with HIV — the virus that causes AIDS.
HIV is spread during sex through semen (cum), blood, and vaginal fluids.
Always protect yourself.

USE CONDOMS EVERY TIME!

Health Education Resource Organization, USA

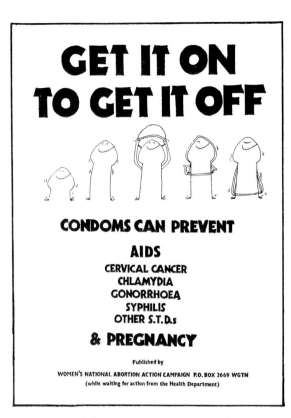

GET IT ON
TO GET IT OFF

CONDOMS CAN PREVENT

AIDS

CERVICAL CANCER
CHLAMYDIA
GONORRHOEA
SYPHILIS
OTHER S.T.D.s

& PREGNANCY

Published by
WOMEN'S NATIONAL ABORTION ACTION CAMPAIGN P.O. BOX 2669 WGTN
(while waiting for action from the Health Department)

Women's National Abortion Action Campaign, New Zealand

There is a very different balance of risk if abortion is illegal/unsafe. Abortion morbidity and mortality could rise as an unintended consequence of promoting condom-only use. Campaigns for safe, legal abortion would need to be intensified.

Using condoms plus another contraceptive

For anyone unwilling or unable to depend on condoms alone, condoms in combination with another contraceptive method is the safest alternative. Both the pregnancy risk and the risk of STD/HIV infection are minimized.

Whatever contraceptive method people would feel most comfortable with and use most effectively is still their method of choice. The addition of condoms is the real issue.

The International Planned Parenthood Federation (IPPF) first recommended doubling-up methods in 1988. Will most people use two methods? Some people are, but no one knows how many. Published studies are almost nonexistent at this time of writing.

Of 54 HIV-positive women in 1989–90 in Scotland, 21 were not using contraception. Of those, seven had no sexual partner and eight were pregnant. Of those using contraception, eight were using condoms only, 20 were using a non-barrier contraceptive only, and five were using both condoms and another contraceptive method. Only half of the women who were using condoms were happy with them. In most cases, it was the women who got the condoms. When asked if they had received enough advice on contraception, nine of the women said they had not, ten said they did not know anywhere where they could obtain free condoms, while many others said they had received too much advice.[7]

Clearly, a doubling up of methods doubles the potential problems. There are tremendous challenges involved.

Many women at risk of both unwanted pregnancy and HIV/STD infection do not currently use contraception or condoms, or only use them intermittently. Their need for information and services to prevent infection may be addressed while their need for contraception may be ignored, or vice versa, if programmes are separate.

Married women, young women, migrant women, street children, sex workers and others who support themselves through sexual services for men, are considered at particular risk in one or other category, but sometimes not in both.

Women in prison or with partners in prison with conjugal visiting rights get very little attention from services of any kind. In a São Paulo prison holding 7,000 men, about 2,500 received lovers and wives at weekends in their cells. Seventeen per cent of the men were HIV-positive in 1990. Yet no condoms were provided.[8]

Women using drugs often do not seek contraceptive services, and providers may not know their specific problems and needs. One combined family planning/drug treatment programme in the USA followed two models. In one model, contraceptive counselling, education and methods were all provided at drug-treatment centres. In the other, counselling and education were provided at the drug treatment centres, and women were referred to nearby family planning clinics to obtain methods. In the first six months, 245 out of 600 women took advantage of one of these two options.[9]

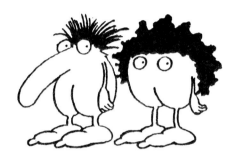

P. Mayle and A. Robins

Safe, effective condom use

People need to know a lot about condoms to use them safely. Many men and women have never even seen a condom, let alone put one on. Most have never been taught how to use them.

Instructional leaflets

Condom instructions are often not clear enough or use words or a style that people cannot understand. Poorly thought out visuals can be most confusing of all. The accuracy and ease of adaptability of many leaflets to different cultures varies dramatically.

Consequently, the World Health Organization (WHO), with technical assistance from the Programme for Appropriate Technology in Health (PATH), created an easily adaptable flyer with visuals and instructions about proper condom use. These are part of a packet that includes step-by-step guidelines on how to adapt the flyer to local conditions. Copies of the packet have been sent to 60 countries whose National AIDS Programmes requested condoms from WHO for prevention of HIV transmission. They are available from the WHO Global Programme on AIDS in Geneva.

This packet was developed following a thorough review of more than 200 existing condom instructions. The best written and pictorial elements were selected and pre-tested in Kenya, Mexico, the Philippines and Rwanda, with literate and semi-literate men and women, and subsequently improved.[10]

Demonstrating how to use condoms

Hands-on instruction can increase condom use and reduce failure rates, as with the diaphragm. With the diaphragm, women are taught how to insert and remove it, and then given one to take home for practice for several weeks. Then they return to the clinic and insert the diaphragm with the provider checking that it is in the right place, before they are expected to rely on it. A comparable procedure might be instituted with condoms.

In Trinidad & Tobago, some male patients at an STD clinic were taught to use a condom and practised on a model of a penis. Others were only given an information brochure. The first group used condoms more often and made fewer mistakes than the second group. Fewer men in the second group used a condom in the following month, and those who did reported a higher rate of breakage and spillage incidents. The only advantage of giving a brochure alone was that it saved staff time and resources.[11]

People need to know:
- when and how to put condoms on, leaving space at the tip for semen;

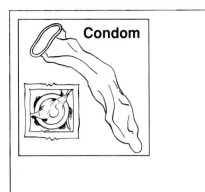
Condom

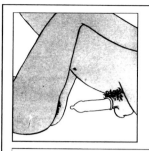

Always put condom on before entering partner.

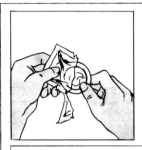

Carefully open package so condom does not tear.
Do not unroll condom before putting it on.

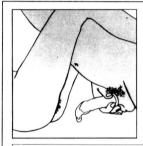

After ejaculation (coming), hold rim of condom and pull penis out before penis gets soft.

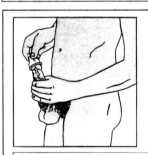

If not circumcised, pull foreskin back. Squeeze tip of condom and put it on end of hard penis.

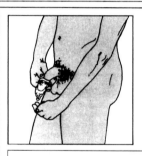

Slide condom off without spilling liquid (semen) inside.

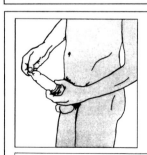

Continue squeezing tip while unrolling condom until it covers all of penis.

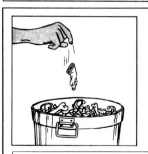

Throw away or bury the condom.

World Health
Organization

- when and how to remove them;
- not to use them after the expiry date;
- not to re-use them;
- not to use the same one anally and then vaginally;
- what lubricants can be used;
- where to obtain a regular, affordable supply;
- the differences between brands and sizes if available;
- safe use of spermicides vaginally;
- how to store them.

When condoms should be used

Condoms should be used with all partners, not just casual ones, and for all vaginal and anal intercourse.

The risk of pregnancy through non-use is highest on fertile days of the cycle. This means teaching fertility awareness.

With STD/HIV prevention, every day is the same. For those who think they might lapse at times, consistent use at least during fertile days, in the presence of an RTI, and during menstruation should be stressed.

Preventing condom failure

The most common reasons for condom failure and breakage and how to avoid these should be described.

Any substances or practices that could damage the condom itself should be discussed, and acceptable alternatives found. Oil-based lubricants can damage a latex condom in less than a minute.

Studies of condom breakage in the USA and Australia found a less than one per cent incidence among experienced users, including sex workers,[12] but rates as high as 15 or 20 per cent have been found among less skilled users. In one Caribbean study, men who had used condoms for many years reported a breakage rate of 10–13 per cent. Ninety per cent

---

Reasons for Condom Failure

The reasons condoms fail to prevent HIV transmission are similar to those in pregnancy prevention:

- failure to use one;
- female genital contact with semen before or after use;
- starting intercourse before putting one on;
- putting it on starting with the rolled rim facing the body instead of away from the body, which makes it more likely to break;
- not rolling it fully open to cover the penis so that it slips off easily during intercourse;
- tearing it with rings, rough fingernails or skin;
- spillage of semen into the vagina after ejaculation because no empty space was left at the tip when putting it on;
- breakage because the condom was too small, too thin, of poor quality, past the expiry date, stored in damaging conditions, or defective;
- breakage because an oil-based lubricant or other agent weakened the latex;
- allowing semen into the vagina during withdrawal by not holding the base of the condom.

Breakage or spillage outside the vagina/rectum does not affect protection.[4,12]

occurred in the woman's vagina, with about half occurring around the time of ejaculation.[13]

Extensive research into the reasons for condom breakage is in progress but not yet published.[14]

Disposal of condoms

Used condoms may contain infected semen.[15] Safe disposal in rubbish containers, a pit latrine or a hole in the ground is preferable. A knot should be tied in the condom before disposal. Condoms should not be put down the toilet because they can block the toilet and sewage system.

Used condoms should not be tossed away outside where children can pick them up and play with them. Condom campaigns encourage people to blow up condoms like balloons so that they handle and become familiar with them. Children too need to become familiar with condoms, but they may try to blow up used condoms they find lying around.

Negotiating condom use

Both women and men may appreciate help in approaching unwilling partners. Women may feel more comfortable talking to their partners about using condoms for contraception and protection from infertility than for HIV/STD protection, for example.[4] Anticipating negative responses and finding ways to overcome these through role play techniques has proved very helpful.

An AIDS educator in Brazil has said: 'When we train women, we not only have to teach them what the condom is and how to place one on their partners, we have to teach subversive techniques. We teach them skills in seducing their partners into wearing the condom. What I call the American assertive woman model says, "Baby, you wear that condom or you're not going to have anything." If a Latina woman says that to a man, the man says, "Well, tough luck, I'm not going to have anything with you." He goes off with another woman or simply smacks her. Traditionally, anything a Latina woman gets from a man is through seduction. I hate to say this. I ask myself where did my feminism go. But we're not working in ideal situations, so we have to take attitudes that are not ideal. Maybe some day men will learn to take care of themselves, but so far they expect the woman to take care of them. And so women have to develop these techniques . . .'[16]

One Scottish woman told her doctor that when her partner first learned he had HIV, he was distressed that no one would love him or come near him anymore, and he felt unclean. She was unable to ask him to use condoms, as she was afraid he would take this as a sign that she no longer loved him. The doctor talked with her about other ways she could show her love, and they tried out ways for her to ask him to use condoms. She was then able to talk to him, and they began using condoms.[17]

Experienced sex workers have taught each other how to put a condom on a man without him even noticing. They discreetly put the condom in their mouths before oral sex and with tongue and lips and then hands, roll it on to the man's penis.[18] This is not a professional secret if all else fails.

Exploring beliefs, worries and misconceptions

People's beliefs and worries about condoms should be explored. For example, some believe that condoms may stay inside a woman's vagina, which they may, and get lost, which they cannot. Others fear that 'rough' sex can damage them, and they may or may not be right.

Certain beliefs and practices may conflict with using condoms. In Rwanda, for example, the flow of fluids between a man and woman during sexual intercourse and in pregnancy is considered important. In Zaïre, it is believed that regular doses of semen are necessary to make a foetus grow, as a man's contribution to pregnancy. Condoms are seen as a blockage of this flow and interpreted as a health risk.[19,20]

There are probably many other beliefs and worries, not all of them misconceptions, which need exploring and responding to in appropriate ways, to overcome condom rejection.

Linking reproductive health and HIV/AIDS work

There is a worldwide network of women's groups, professional agencies and organizations devoted to the promotion of safe motherhood, contraception and abortion rights, alongside a worldwide network for AIDS prevention and control. Their respective goals can be promoted by more sharing of experience and information, and joint training and activities.

Family planning services are the first line of health care for many sexually active women and some men. Many family planning providers are taking on a large role in AIDS education. To this, they bring long experience in advocacy, programme planning, media work, training, service promotion, counselling and sex education. The IPPF AIDS Unit was set up to promote HIV/AIDS prevention through family planning services.

Many national family planning associations are contributing to national AIDS planning; training staff to respond to clients' questions and concerns about sexuality and to minimize the risk of HIV transmission in clinics; providing training and resources for other health care workers and professionals; providing HIV testing and counselling; talking about safer sex with clients; providing condoms; and setting up community-based programmes for people at higher risk, including sex workers, women using drugs, workers in the tourist industry, migrant workers, and gay men.[21]

For example, the Planned Parenthood Association of the Western Cape in South Africa designed a programme of combined family planning and AIDS education for unemployed, homeless young adults living in squatter communities. The programme focused on the community's concern about changing sexual practices leading to prostitution, teenage pregnancies, high birth rates and infant mortality. Volunteers from the community were taught about contraception, sexually transmitted diseases and AIDS, and in turn were teaching others in the community.[22] Many national associations, however, are still doing little or nothing along these lines.

Promotion of safer sex and condom use among those at risk of HIV is universal policy in AIDS education and services. The same is not true in all maternal health, family planning, infertility or abortion services. National associations and clinics need to examine their policies in this light.

Reproductive health service providers are as reluctant to talk about sex as anyone else. Training is widely recommended and increasingly being given for staff in many clinics. This can prove a difficult challenge where staff are mostly part-time and working on a sessional basis with limited overall training.

Safer sex as a subject of all counselling can be done individually or with groups of clients who are waiting for individual counselling. Some clinics show videos about safer sex in waiting-rooms. Safer sex workshops can also be offered to women's groups and at community level.

Condoms should be shown and suggested to everyone. If clients protest that they do not need condoms, some providers respond: 'That's all right. Take them anyway and give them to someone who does need them.'[4]

Service providers' biases against condoms also need to be explored and challenged. Several generations of providers have been taught that condoms are not a method of choice, because of their potentially high failure rate. Many clinics do not even stock condoms, let alone show and suggest them to most people.

The IPPF advise that service providers should be specifically trained to teach people how to use condoms correctly and consistently.[15] Models for demonstrating this are needed for teaching both staff and clinic attenders, with a supply of condoms specifically for practice sessions. Both men and women need to learn how to use condoms, and teachers of both sexes need to be available for this, to avoid embarrassment.

Leaflets, posters and other material on safer sex should be visible and available. Materials promoting contraception plus condom use should also be available, as well as those on HIV and other RTIs. All reproductive health services have leaflets describing the methods and services they offer. Instead of having separate leaflets about condoms only, information about condoms could be included in all leaflets.

If possible, more than one condom brand should be available. Condoms recommended for anal intercourse and condoms without spermicides should be among these.

The number of condoms given out at each visit should be based on clients' expressed needs and how often they can return for a new supply. In the UK, for example, the number of condoms a family planning clinic can give out per visit is fixed. This does not promote safer sex.

And from the other side, HIV/AIDS education and services need to take reproductive health issues on board as they promote safer sex.

Reaching men: the most difficult challenge

Through family planning services

Family planning services were set up in most countries between 1960 and 1980. Condoms were among the least favoured contraceptive methods during that time, and vasectomies rare in most countries. Women need contraception the most and most methods are used by women, so services are overwhelmingly visited by and promoted to women.

Surveys often show that an important factor in women's decision whether to use contraception is their partner's approval.[23] The same is true of condom use. Heterosexual men are notorious for their unwillingness to take responsibility for other contraception or condoms. However, when men are targeted in ways that appeal to them, this unwillingness can disappear.

Ideally, there should be as many men visiting family-planning clinics as women. Clinics are increasingly trying to find ways of getting men to attend on their own and with their women partners. Many strategies are being tried. Targeting men separately seems to work well, at least initially. Public demonstrations of condoms – in meetings, in classrooms, in marketplaces, and on television – have been given. Condoms are handed out and men encouraged to attend a clinic.

Men-only sessions are offered at clinics because men feel intimidated sitting in a waiting area full of women. Public campaigns such as the 'Men Too' campaign of the Family Planning Association in the UK have been launched, with leaflets directed at men.

Using satisfied male clients to reach other men also seems to work effectively, as vasectomy promotion campaigns have learned. In Colombia, Profamilia, the national FPA, opened a clinic for men in 1985. They provide vasectomies, testing and treatment for urological problems, sexual problems, infertility and STDs, as well as general physical examinations, condoms, and family planning education. They had few clients at first so they mounted a radio campaign and later also advertised on television.

They began by training men to interview clients, but now use both men and women, as the men do not seem to mind talking to women as long as they are made to feel at ease and privacy is respected. Between 1985 and 1990 they saw 80,000 men.[24] Such a clinic is an ideal place to educate men about safer sex and condom use, and to train them as peer educators.

Clinics could work with gay men's organizations to target bisexual men as well.

Through public education

Public education campaigns work too, but they require long-term commitment to reach their goals. The Swiss STOP AIDS campaign began in 1986 with a steady flow of preventive messages through various media. A representative sample of 1,200 men were interviewed about 'occasional relations' for the next three years. Every-time condom use increased among men aged 27–30 from 8 per cent, to 17 per cent, to 29 per cent, to 48 per cent over this period. Among men aged 31–45, condom use remained at 20 per cent over the same period. Younger men were more amenable to change.[25]

Individual attention in the context of public campaigns is important too. One project in southern Africa that is no longer active trained men volunteers to educate other men about AIDS prevention, condom use and contraception in the community, the workplace and marketplace. They used one-to-one discussion with men in factories, bars, hotels, clubs and neighbourhoods. They convinced one night-club owner to install a condom-vending machine in the men's toilet and then went back to get him to include the women's toilet. They held a sponsored breakfast for employers and challenged them to buy one pack of condoms for each of their employees and install vending machines in their workplaces. They described this as preventive medicine, to decrease absenteeism and the cost of medical insurance. They also trained unemployed young men to sell condoms part-time to earn money including at concerts and similar events.[26]

Combining public and individual attention is the optimum goal. One model for this comes from activities organized for the International Day of Action for Women's Health. In 1988, a group of social scientists at the University of Sokoto in Nigeria organized a campaign on the prevention of maternal mortality, with the theme: 'Your wife's health is important. Look after her.' Two discussions on this theme were broadcast on radio several times and a television programme was made in which a nurse-midwife, home economist and local women's leader were involved. At the same time, posters were distributed throughout the state with assistance from the state government. One department provided a vehicle with an efficient public-address system to visit a number of villages. With village heads as guides and help from religious leaders, they were able to visit ten districts where they addressed the men in public places and gave out posters.[27]

Through workplace programmes

Men are being reached at their workplaces as well. Construction and other companies bring large numbers of young men on to sites in remote rural areas, e.g. to build roads or dams. Women also come to these sites to provide sexual services. The managers of a rural construction project in Malawi found out that in the wake of one such project, the rate of HIV infection in the local population had risen. In

1987 they began informing their staff about the risk of HIV infection and providing free condoms with pay packets. By 1990, there was a big decrease in STDs.

They contacted another international construction company responsible for a large road-building project to suggest they do the same. That company said that their budget would not allow it.[28] Donors who fund such projects, who often also fund AIDS prevention from other budgets, could require contractors to include prevention of HIV infection in development projects.

In Zimbabwe, the Commercial Farmers Union met with village leaders to talk about AIDS and condom distribution among farmworkers. They then met with farmworkers and proposed to give out condoms with their pay packets. As these were well received, they gave back-up supplies to a woman health worker and to several male workers in the village, and these also were used. Condoms were then also placed in the farm butchery, store and beer-hall, to widen the number of sources. Because all the men were receiving condoms, no one had to be embarrassed about having them. Demand increased, so a supply was included at other commercial outlets and at the post office.

To increase awareness of risk, an AIDS Committee that included both men and women was elected in the village. The Union sent them on training courses and made informational material, videos and drama group performances available. Treatment for STDs dropped, there were fewer family rows, women's work attendance for farm work increased, and condom use became sustained. There is considerable community pride in these achievements.[29]

Reaching couples

AIDS educators in the Philippines, Tanzania and many other places have said how important it is to counsel people together in couples and give AIDS education talks or seminars to mixed audiences. If women hear the information alone, they will not be able to convince their husbands to take what they have learned seriously. If men hear it alone, they can choose to ignore it. If both hear it together, it is more difficult to ignore.[30,31] Individually or publicly, this is an important way of supporting women so that they do not have to deal with men alone.

Approaching people as couples may best be done in several stages, however, rather than immediately. In Tanzania, during a number of AIDS education seminars for couples, the women remained silent and deferred to the men. A number of times, various men would make the statement: 'If you can tell me how to control my sexual urges, then I will stick to one partner.' This would be met by laughter and hand clapping from other men on each such occasion.

One time, a woman spoke up and said that she was sure her husband had other partners when he went away on business. She asked if she could ask him to wear condoms with her. Some people in the audience said yes, but the majority, including the other women present, said no. Once the seminars were over, however, many women would come to the front and ask the same question again and again: 'What are we to do about our husbands?'[31] This suggests that separate sessions are also needed.

Focus group discussions on contraception in rural Kenya support this. Men interviewed separately from women said they wanted more children than the women, because approval from other men comes from large family size. However, the men were very interested in knowing more about contraception, and in learning how the body works. They also wanted to know why contraception was now necessary when before it was not. They felt that it was inevitable that they would accept the use of contraception, but that it would take time to convince them. They wanted to be taught about contraception in single-sex groups.

The women expressed similar interest in being given information. They preferred this to be provided by someone knowledgeable and from their own area, both for familiarity and to save the time and cost of travel to a clinic. They wanted plenty of opportunity to ask questions in small groups with other women. They also felt that far more energy and effort had to be spent on talking to the men about using contraception and having fewer children. Once they had the information they needed, they wanted to have counselling with their partners. They also preferred community distribution of methods and if possible, done by the same woman who had taught them about the methods. [5]

Promoting contraception and condoms: some pre-conditions

Before individuals can be expected to take up safer sex as it has been defined here, many pre-conditions need to be met at the macro-level.

Removing legal and trade restrictions

Some countries have restrictions which prevent the easy import or use of condoms. Laws may prohibit use of contraception altogether, or restrict its use to married couples.

There may be restrictions on publicizing, advertizing, supplying, or providing condoms. Publicity in the media may be more acceptable if generic advertisements rather than those for named brands are utilized. [4]

In 1990, the Irish Family Planning Association was fined for selling condoms in a record store. By law, condoms are only available in the Irish Republic from pharmacies, doctors, STD and family planning clinics. Changing this law is taking years to achieve. [32]

In some countries, carrying condoms may be considered legal evidence of prostitution and grounds for arrest and trial. The case of a woman who was arrested for carrying condoms at an airport customs hall, as she tried to enter Spain as a tourist, was widely reported not long ago. Sex workers face this kind of arrest and harassment on a daily basis.

Trade restrictions such as high import duties greatly increase prices. In Mexico, condom import duties were 45 per cent in 1988. They were reduced in three stages to 10 per cent by 1991. [4] Bureaucratic delays in clearance procedures can mean that condoms sit for months deteriorating in customs warehouses.

Innovations in condom names, packaging and promotion

Public figures can play a crucial role in promoting condom and contraceptive use. In 1991 a public statement by President Museveni of Uganda promoting condom use was given widespread media coverage and was expected to have a lot of influence. [33] President Kaunda of Zambia spoke out on this issue much earlier, when his family was personally affected by AIDS.

Condoms have been gaining legitimacy in Paraguay ever since the Catholic Church started speaking out against them. [34] As public relations experts say, any publicity is better than no publicity at all.

Songwriters and singers have been involved in campaigns in many countries. For comedians, sex is a ripe field for humour that can be used to good effect.

Nana, the brothel owner in Uruguay, proposed to the Uruguayan government that sports figures, singers, artists and many other public figures should be featured on television and in advertisements to promote condoms, using her slogan: 'Camisinha, por favor.' She believes that the usual dry words for 'condom' turn many people off, especially women who consider themselves respectable. She proposed giving the condom a new image through a nicer, more appealing name. In Spanish and Portuguese, 'camisinha' (which translates roughly to mean little sleeve, wrapper or cover) has been promoted and become widely known in Latin America.[35]

The brand name Durex is often used to mean condom. Social research on condoms has led to other attractive names and packaging, with sophisticated promotion campaigns to accompany them. For example, the brand name Prudence has become a generic term for condom in French-speaking Africa.[36]

In deciding which brand to buy, men in Barbados and St Lucia took into account recommendations from friends most often. But advertising, packaging and price also mattered. The majority had used four or five different brands; some had used up to twelve brands.[13]

Condom advertisements have been designed to appeal to various target groups, sometimes using different messages for each. Humour in Sweden and Thailand has worked well.[37] Many campaigns use posters, pocket calendars, beer mats, stickers, badges and T-shirts with a logo and slogans, as well as condom packaging and leaflets.[36]

In the Caribbean, extensive research by one FPA into culturally appropriate themes and images led to a campaign focused on lifestyle issues, rather than AIDS, family planning, or health-related behaviour. The campaign was based around the slogan: 'Condoms . . . Because You Care'. Positive, relational and social aspects were stressed through images on display boxes, condom symbols and promotional posters.[38]

More women are buying condoms, so advertising and campaigns have begun to target women as well.[13] Brand names such as Mates, from the UK, appeal to both sexes, depending on the packaging. However, few brands of condoms have both names and packaging which appeal primarily or equally to women. In fact, many have a very macho image. The slogan 'Love with Prudence' appeals to caring, caution and responsibility, which both women and men can relate to.[36] Yet the logo is a stalking panther.

In Uganda, the brand name Protector was chosen specifically because it sounds macho.[33] Brand names in Japan include: 'Here Come the Giants' and 'Almighty'.[39] In the Caribbean brand names like Panther, Rough Rider, and Sultan are popular.[13] These all appeal to male sexual prowess and domination but hardly serve the empowerment of women.

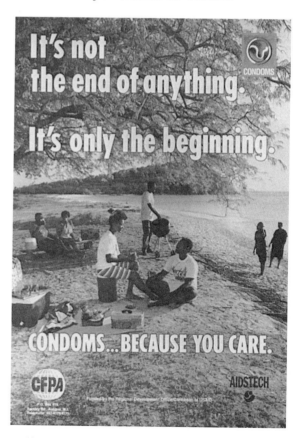

Caribbean Family Planning Association, Antigua

In the Philippines, one company has put out a condom called 'Sensation'. On the packaging it says: 'For her pleasure'. This appeals both to male competence and men's desire to please women sexually, and is considered good marketing there. However, there was negative feedback from the gay community.[30]

Advertising and packaging should not only be attractive in a culturally appropriate way, but directed at both sexes and all sexual preferences.

Ideas for promoting contraceptives and condoms together have barely been considered. For example, a month's supply of condoms could be included in each birth control pill packet. A sample of condoms and a promotional leaflet could accompany other methods.

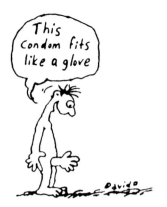

David

Increasing condom sales

Pharmacies are a standard outlet for condoms, but they may not necessarily make customers feel at ease about their purchase. A survey of pharmacies in Concepción, Chile, found that 56 per cent of pharmacy staff who sold condoms were men and 44 per cent women, while 86 per cent of buyers were men. Forty-four per cent of staff said they felt uncomfortable when they were asked if they sold condoms. Another twelve per cent said they felt embarrassed. Four per cent said they made ironic comments to buyers. When volunteers went into pharmacies pretending to be buyers, they were often given suspicious looks.[40]

If men are made to feel bad, what about women. In Paraguay, the following women's joke is circulating:

'I prefer to buy surgical gloves instead of condoms. I'm not embarrassed to ask for them in the pharmacy, I can use them ten times and I get all those different sizes!'[34]

Condom sales in Japan have for some time been done door-to-door by saleswomen, targeting housewives during the day while children are at school and husbands out at work. The saleswomen also teach women how to use condoms.[39]

In Zaïre, it was found that many sex workers and their clients ride the river barges on the Zaïre River. Prudence salesmen took to the docks and boats, some of them riding to the interior of the country to teach and promote condom use along the way.[36]

There are an increasing range of accessible outlets for selling or giving away condoms, e.g. pharmacies, outpatient clinics and health centres, shops, market stalls, hotels and motels, restaurants, clubs, bars, barbers, hairdressers, supermarkets, garages, ferries, theatres and cinemas, schools, men's and women's toilets, military, police and many other sites.

Increasing condom production, distribution and availability

In many countries condoms are still available only in cities and from commercial outlets, and supplies are often not consistent.

Most developing countries import contraceptives and condoms, or do not produce enough themselves to meet national demand. The industry is expanding everywhere to increase production, but it would have to expand at least three times globally to supply the majority of heterosexual couples and gay men using condoms worldwide. New industries would have to be built in more countries, and distribution, storage facilities and infrastructure greatly improved. Ecologically, the problems of disposal would increase.[4]

On the other hand, developing countries may produce enough condoms but not promote them. Indonesia, for example, is a net exporter of high-quality condoms, and has the largest condom factory in southeast Asia, producing 130 million condoms annually. Yet the national family planning programme estimates national usage at only 3 per cent, and high-quality condoms are expensive.[41]

One of the consequences of the shortage of condoms is that those who manage to get them may sell them for income rather than use them. This was found to occur in Indonesia among transvestite sex workers and entertainers.[41] And Pro-Pater, a clinic for men in Brazil, does not give out condoms for fear of this.[24]

Improving condom quality control

Most developed countries require quality testing of condoms by manufacturers. International and many national standards exist.[44] But people need to be able to identify brands that meet these standards. An easily recognizable international symbol is required.[14]

Untested or defective brands should be removed from the market. In practice, this may not occur. A random study in Australia found that batches of some brands, marked as tested, were faulty.[42] Regular checks are needed.

In developing countries, even fewer controls operate. In the lower price range, brands can be very poor in quality. The cheapest condoms in Indonesia are said to break easily and smell of gasoline.[41] Removing sub-standard condoms

from the market in the absence of alternatives people can afford would create as many problems as it solved.

Reducing the cost of contraceptives and condoms

For many people, the cost of both contraception and good quality condoms is out of reach. Affordable contraception seems to be the exception rather than the rule in developing countries. Typically, less than half the population has ready access to a choice of methods from either the public or private sector.

In the Netherlands, France, Norway and Singapore, contraceptives and condoms are available to 100 per cent of the population from public-sector sources at low cost.[2] In the UK, there is a requirement on the health service to provide contraceptives free, yet there is very limited or no access to condoms under this policy for the majority of contraceptive users.[32] In other developed countries, such as the USA, low-cost or free contraception is subsidized for part of the population and expensive for everyone else.

In some developing countries, low-cost government programmes are subsidized from national budgets and/or by foreign donors. In Africa, only Botswana, Burundi, Egypt and Morocco provided low-cost contraception to more than 60 per cent of the population up to 1991. The percentage was considerably less in most other countries.

Many countries have yet to commit themselves to subsidizing contraceptive or condom costs. At the same time, where government subsidy is extensive, ways to reduce subsidy are being sought. If these services are forced to be self-supporting, most methods will become or remain inaccessible to the poor.[2]

A concern in developing countries is that if subsidies come from international donors, there is no guarantee that the funds are secure. Loss of subsidy would mean sharp price rises, and may lead to discontinuation of use.[41]

Research suggests that one per cent of income is as much as anyone should have to pay for contraception. In developed countries, the annual cost of pills, IUDs and condoms is in line with this general rule, while female sterilization is under five per cent of average per capita income.

In a few developing countries, subsidies keep costs down to a similar level. In Bangladesh, for example, most couples can buy a year's supply of pills or 100 condoms for less than one per cent of average per capita income. But price increases of over 60 per cent in 1990 caused a drop in condom sales of 35 per cent and in pill sales of over 10 per cent.

In Ethiopia, an annual supply of condoms costs 30 per cent of average per capita income, and subsidized prices are available to only 30 per cent of men. In Uganda, public sector condom distribution reached only six per cent of the population up to 1991. In Kenya, the private sector charges 37 per cent of average per capita income for the pill and 89 per cent for female sterilization.

In 29 African countries from whom data was available, an annual supply of condoms costs more than ten per cent of average per capita income. Ten other countries are keeping the cost of condoms below five per cent of average per capita income through social marketing programmes.

Improving this situation is within the bounds of almost every government. It has been calculated that the entire developing world could provide universally accessible contraception for only $10 billion per year by the year 2000, by combining subsidies in the private sector with free contraception to those who cannot afford it. If this seems a lot, it should be noted that the developing world spends nearly $150 billion annually on weapons.[2]

The solution that is increasingly used by many governments is large-scale social marketing. These programmes involve the private sector in the delivery of methods and recovery of the costs of subsidized services through modest charges. Zaïre began a successful social marketing programme for condoms in 1989, for example.[20] The cost of a dozen Prudence condoms is about half the price of a bottle of beer, which is substantially less than other brands sold in pharmacies.[36] In Malaysia, a newly formed company is working with international donors and the national government on social marketing of condoms for both contraceptive and prophylactic purposes, including for people who are hard to reach.[41]

If governments and national AIDS committees are serious about supporting women's right to decide the number and spacing of children, safe motherhood, and STD/HIV prevention and control, then the first order of business on their agendas should be to make free or cheap contraceptives and condoms and safe abortion available to everyone.

If people cannot get access to these, if they cannot afford to pay for them, or if the cost is a drain on their income, AIDS-prevention campaigns are a waste of time and money.

Developing new barrier methods

HIV/AIDS demand a serious re-examination of contraceptive and prophylactic research and development priorities. Many new contraceptive methods and devices are on the market or in clinical trials, e.g. Norplant, the female condom, hormone-releasing vaginal rings, once-a-month injectables, new IUDs, vaccines, new post-coital pills, a male pill, and non-surgical sterilization.[1] Only the female has any value for protection against HIV and RTIs.

Neglect of research into barrier methods of protection has not ended in spite of a decade of HIV/AIDS.

The WHO Human Reproduction Programme in Geneva are coordinating non-commercial contraceptive research and development worldwide, as well as working with the commercial sector. Because of HIV/AIDS, they have been:

- assessing existing spermicides for their bacteria- and virus-killing activity;
- carrying out acceptability studies of the female condom;
- assessing a non-reusable injection system for injectable contraceptives;
- watching for possible effects of contraceptive vaccines on the immune system in clinical trials;
- studying whether oral contraception influences the risk of HIV transmission. [1,43,44]

But the vast majority of their work and resources continue to be spent on methods with contraceptive but no prophylactic value.

Encouraging people to use contraception has been greatly facilitated by the existence of a range of methods. The world could do with a wider variety of barrier methods, to appeal to the varying tastes of the hundreds of millions of people who will hopefully be convinced to use them over the coming decades. Innovations could take three forms: better female barrier methods, new variations in male condoms, and virucide preparations.

Many women have been called for the development of a 'virucide' which would kill HIV but not act as an irritant to genital tissue. Some are even calling for a virucide that would not kill sperm, for women trying to get pregnant. The WHO Reproduction Programme, the Population Council and others are investigating these possibilities. [45] At the moment, it is an open question whether these hopes are realistic and it will be several years or longer before research and clinical trials could bring new preparations to the market.

Nonoxynol-9 in spermicide is a virucide and has not yet been shown to be effective against HIV *in vivo*. Anything capable of killing HIV is very likely to kill sperm and potentially irritate tissue as well. [14,46] And as HIV appears to be able to live on sperm, there may be no protection for women trying to get pregnant with a virucide that is not also a spermicide.

However, even the most cautious experts on this subject support research and trials of potential virucides, since an effective preparation would offer couples who reject condoms an alternative. On the other hand, even though a virucide would be used by women, the decision would not necessarily be controlled by women alone. Campaigns would still need to encourage those who reject all barrier methods to give them a chance, and not just provide an alternative for those already willing to use condoms.

One successful innovation has been female condoms, which are now coming on the market. In early 1992, a brand made of polyurethane called Femidom was made available in Swiss pharmacies. In two weeks, 25,000 were sold. [47] Then sales dropped sharply. The level of sustained use remains to be seen. This brand is likely to be approved for use in most European countries by 1993. [48] It costs three or four times more than a male condom, one of its main disadvantages. Another brand made of latex, called Women's Choice, is due out in the USA.

Research during the development of the female condom showed that polyurethane is as effective as latex in preventing HIV transmission, at least in the laboratory. [49] As condom use increases and health workers demand increased supplies of latex gloves, rubber products may not be able to keep up with demand. Polyurethane products, if developed, could help to solve this problem.

The commercial sector has already introduced many innovations in male condoms. There are thinner and thicker brands, brands said to be better for anal intercourse, lubricated condoms, fruit-flavoured condoms, different coloured condoms, condoms with special features such as nobbles as sex aids, and, most importantly, condoms of more than one size.

Certainly the least that can be expected is for condoms to come in more than one size. USAID supplied huge quantities of inexpensive condoms manufactured in Australia to African countries in the late 1980s, but many men complained that they were too tight and they would not use them.[20] On the other hand, Indonesian men have complained that imported condoms produced in the West are too large.[41] Without pandering to ridiculous stereotypes, penises (like vaginas) do come in many sizes, and condoms (like diaphragms) should too.

Products still at the development stage for men include looser condoms that fit tight at the base and ones with balloon ends.[14] For women, a latex panty with a built-in condom is also being researched.[4]

One very major advance would be male and female condoms that are washable and reusable, as diaphragms and caps are. In the past, some condoms were reusable. They would be unacceptable by today's standards, but that does not make the idea impossible. Reusable condoms would be ecologically preferable and much more accessible to those with limited purchasing power.

It is important to find out what people do not like about available brands. Comfort was one of the things men most commonly asked about when buying condoms in a Chilean city.[40] In New York City some men liked the size of the female condom because it gave them more room for movement.[50] If

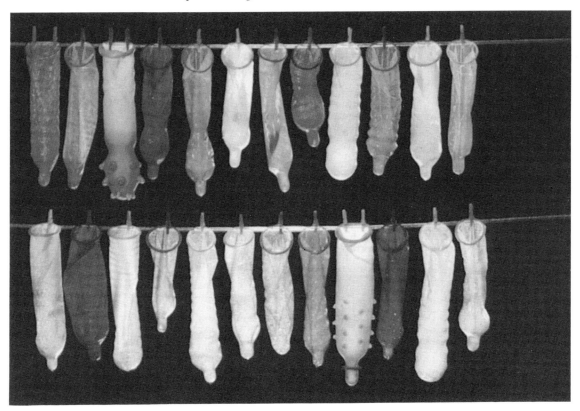

Charles Papavoine

complaints about condoms were taken into account, research might take off down new paths.

A history of the condom over the centuries reveals that condoms used to come in all sorts of shapes and sizes, and could therefore do so again.[51] There is room for much creative work.

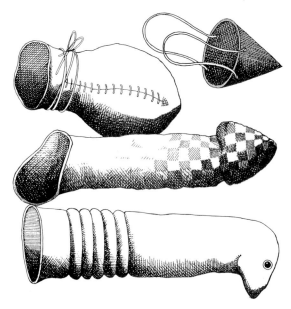

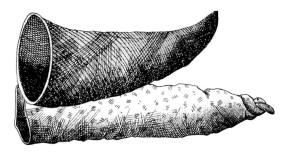

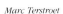
Marc Terstroet

The female condom

by Barbara James and Patricia Wejr

The idea of a female condom has been around for a long time. One type was launched in Britain in 1920. Promotion and research was then abandoned until about ten years ago when a Danish medical team produced a new version. This version was shelved until a British company, Chartex International, bought the rights, did further work and launched the brand called 'Femidom' in the UK and Switzerland, 'Reality' in the USA and 'Femi' in some other countries.

Femidom combines features of both the diaphragm and the male condom. It is a loose-fitting polyurethane sheath about three times the diameter of a male condom, with a flexible ring at either end. The original design had one ring around the open end, but there were difficulties with insertion. A second ring was then added inside the closed end of the sheath. This ring is used for insertion and then helps to keep the sheath in place. It is inserted in the same way as a diaphragm, but the ring does not have to be around the cervix. The ring on the open end remains outside the vagina.

Polyurethane has been shown to act as an effective barrier against HIV and other sexually transmitted diseases in vitro. Femidom was found in clinical trials to be about as effective in preventing pregnancy as the male condom. Inconsistent use as well as method failure have both been found to lead to pregnancy. Post-marketing research with larger numbers of varyingly motivated people remains to be done.

If the female condom reaches the market widely, it would become the only available barrier method controlled by women to provide as much protection as male condoms against STDs and HIV. This would be its main advantage. By mid-1992 Femidom/Reality had been approved by Switzerland, the USA and the UK. There has been some debate over the wisdom of doing this too quickly, however, because of the lack of large studies evaluating pregnancy rates with it, let alone level of protection against HIV.

More information about the female condom's disadvantages is beginning to appear. In a clinical trial of Femidom in Britain,[52] 34 of 106 self-selected couple-participants found that the entire device was accidentally pushed into the woman's vagina on at least one occasion. This was often not noticed until after ejaculation. Twenty-six of the women said that the man's penis needed to

be guided carefully into the condom. Otherwise, he could accidentally bypass it on penetration, which happened to each of them at least once during the study. To avoid this, they had to hold the device in place for penetration. However, those who used the method for a year experienced fewer insertion problems over time.

Twenty-three of the women found that the condom either slipped out of the vagina or was drawn out with the penis during repeated penetration. It was also reported to make a variety of unappealing noises during intercourse.

Fifty-seven women reported adverse effects, such as soreness caused by the outer ring and discomfort for both the woman and the man from the inner ring. Further, the method is currently available in only one length (17cm). For some women, the outer ring hangs loosely at the vulva when first inserted, which is sexually unappealing and could discourage its use. If it is inserted in advance of intercourse, oral sex could be unpleasant or difficult. The method also requires a woman to have some degree of ease in touching her genitals and inserting things into her vagina.

For women at high risk for HIV and other STDs, it may well be worth the time it takes to

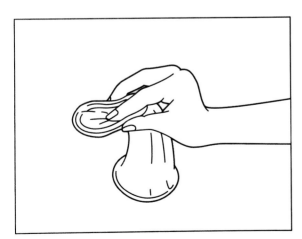
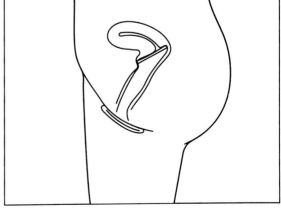

Chartex International

learn to use the female condom well. In several trials by sex workers, a majority found the female condom a valuable method of protection, particularly because it was under their control. Some sex workers have said anecdotally that it is easier to insert if the inner ring is removed and the condom put over the penis prior to penetration. The manufacturers do not recommend this, however, as the effectiveness has not been evaluated.

One of the main problems is how much they cost, roughly three times more than male condoms. This might tempt women to reuse them, which is also not recommended. In addition, male cooperation remains as essential as with male condoms.

Although the majority of the participants in the British trial did not find the method acceptable and dropped out during the course of the study, there were a significant number of couples who did like it. Other advantages were also apparent. Loss of erection did not affect the efficiency of the condom and immediate withdrawal of the penis after ejaculation was not necessary. It could be inserted in advance of intercourse, potentially increasing spontaneity, though most couples did not do this. The polyurethane is less likely to cause allergic reactions and it rarely ruptured. It warms quickly to body temperature, which makes it more comfortable. Increased sensitivity was reported, compared to the male condom. And the method does not have to be fitted by a health professional.

The British report recommends that its acceptability might be increased if the method came in more than one size, if the rings and lubrication were improved and if the 'noises' could be reduced.

Many women are interested in the female condom. It seems to be a product with a lot of potential but needing further work. At its best, it could be an important addition to the list of available barrier methods, and a welcome one for safer sex. Only time and trial will tell.

Workshops on counselling, quality of care, sexuality and AIDS

by Elvira Lutz

In Uruguay, 'safe sex' in the proper sense of the word is nothing new. The Uruguayan Family Planning Association and other similar organizations, including the Uruguayan Sexology Society, have always supported the need to promote safe sex, while taking into account the undesirable consequences of unwanted pregnancy.

However, we are all aware of the enormous opposition to the idea of giving proper sex education. Our work over 15 years and the obstacles which have stood in our way are reliable proof of the strength of this resistance.

Paradoxically, thanks to the emergence of AIDS, doors have started to open which had previously remained tightly shut. Ironically, it was not the proposal of 'sexual health for all by the year 2000' which made it possible to introduce sex education, but terror in the face of the AIDS scourge.

All of us who work in family planning have one advantage when it comes to tackling this new disease – we are in touch with the issues of sexuality and prevention of STDs. We are the sexual confidantes of our clients, most of whom are young and sexually active. We can help by providing information and education and in preventing STDs, particularly AIDS. However we are not ready to talk about them naturally.

So we decided to hold a series of eight workshops between August and December 1989 to discuss these issues. It was the first time that workshops of this kind had been held in our country.

Information about the workshops was sent to the different authorities and they were asked to choose members of staff to attend – preferably people who would find it easy to communicate, who were motivated and who held key posts so that the workshops could be repeated afterwards.

Each workshop lasted three days, eight hours each, and was attended by an average of 40 participants. The participants included members of our staff (doctors, nurses, midwives), delegates appointed by the National Anti-Aids Programme of the Ministry of Health, staff from the Ministry of Education and Culture and the National Youth Institute, health personnel connected with family planning services in the interior of the country, and representatives of different non-governmental organizations and organized women's groups.

Throughout the workshops we concentrated on personal involvement and encouraged a warm and open atmosphere. This enabled the participants to share their feelings, experience and knowledge about the different issues.

The participants from the interior of the country were given teaching material and information so that they could distribute it in their communities through outreach work.

Equal priority was given to the following issues and the links between them: quality of care, contraception, condoms, sexuality, masturbation, homosexuality, STDs and AIDS. There were some formal presentations. The rest of the time, we worked in groups with activities and discussion. We used questionnaires, sketches, role play, dramatization, leaflets, videos and a variety of group exercises, including relaxation to music, sensitization through reading and interpretation of poems and texts. These were used to explore the level of knowledge, detect and break down myths, clarify values, encourage a change in attitudes, compare ideas, and encourage a close dynamic within the groups.

The groups were asked to discuss the relationship between AIDS, sexuality and contraception and to report back to the plenary. Exercises were done on the importance of condoms in preventing STDs and AIDS. We tried to encourage the participants not to discriminate against people with AIDS, emphasizing that AIDS is an illness and not a punishment and that it is not exclusive to certain groups but can affect anyone.

Evaluation by the participants was done at the end of each workshop, each day, and at the end of the sessions. Participants were asked to write down what they were feeling at that moment, and what they wanted to say to the group and the facilitators.

Two years of workshops, but where were the men?

Since these first workshops, we have done many others in the past two years. More than 1,000 participants have attended, including:

health care workers (doctors, midwives, nurses), teachers, community leaders, young people, sex workers, lesbians, health educators, gay men, priests and other clergymen. We have seen many come with misconceptions and blocked thinking, and who progressively open up and want to know and understand more.

However, one fact was true in the very first workshops and has remained true subsequently. The overwhelming majority of people who have participated in these workshops, 95 per cent of them, have been women. Without exaggeration, the average number of men who have attended, in two years, is less than five per cent. Yet these workshops were always equally open to men and women.

Why this tremendous presence of committed women and this eloquent absence of men? In the fight against AIDS, men occupy as ever the leadership in the Ministries, the institutions which control the important programmes, and in the research community, where they organize the struggle against this enemy in an almost military fashion. They are not involved, however, in either the work of prevention or education.

It would seem that these are considered the proper sphere of women, too maternal and passive for the warriors of science and health. Yet according to all the evidence, HIV – the intelligent virus – is playing dirty tricks on them and still winning the game after ten years in the laboratory. Ten years in which the only recourse we have had is prevention and education. And yet it would seem that it is only women who are interested in these, women who have the most important role to play and the most difficult – to change the ideology of sexuality that alienates us.

Translation from Spanish by Ruth Mahnen.

Safer relationships

There is an enormous gap between women's lived experience and what most women want sexual practice and relationships to be. This is perhaps the central issue of sexuality for women. HIV did not invent it. HIV has been able to thrive on the actuality of women's sexual experience.

What is sexuality?

Sexuality is more than sexual practices and cannot be separated from the relationships in which it is expressed. Sexual relationships may or may not be well thought out, rational, planned, mutual or mutually satisfying. Women's reasons for having sex may be different from or in conflict with their partners'. Pleasure, pain and power are expressed through sex. From making love for the first time or as part of a long-term relationship, or having sex for its own sake, or in order to become pregnant, get affection and emotional closeness, to sex as a duty, service or profession, or to secure survival, a favour or a socially acceptable position, to sexual harassment, rape and sexual abuse – women's experience covers them all.

How can we address these issues all at once, and in a coherent way?

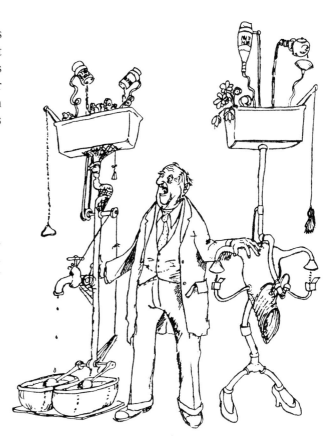

HUMAN SEXUAL RELATIONS CAN BEST BE UNDERSTOOD BY REFERENCE TO THE MODELS I HAVE HERE

Neil Phillips

Using research

Many studies of sexuality and HIV risk only crudely describe risk-related sexual practices and condom usage. Sometimes they have as little to do with sexual relationships as the curriculum of many sex education courses. Although the data prove risk exists, only an insight into the complexity and multi-level character of sexuality in relationships can explain why. Attempts to substitute 'safe' for 'unsafe' practices depend on the meanings those practices have for people and the degree to which new practices provide emotional satisfaction and find social support.[1]

Sexual expectations and rituals can differ greatly from one culture or ethnic group to another. In Uganda, for example, Bantu groups stress mutual satisfaction between sexual partners, including touching and stroking of genitals and mutual masturbation, and have some expectation that women should enjoy sex. In contrast, Nilotic groups give little recognition to female consent or mutual satisfaction. The sex act stresses female resistance, male aggression and mutual antagonism. There are taboos against women touching men's genitals and in some cases, their own. Safer sex campaigns which stress consent and mutual satisfaction would be appropriate in the former but not the latter circumstances.[2,3]

A study among gay men in Australia showed that people may or may not enjoy doing certain things, which affects how often they do them when they have a choice. It showed that people may do risky things with a regular partner but not a casual one, or vice versa, and that the frequency of this risky behaviour can be intermittent or often. It showed that people may like having things done to them, but may not like doing them to someone else. And that what people find physically satisfying may not be the same as what they find emotionally satisfying.[1]

Only with studies like these does it become possible to explore directions for change in a meaningful way.

Safer sex education

The meaning of 'safe'

What is the meaning of 'safe' in the context of sexual relationships? The very concept implies women having control over their lives and wellbeing. How can women who are in safe relationships teach and learn from those who are not, and help each other?

All of these questions and issues have implications for practising safer sex. There are many, many myths to shatter and painful experiences to overcome as women sit together to talk about sexuality, relationships and HIV. There is much laughter, enjoyment and pleasure to share as well.

Most people have barely begun to think about how to achieve safer relationships, both individually and at a social level. Different women are going to want very different things and at different points in their lives. Building self-confidence and achieving fundamental changes take time.

Every society has ways of teaching the young about sexuality, whether it is done by parents, aunts and uncles, or through sex education in schools. Some societies leave the young in ignorance, to find out about sexuality through trial and error on their own, from friends, or from films, magazines, books and the consumerist messages of the advertising media.

Sex education in schools often consists only of a few basic lessons in anatomy and reproduction, and more recently, basic information about HIV transmission and prevention. Excellent models and programmes for sex education exist in Scandinavia, the Netherlands and in isolated programmes in many countries, as well as in published

If you think sex education is dangerous

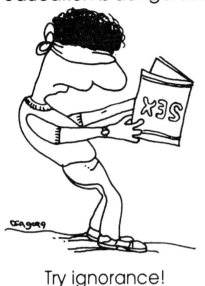

Try ignorance!

South Pacific Commission

material. Yet attempts to implement better programmes, train staff and reach young people in most countries are the subject of heated debate.

It is very difficult to implement a national programme of sex education for young people when parents, religious leaders, policymakers, teachers, feminists, and young people themselves have conflicting views and values regarding sexuality and therefore, about what should be taught.

The director of Family Life for the Roman Catholic Archdiocese of New York City has said: 'We don't say "Smoke carefully." We say, "Don't smoke." A huge campaign could work to stop kids from having sex. We don't water down principles. AIDS was caused in this country by promiscuity and casual sex. It is not traditional values that have brought us where we are.' While the director of a service centre for young gays and lesbians in New York responds: 'If you deny young people information based on your morality, you are

sentencing them to death. Nothing is more immoral than that.'[4]

Debates about sexuality and morality go beyond what is right for the young, however, and even the priests don't agree with each other. A bishop from Tonga condemned the use of condoms to combat AIDS. 'In our enlightened age, do we have to be satisfied with giving our people the lethal rubbish of western civilization, and sit back and watch them become addicts of the permissive society with just a bit of rubber between themselves and death? We have to rebuild our people's cultural respect for themselves . . . and build a society based on sound morality. Encourage a permissive society in the Pacific with the western condom culture – a con culture really – and you are counting not only on physical death, but also the death of the spirit of the people. You are also promoting a host of social ills, as well as much economic burden.'[5]

While a priest in the Bahamas described condoms not as a contraceptive, but as a 'contramortive' – not against life but against death.[6]

In Uganda, the churches are very involved in the campaigns of the AIDS Control Programme. The message of 'Love Faithfully' was devised by them together for people who are and want to be monogamous. For others, they offer a 'Love Carefully' message.[7] Compromises such as this provide a way forward, acknowledging that what people do goes beyond disagreements about what they ought to do.

Whatever their views, people of all ages need safer sex education. Creating spaces where both women and men can talk about sexuality and relationships without fear, separately or together – individually, as partners or in groups – is crucial. One session is not enough. People need time to open up, to talk to their partners and their children, and to be able to come back to discuss what happened and get feedback and support.

More and more such workshops are being organized. In the USA, SisterLove: Women's AIDS Project in Atlanta run 'Healthy Love Parties' and the Chicago Women's AIDS Project have 'Girls Night Out – Safer Sex Workshops for Women'. The coordinator of SisterLove went to Nigeria in 1991 to train women's groups to run safer sex workshops as well.[8]

The aim of workshops like these is to give women information about HIV/AIDS and safer sex, and for them to create and share their own safer sex alternatives in an informal and enjoyable way. The facilitator ensures that women are aware of their risk of infection, understand the value and meaning of safer sex, and realize the importance of self in decisions about themselves and others. Then women get the chance to do roleplays to practise talking with partners about safer sex.

SisterLove's parties are organized in the home of one woman, who invites other women friends, family and acquaintances to come. Such groups can also be held in community centres and other places where women meet.

In the Chicago workshops, during round-the-room introductions, women are asked to name positive things about being a woman, so that work on self-image begins from the start. Next they do body awareness. Taking the words vagina, penis, intercourse, oral sex, semen, and masturbation, women are asked to come up with street/slang terms for them, which leads to wide-ranging discussion. Then they are given a drawing of the reproductive system and talk about the various parts of the body, followed by basic AIDS information.

In the SisterLove parties, members of the group read out from cards a set of questions and answers about safer sex, to stimulate discussion. A safer-sex survival kit is then shown. It contains lubricants, latex finger-cots, latex gloves, condoms, latex squares, and bleach. The purpose of each is demonstrated and described, and they are handed round.

The women then try using condoms on bananas or cucumbers, and latex squares on their thighs at the knee-joint or hands at thumb-joint. Volunteers are asked to role play various couples negotiating safer sex. After each, the women discuss whether the strategy would work for them or not.

Next, a 'Box of Safe, Erotic Potential' is brought out, containing household and erotic items. Each woman draws one item out of the box and describes how she would use it erotically and safely for sex with a partner. Lastly, each woman gets a chance to offer comments and concerns about the party and about safer sex. An evaluation form is filled out. Women are encouraged to go home and try out what they have learned at the party with their partners, and come back for a follow-up party to talk over their successes and problems.[8,9]

In the Chicago workshops, they also have a race in which small groups have to pass a banana along and each woman puts a condom on it and takes it off, to see which group can do it the fastest. Condoms are discussed as both contraceptives and prophylactics.

The risks of alcohol and drug use, injecting drugs and sharing needles, and reproductive tract infections are discussed in relation to HIV transmission. The continuum from low to high risk is explained, using a drawing of a thermometer. There is a discussion about choices, having the right information and sharing it with others.

At the end, women are given a 'personal pledge card' on which they write down the changes they are willing to make in sexual decision-making and practices to take care of themselves and help their communities to understand and deal with AIDS. They can share these if they want to. Women from the group are asked to volunteer to host or run future workshops.[10]

A sex therapist in Mexico has been conducting safer sex workshops for several years. Eroticizing and de-genitalizing sexuality are the most important aspects she tries to bring to these. She gets excellent results with young people, but has problems reaching them. She finds that people aged over 30, however, are accustomed to certain ways of relating and do not change easily.

She has found that women have almost no idea about the risk of AIDS. Many women have a very hard time achieving a sense of their own sexuality, and AIDS has made this worse. She has seen many women who have stopped any sexual activity, lost desire and become depressed, which has badly affected their relationships. She suggests that they continue to do the same things they used to do sexually, without exchanging semen and vaginal/anal mucus.

Most of the women who have already attended have been middle class, but she has held some workshops for women in poor neighbourhoods. Men have also attended, but heterosexual men seem to be the least receptive. Women and gay men are more open and willing to learn, yet their receptivity goes down when heterosexual men are present. However, she finds that if only women attend, the workshop may not have any effect. They may go home with new ideas that their partners will not share. She believes that the real problems of AIDS can only be understood if both partners attend such workshops. [11]

Young women's experiences

How do women learn about and first experience sexuality and sex – not only intercourse, but touching themselves, masturbating, kissing, petting, touching others and being touched?

In the USA, among 300 white, black, and Latina adolescent girls, more were having intercourse in the late 1970s and 1980s. Prior to that time, petting had been the furthest young women often went. Then, 'going all the way' became something that had to be experienced, as 'the real thing'. In the 1980s the girls' first experiences of intercourse fell into two main categories.

For about 75 per cent, the experience just happened. They do not know how it happened. The facts they had learned about the biology of sex had not sunk in. It happened very quickly and then it was over. Many had expected intercourse to hurt, and it did. One described it as 'putting a big thing into a little hole'. While they did not feel they were coerced, they also did not feel they chose to do it. They did not enjoy it. In fact, they were often bored by it and did not see what all the fuss was about. Some resisted penetration and told hilarious stories about this. These girls felt disappointed, both physically and romantically. They often blamed themselves for this. But they also often thought it was worth it, because it proved they had courage, were mature, had 'done it'.

Afterwards, they often decided never to have sex again or to wait a long time. The waiting was usually for desire or a better partner to appear. They waited, then tried again, then waited again. It took some time before they realized they were very likely to keep doing it and to prepare for this by obtaining contraception. They often said they thought first intercourse for girls should be at an older age than their own had been.

About 25 per cent told of sexual curiosity, exploration and pleasure leading to first intercourse. They often initiated both petting and intercourse, and had had experiences alone that awoke them to the possibility of pleasure.

J: I discovered [first with water in the shower] that I could rub my clitoris and it did feel good. And so I would masturbate in bed at night. Which meant I didn't get to sleep for ages.

Q: And which meant you didn't have any trouble, in fact, figuring out how to have an orgasm.

J: No, actually I didn't. No. Has my life been too simple?

This group of young women frequently talked about their mothers and other women around them as always being open about sex and adult life. When they were ready to try sex, they already expected pleasure. They knew what they wanted to try and what not, and they were often prepared with contraception. They moved gradually through petting to intercourse and erotic understanding. Some had pain at first intercourse, and not all experienced orgasm. But their experiences were positive and they went on to improve on them. Lesbian relationships were among the most charged emotionally.

This study concludes that:

• anti-erotic sex education remains the experience for the majority of young women;
• teaching young women only to say 'no' or 'not just now' sabotages their sense of sexual confidence;
• pleasure, effective contraception and safer sex depend on sexual self-confidence;
• to take possession of sexuality, young women need an erotic education.

A workshop or brochure that addresses young women's early sexual experience in an erotic way might ask:

– Do you get wet when you have a romantic or sexual daydream? When you think about kissing or petting? Do your genitals become warm and feel pleasure?
– Do you know where your clitoris is? Have you touched it? Excited it?
– Are you sexually excited when you and your partner are together, kissing or petting? That is, does your heart beat differently? Is your clitoris warm, pulsing, swollen? Is your mouth watering? Is your vagina moist, warm, contracting and opening or fluttering? Are your toes curling or spreading? Are your nipples stiff, sensitive, quick to pleasure?
– Do you have an idea what an orgasm is? Have you tried to give yourself one?
– Have you visualized or imagined what it will be like to be naked with someone? To kiss or pet without clothes on? Have you tried it?
– Have you touched your breasts and genitals? Have you touched yourself inside? Have you imagined someone else doing it? Have you imagined touching someone else?
– If you are considering having intercourse, have you imagined what penetration may feel like?
– Have you looked into various forms of contraception? Obtained a method? Tried using it?
– Have you handled a condom? Do you know how to use them?
– Does the idea of having sex with your partner excite you?
– Does the touch of that person excite or pleasure you?
– Do you think your partner will take the time to pleasure you, or to learn how? To practise sex safely with you? To stop whatever he or she is doing if you want to stop? To continue until you want to stop?[12]

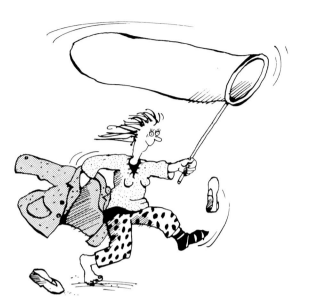

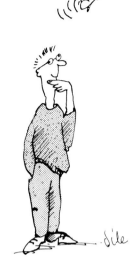

Swiss AIDS Foundation

Communicating about sexuality

In many places, discussion of sex and sexuality is prohibited or perceived to be prohibited. In some cases there are specific prohibitions on discussion between mothers and daughters, or fathers and sons, or relatives of the opposite sex. But this can change and women are beginning to talk with each other and their partners. Following workshops organized for women's groups in New Caledonia and Papua New Guinea, women have become involved in STD/HIV education and prevention work with other women. [13], [14]

Women sex workers, interviewed on Spanish-speaking television in the USA, said that married men come to them because 'their wives do not give them what they want'. In contrast, a male sex worker said that his services were highly sought by women, especially married women aged 45–59. Their main pleasure consisted in being with someone they could talk to, who would show them some tenderness, who would listen to them and to whom they could tell what gives

them pleasure. He said that these 'new women' demanded a special quality from their partners – communication. [15]

Women do not easily talk about their own capacity for sexual pleasure, what they like and do not like to do sexually. It needs a lot of courage to say these things to and hear them from partners. There is often embarrassment, shyness, insecurity, and lack of trust, confidence, or experience to overcome.

Often people do much more sexually than they will describe or admit to in words, a measure of how little they acknowledge or like themselves as sexual beings, and of how much they have distanced themselves from sex.

A study among young women in Britain found that embarrassment was one of the most potent barriers to practising safer sex. As one girl said: 'If I don't die of ignorance, I will die of embarrassment instead.' Anything that made them feel uncomfortable, uncertain, or ambivalent was embarrassing. This ranged from feelings of strong physical attraction, to fear of losing control, to being rejected, looking silly or being laughed at if they asked for condoms to be used or to have non-penetrative sex.[16]

Women have had many negative experiences of sex as well as positive ones, which cannot be ignored. Some women prefer not to have sexual relations at all, and may be made to suffer a great deal for this, not only by their partners but by their families, other women and the society around them.

For women with HIV or with partners with HIV, these problems are not different, but the presence of HIV may complicate and exacerbate them, and make them more difficult to solve.

Examining traditions and taboos

Many taboos and traditions regulate sexuality and reproduction, such as not having sex during pregnancy, menstrual periods, breastfeeding, mourning, or on certain religious holidays. How much are these observed or ignored in practice? Are they protective of health and involve safer sex, or not?

In India, traditionally, economics, religion and sex were seen as the three core aspects of life. The *Kamasutra*, written in the fourth century, treated sex as a source of pleasure for men and women rather than for reproduction only. Sexual life was considered sacred and sexual pleasure important. Now, the image of women as passive, submissive and chaste is promoted. Yet women are also seen as a volcano of uncontrollable urges, to be controlled by others.

Groups such as Chetna in Ahmedabad, the Women's Development Programme in Jaipur, and Streehitakarini in Bombay have evolved culturally acceptable ways of providing sex education to poor and non-literate women. But most efforts are restricted to women of reproductive age and focus on reproduction. There are indigenous media that are oriented to the subject of sex, such as the 'tamasha' of Maharashtra and the 'nautanki' of the North, but these are mainly for men. Pre-marriage and marriage songs often centre around the theme of sex. These could be examined for their potential as tools for a more broad-based sex education.[17]

In Tanzania, contraception is still not an open subject or widely used and some women practice it in secret. Many women use breastfeeding and sexual abstinence to prevent pregnancy. In the past, husbands had sexual relations with other women during this time, usually single, divorced or widowed women in their village. As long as this was discreet, it was allowed. With AIDS, this practice is said to be diminishing. More men are turning to their wives for sex, and women are getting pregnant more often.[18] In response, in 1991 the Union of Women of Tanzania began a three-year project to promote contraception.[19] But such a campaign, useful as it is, assumes that men will continue to remain faithful to their wives out of fear.

In Ghana until 100 years ago, there was an initiation rite called 'dipo' for girls aged 14–20 which lasted over a year and included tuition in housework, cooking and parenting, and a series of tests to prove they had learned well. At the end of this period, the girls were ready to be courted by young men and married. Scarification marks signified that the girl could be courted. Without them, she had to be left alone. If she became pregnant before dipo, she was banished from her tribe. This practice was banned by the British in 1892 and went underground. By 1950, dipo lasted only two weeks and involved girls as young as eight. Today, only the Krobo people practise dipo in a symbolic form for five days at a mass ceremony. With girls taking dipo even before puberty, early sexual activity and pregnancy is no longer frowned upon. The advent of AIDS has led the Krobo to realize that this practice used to promote safer sex and now promotes its opposite.[20]

The Kikuyu in Kenya used to teach young, unmarried men and women to practise a form of controlled sex, in which they were able to sleep together and achieve sexual satisfaction without intercourse. This practice disappeared because Christian missionaries forbade it, along with initiation ceremonies.[21]

In France today, among 16- and 17-year-olds attending vocational colleges, 17 per cent were at the kissing stage, 38 per cent had begun petting, while 73 per cent of the boys and 36 per cent of the girls had experienced inter-course.[22] Sex education that encouraged young people to stay at the kissing and petting stage longer, and older people to return to these practices, would fit existing practice while promoting safer sex.

The power imbalance between men and women

The imbalance in power between men and women – economically, socially and physically – is responsible for much of the lack of safety in sexual relationships. The gender role of 'woman' affects marriages, non-marital rela-tionships and commercial sex as well. Women are taught to be and are treated as the second sex by their families, religions, schools, employers and government policies.[23]

A study in Switzerland found that men approach the buying of sex in the same way as the approach all sexual relationships – as the ones in control. The reasons why male clients of sex workers often refuse to use condoms comes from that differential in power. Men have the money, the physical strength, and the gender-defined right to demand specific sexual practices. Each puts women at a disadvantage if they demand safe sex or condom use.[24] Tactics include:

- Questioning her judgement: 'Surely you can trust me?'

- Humiliation: 'Why a condom? Are you ill?'
- Playing women off against each other: 'Last week, down the street, I didn't have to use one.'
- Offering more money or threatening to leave.
- Agreeing to use a condom and then being faster than the sex worker and doing it without.
- Having a threatening appearance.
- Threatening violence.
- Using violence and force.[25]

Most, if not all, of these tactics will be familiar to women who are not sex workers. Violence, threats of violence and fear of violence have been commonly reported by both married and single women in all regions as the reason why they do not ask for or insist on safer sex, even when they know there is a risk of HIV infection.

Rape, sexual abuse, sexual assault, forced prostitution, and other violence against women and children, including in marriage and families, occur in all countries and social settings. In Belgium, it is estimated that 6–12 per cent of girls have been exposed to abuse. In Ireland, it is estimated that 6 per cent of adults were abused as children. In Denmark, a survey indicated that about 13 per cent of women have been exposed to sexual abuse. In Norway in the mid-1980s, 10–14 per cent of children under 18 had been sexually abused, two-thirds of them girls.[26] In Puerto Rico, in a six-month period following the passage of a law allowing police intervention into domestic violence, 7,000 incidents were reported, 95 per cent of them by women.[23]

Many children and adult women are forced into prostitution because of poverty. Evidence of forced and child prostitution is widespread in the Philippines, India and Thailand. Parents may hand girls and young women to agents for money when they cannot afford to keep them. They are often told the child will do domestic work. Girls may be dedicated to a sect such as Devadasi in India. Women may be conned or sold into 'marriages' or 'domestic work' in their own or other countries by agencies, when in fact they are being sold for unlimited sexual access.[27,28,29,30]

These crimes are a damning indication of how men can and do express their power over women and children sexually. Even though the majority of men do not commit them, male sexual culture at its worst encourages them and at its best does not condemn them. The ever-present threat of violence serves to keep women passive, and allows men to retain control of decisions about sexual relations.

Sexual violence and rape have implications during an epidemic of a sexually transmitted disease. They are a source of transmission of HIV. They are used to express anger against and blame women for being the source of infection and for any restrictions imposed on men's sexual lives in the name of safer sex. And they are used to silence women's efforts to practise safer sex.

The widespread rape of women by soldiers was thought to be a major factor in the spread of HIV in the north of Uganda during the civil war from 1986. Reported rates of HIV infection among soldiers were one in three at the time.

It has also been reported in Uganda that men with AIDS, whose wives have left them, have become 'desperate' for sexual partners and have resorted to capturing or raping young girls. One such elderly man had a reputation for snatching schoolgirls as they passed by his house to and from school. Another supposedly 'sexually starved' man with AIDS took advantage of wedding and funeral ceremonies to snatch girls returning late to their homes.

Fear of AIDS has also triggered marital sexual violence. In some quarters in Uganda, men who had been used to constant extra-marital sex and were then confined to their wives have been reported to be increasingly sexually violent with their wives as a catharsis for their frustrations. Others have accused their wives of provoking aggression by refusing to have unprotected intercourse.[31]

There appears to be a clear relationship between sexual and physical abuse of women and women's use of drugs. Among 30 women who were representative of the women in a New York drug treatment programme, including Latina, black, and white women, 20 per cent had mothers who were physically or sexually abused and many of the women had been abused themselves as children – 30 per cent had been physically abused by a parent, 23 per cent had been sexually abused by a family member, and 10 per cent had been victims of incest. As adults, 63 per cent of the women were physically abused and 13 per cent were sexually abused. The damage to self-esteem leaves many women believing they cannot control their lives or bodies, especially in sexual relationships with men.[32]

In Nigeria, a high level of sexual harassment of girls and women either seeking or attempting to retain employment has been reported. Girls in school are being pressured into giving sex to older men in return for school fees or to teachers to get pass grades. As a result, a commission was set up to deal with this issue.[3] The Tanzania Media Women's Association have also taken up these issues.[18]

There are campaigns against violence against women all over the world, by women's groups, health organizations, sex workers' rights groups, and church groups.

Prosecution of these crimes often punishes the victims at least as much as the perpetrators, and women are working to change this. In some countries the police have begun to improve how they deal with victims and prosecutions. In some, court procedures have been slightly improved.

Laws are being passed in some European and Latin American countries against rape and forced sex within marriage. As these laws begin to affect individual and social norms, it may

STOP OLDER MEN FROM HAVING SEX WITH SCHOOL GIRLS

Speak, South Africa

Challenging male sexual norms

Women are in a period of tremendous transition – challenging ideologies of biology-as-destiny, submission and obedience, fighting for and winning a tremendous range of laws and services, becoming more educated, and entering more jobs and professions – in the face of inequality, injustice and opposition on the part of institutions and individuals.

It would be wrong to ignore these changes in any discussion of women and sexuality. Yet many AIDS activists are doing exactly that when they assert that women have little or no power in sexual relations with men and go no further. Many criticize the fact that women are being asked to take responsibility for safer sex with men, as with birth control. As if responsibility were not power. As if women could become empowered without taking responsibility.

> . . . it is important to guard against the danger of overemphasizing women as victims. That reinforces the helpless, passive image of women, which we strongly oppose. The image that we prefer to encourage is the one we ourselves are using: women as active participants in this struggle, taking active roles in supporting each other and in fighting against HIV/AIDS. The use of that approach depends on women's ability to feel strong and confident. So long as a helpless, passive image continues, women feel unable to assert themselves in the ways that are necessary to make the effort to overcome their problems.[34]

While there are many cases of women who deny the risks they face and find it impossible to protect themselves from HIV, others are challenging gender and sexual roles.[35] Concentrating only on cases of women who have not yet managed to overcome the obstacles can help to make the image of women as victims a self-perpetuating one.

become more possible for women to demand safer sex within marriage, and to say no to unwanted sex.

There are national and regional campaigns against forced and child prostitution in Asia. Many groups are now making links between prevention of rape and of HIV infection, as the Women's Crisis Centre in Fiji is doing.[27,29,30,33]

Many women are learning self-defence, and the younger the better. Legal and support services for abused, raped and battered women in many countries are speaking out for women who have experienced violence because they asked for safer sex.

Eliminating the threat of violence and sexual violence from women's lives would be the best sign that safer sexual relationships might be possible for women.[23]

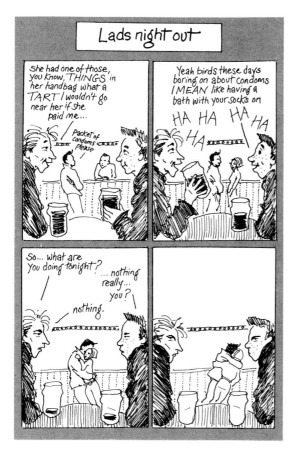

Clara Vulliamy

At the same time, it is male sexual norms which need to change, and men who have to take responsibility as well.

More than one lifetime partner

Sexual relationships, particularly for women, are to do with finding partners and for most, living with them and having children. They are about love, companionship, affection, security, support and survival, as well as sexual pleasure. Few women or men are lucky enough to find one partner willing and able to fill all these needs for life.

Women have begun to question monogamy as well as polygamy, and what it means to them as women, with and without children. Is it fear of condemnation, lack of opportunity and independent resources, or fear of being alone that often make women more monogamous than men? Or are women more monogamous and men less monogamous by nature?

Both women and men sometimes live with one person but have other partners; others have more than one partner or practise serial monogamy. How do women feel about this? What is good and bad about greater sexual freedom? Should people be open and honest about what they are doing, or is it better not to?

Whether people are married or single, heterosexual, bisexual or homosexual, younger or older, most have had more than one lifetime sexual partner or have partners who have done so. This is one of society's biggest secrets from itself. AIDS has forced us to acknowledge and face the implications of our relationships and re-examine our values.

Early intercourse

The minimum legal age of marriage and the average age at marriage are rising in many cultures. More young people are having sex and children before marriage. With or without marriage at an early age, sexual relations begin very young for many women.

In Norway, a population-based survey found that almost ten per cent of girls had had first intercourse by age 15, and almost 46 per cent by age 17.[36] Sexual activity for many inner city girls in New York City begins during pre-adolescence and early adolescence.[37]

In Nigeria, a woman's pre-marital virginity is no longer considered important by many, more so in urban areas. Many young women have sex as a preparation for marriage, which may include becoming pregnant as proof of fertility. Others have sex to satisfy sexual curiosity, and for fun, love and enjoyment.[38]

In a community-based study of gynae-cological diseases in two rural villages in India, it was found that 47 per cent of the unmarried girls in the study had had sexual intercourse.[39]

Earlier sexual activity tends to mean more partners overall, which in turn means potentially more exposure to infection. In Ethiopia, unpublished data showed that the younger the age at first marriage, the shorter the marriage and the greater the likelihood of divorce, remarriage, or the need to sell sex for support.[40]

These facts do not argue against a higher age at marriage. They argue for the elimination of poverty and for safer sex education, access to contraception and condoms at an early age. Young women would not be at increased risk of unwanted pregnancy, RTIs or HIV, if these needs were not neglected.

Marriage

Marriage is the norm in all societies, but it is not a static structure. Nor does it involve only one form of sexual practice or access.[2] In some cultures, marriage is an economic union and a way to ensure that children will be born. Financial support, rather than faithfulness, may be expected from men,[41] while in others, faithfulness between partners is expected.

In spite of this variety, in most cultures a married woman is expected to be faithful and sexually available to her husband. Adultery, especially by women, can be severely punished. Stoning and even death still occur in some Muslim countries, but in most others, separation, divorce and social ostracism are common.

Traditionally, women are supposed to depend on men for economic support for themselves and their children. This is to some extent a myth, since women have always worked to provide for themselves and their families. However, marriage is a source of economic support for millions of women, who

may or may not have paid work outside their homes. Love, position, and economic support cannot be ignored when we talk about sexuality.

The social and economic dependence of women on their partners militates against any demand that can be perceived as threatening to the relationship. Safer sex may be one of them, whether or not women have a lot to say about other family and household matters.[42]

Marriage traditions are being affected by HIV and changes are being proposed which may appear to increase safety, but have unintended disadvantages. From fear of HIV, some men are reasserting the traditional demand to marry a virgin, to ensure that she is not HIV-positive. There is evidence in Uganda that the age at marriage for girls may be falling because of this, thus reducing girls' chances of completing their education and getting properly paid employment. Young women may still be at risk, however, since male virginity is not required.[43]

High bride-prices have prevented young people from marrying, sometimes for many years. This encourages seeking other partners in the meantime. Will lowering the bride price, as some local leaders in Uganda have suggested, help to ensure greater fidelity or safety in the long run?[20,43]

Meanwhile, married women do claim the right to say no. Culturally accepted images of male machismo and female obedience among Puerto Rican men and women are only part of the reality, for example. In fact, women have a dual role, not only as dedicated, self-sacrificing, obedient and faithful wives and mothers, but as women with perseverance, ambition and a sense of determination to achieve personal goals. Thus, while a woman is expected to live with one man all her life and tolerate his infidelity and abuse, she also claims the right to decide whether a man is going to live with her. She may choose to kick him out if he drinks too much, is not a good provider, abuses her or their children, or puts them at risk of HIV infection through drug use and refusal to use condoms.

One Puerto Rican woman in New York, with no friends or family nearby, left her husband when her last baby was born because he was putting them at risk. This man, contrary to the macho stereotype, had begun using drugs while in the army, because he was distraught at having to be separated from his wife and children. She took it upon herself to learn about AIDS and to protect herself. In spite of his behaviour, she still loves him and sleeps with him occasionally – and always makes him use condoms.[35]

Women in Uganda are taking dramatic steps to respond to the AIDS crisis, in spite of cultural and socio-economic pressures. A man who was dying of AIDS demanded that his senior wife leave their city home and help care for him in his village. She refused, not only because he had three other wives in the village to look after him, but because he still expected her to have sex with him and she would not. Her stance left her extremely vulnerable to condemnation from his relatives, who took all their possessions, everything from the business they had run together, and their house when he died. But she went to FIDA, a voluntary association of women lawyers in Uganda, who helped her to move back into her house and to fight a forged will the relatives drew up against her.[44]

FIDA provide legal education and free legal aid to disadvantaged and poor women, most of whom are widows. Under the national non-molestation and separation law codes, they also provide protection for women who decide to leave husbands who refuse to change their sexual behaviour when there is a risk of HIV infection.

When her husband took a second wife, a Muslim woman from Mukono district objected and refused to have sex with him. When the husband tried to reassert his conjugal rights,

she called her neighbours in. They took her side, as he had another source of sexual satisfaction. She wanted to stay in her marriage, because she didn't want her children to be raised by another woman and she was not financially able to raise them alone. She also sought external support and protection from FIDA.[45]

FIDA are finding that they have more referrals for cases involving women's sexual rights and AIDS than any other issue. Women who have refused to have sex with phil-andering husbands sometimes send their husbands to the Association's offices to be talked to. The men demand what they consider to be their sexual rights in return for continuing economic support. But the women are standing firm, because the men can and do get sex elsewhere.

FIDA sometimes recommend that women leave their husbands and seek employment, and refer them to a women's credit fund for help in setting up a small business. Others such as TASO (The AIDS Support Organization), argue that women should stay in their homes. TASO have found that if women leave, they will only look for another man – jumping from the frying pan into the fire.[44]

Women's affairs officers of 335 resistance committees from Rakai district in Uganda recently passed the following resolution:

'If our husbands go with other women, we should be protected by law so that we can abstain from sexual relations with them, but remain in our homes enjoying the same rights and privileges.'[45]

In marriages where both partners are financially independent, the balance of power in sexual relations may be quite different from those in which the woman is economically dependent on the man or the man on the woman. But marriage, no matter how strong a bond it may be, and no matter what the balance of power between partners, is not always the same as having only one partner.

In some societies, polygamy is a socially sanctioned way for a man to satisfy his desire for more than one woman and have many children, and is a sign of wealth. Polygamy where the husband is faithful to his wives and the wives to the husband can be a form of safe sex. In Nigeria, however, it has been found that younger wives often suffer from both sexual and economic neglect by their husbands, who are in most cases considerably older than them. Consequently, the women seek extra-marital relationships to satisfy both their sexual and material needs.[38] Nor does polygamy necessarily stop husbands from seeking partners in addition to their wives.[46]

The All Women's Action Society in Malaysia have noted increased advocacy for and practice of polygamy nationally, linked to the revival of certain interpretations of Islam. They are concerned that this has implications for HIV infection for women.[47]

Divorce

Legal or de facto divorce is now available to both partners in most countries, and the rate of separation and divorce is increasing steadily in many regions. In some developed countries, half of all marriages break up. People who are separated or divorced tend to seek new partners, but finding someone may take some years, particularly for women with children and older women. As often occurs before marriage, women may have a number of partners before remarrying, if they remarry at all. With more marriages breaking up, economic instability and poverty are affecting many women, especially those without education, training and access to jobs that provide adequate support. For women, divorce often brings a loss of status and rights as well as income.

In Zaïre, divorce in many cases is not necessarily a woman's choice. Her parents can also remove her from a marriage because of disputes over dowry, fear that a co-wife will make her suffer, the inability of the woman to cope with heavy work, and inability or irresponsibility of the man to meet her basic needs. Women themselves choose to divorce for these and other reasons, e.g. infrequent sexual relations, impotence in the man, violence by the man, insults to her family by the man, infertility, the death of children because the man failed to support the family, and tribal wars.[48]

In Tanzania, divorce is legally possible. However, if a bride price has been paid, part must be returned if the woman leaves the marriage. If this is impossible, women may be forced to stay in their marriages. Because men are usually better off economically, divorced women may have to leave their children behind if they leave the marriage. Not only do women not want to abandon their children, they also fear ill-treatment by stepmothers. There is a legal clinic in Dar es Salaam to help women with marital problems such as these.[18] But to leave a husband, even because of fear of AIDS, is not easy.

Death of a partner

The death of a partner also leaves women alone and often economically and sexually vulnerable, particularly if she cannot legally inherit her husband's property.

In Uganda, in situations where a husband has died of AIDS, wives have fled to other towns or parts of the country to avoid being stigmatized and to start a new life.[45]

In some cultures, widows are inherited by the brother of a man who has died, and are supposed to be sexually available to them.[3] In some African countries, ritual cleansing of widows after a spouse's death involves intercourse with a member of the spouse's family to purge the spouse's spirit.[49] Because these practices create a risk of HIV transmission, especially when a woman's husband has died of AIDS, they are now being questioned and altered. In 1990 women in Tanzania called for changes in these customary laws and practices.[19] In Zambia, one traditional healer offers condoms for use in ritual cleansing. In many villages, chiefs have banned intercourse for this ritual and replaced it with safe practices based on past traditions.[49]

Economic separation of partners

The combined effects of war, economic recession, structural adjustment policies and political crisis in many countries have led to increasing unemployment, and women are among the worst hit. Not only are jobs disappearing and salaries and wages not keeping up with inflation. In many countries men and women are forced to leave home to seek work. More women, in turn, are having to fend for themselves and their children, or seek other men to support them. Some women are being forced into selling sex both at home where men have left and at men's work sites. Others are only seeing their partners one or two days a month or even less often, with the problems this brings for the relationship.

In Switzerland, there are many seasonal workers from southern European countries. These workers are not permitted to take up residence nor can they bring their families with them. Among a group of Spanish and Portuguese men in this situation, only half described themselves as faithful to their wives, but fidelity had different meanings. For some it meant a commitment to stay with their wives, to whom they would return on visits, but not sexual exclusivity. Some went to sex workers. Others changed partners frequently in order to reduce the chance of emotional involvement.[50]

The migrant labour system that has evolved out of colonialism in Africa is another example of the interplay between sexuality and economics. Interviews with migrant mine-workers in South Africa, for example, showed that frequent and lengthy absences from their homes disrupted their family and sexual relationships. In a lonely and hostile environment and separated for long periods from their wives, some of the men seek sexual relationships in nearby towns. Long absence subjects marriages to great strain, and commonly, divorce and abandonment deprive women of economic support. With access to few opportunities on the labour market, some wives turn to selling sex.[51]

These miners expressed constant anxiety at being separated from their wives and children. As in Switzerland, some of them had no other partners. Others went to sex workers or had short-term relationships with local single or divorced women. Some set up longer-term, though not necessarily permanent relationships with local women, which involved living together some days and domestic obligations on both sides. A complicated network of places where the men meet women exists, which sometimes extends far beyond the mine locality into neighbouring areas.

Longer-term relationships are more likely because the men no longer work on short contracts or return home regularly, as they used to. Many stay at the mines for years and renew their contracts annually. They are forced to take a break in service in order to go home. High unemployment makes them easy to replace and they cannot get their jobs back. Hence, their chances of spending time with their wives can be minimal. Yet employers typically deny that there is a risk of HIV, or merely give directives to the workers to use condoms.[51]

Men who migrate to cities from rural areas or from poorer to richer countries often do not find work. Studies of sexuality and AIDS that take account of such economic issues point out that sexual machismo, 'having' many women, is a common response among poor and unemployed men who have no other way to prove their worth.[35]

Migrant women workers may be the least likely to have access to safer sex education or protection from sexual abuse. Women comprise a fairly large percentage of overseas migrant workers from the Philippines. In jobs such as domestic work, they often have to have sex with the employer in order to stay in employment. Studies in the Philippines have found a higher prevalence of HIV among returning migrant workers than home-based sex workers.[52]

Most migrant labourers are not permitted to reside in the countries and areas where they contribute to the economy and cannot bring their partners and children to live with them. Whole cities and communities are suffering from age and gender imbalances as a result of these restrictions. Sexual relationships and the social structures which maintain them suffer concomitantly. Professional and white-collar workers probably move for their work as often, yet they would never tolerate the living conditions and separations that are forced on migrant labourers and their families.

Government policies are needed to improve migrant labour conditions and employment policies, and give workers the right to bring their families with them, as part of AIDS prevention.

Extra-marital relationships

Extra-marital sex is prohibited or frowned upon in most societies, but many married people have extra-marital relationships.

In 1990 in Thailand among a large group of men and women, most of whom lived in rural areas, 17.2 per cent of men and 0.9 per cent of women with spouses or regular partners reported sex with casual partners in the previous 12 months, while 46.3 per cent of single men and 2.0 per cent of single women reported sex with casual partners.[53]

As Nana, the Uruguayan brothel owner, said: 'Men can afford to be relaxed because they think that their wives do not get up to the same tricks as they do. Don't forget that you're talking to the owner of a brothel, and I know very well what tricks men get up to. They don't lie to me, though they may be able to deceive other women. I know of a whole village that comes to my brothel, and I have 20 girls working round the clock.'[54]

More men admit to having extra-marital partners than women, and they probably do. But men often exaggerate when asked how many sexual partners they have had, while women probably keep this information more secret. In India, for example, one group of rural women said that when they wanted no more children, they preferred to be sterilized themselves rather than for their husbands to have vasectomies, even though vasectomies were safer and easier. They were having extra-marital affairs, and if they fell pregnant as a result, their husbands would know what was going on.[55]

In Nigeria a survey among married women showed that one-third of rural women and 60 per cent of urban women had more than one sexual partner, who was usually also a friend and married himself.[38]

In Rwanda, 86 per cent of women in a large study believed that most married men were not faithful and 44 per cent believed that most married women were not faithful. Sixty-seven per cent of the women said that they had had only one lifetime sexual partner. The women were given a series of scenarios describing sexual relationships and asked if they approved or disapproved:

- A married woman of 30 learns that her husband has taken another wife somewhere else. In revenge, she takes another partner herself – 3 per cent approved.

- A woman has a temporary illness that prevents sexual contact. Her husband takes another partner – 18 per cent approved.
- A woman of 20 knows her boyfriend cannot pay bridewealth and that her father wants her to marry someone else. She tries to get pregnant by her boyfriend – 38 per cent approved.
- A single woman of 25 has one boyfriend who visits her regularly and helps her financially. She has no other partners – 59 per cent approved. [56]

In Zimbabwe, an urban sample of 30 men and 30 women were interviewed about extra-marital sex. Initially, 42 per cent of the men and 27 per cent of the women said extra-marital sex was acceptable for men. Eight per cent of the men and none of the women considered it acceptable for women.

The women were then asked if there were conditions that made extra-marital sex acceptable for women. Eighty per cent of the women said that men took female sexuality for granted, that they no longer cared about exciting their wives sexually, or responding to them when they made efforts to dress up or look attractive. In these situations, it became understandable for women to look elsewhere for gratification.

'After two months of no sex, I tried to arouse my husband sexually and he hastened to tell me that I had a disease of high libido, which my parents had to treat. I was hurt and decided to treat myself.'

All of the men but only 20 per cent of the women thought that married women engaged in extra-marital sex. However, all but two of the men did not think their wives had extra-marital sex, only married women in general. All but one of the men and all the women thought that married men engaged in extra-marital sex. When asked about their own practice, 67 per cent of the men and 3 per cent of the women reported that they sometimes had extra-marital sex. [57]

If safer sex within marriage were to become the social norm, not just outside, all sex would be safer even in the absence of fidelity.

Non-marital heterosexual relationships

More women are living without a steady partner. Some have no partners, others have one or more than one partner at any one time. Many people live together in stable unions without marrying. Are these relationships as monogamous as marriage? Do they break up more easily? We do not know.

What is known is that the number of women-headed households is high in many countries. Kenya is typical, with 36–46 per cent of households headed by women. Generally, women-headed households have less income and fewer resources than those headed by men. [42] Women on their own, usually with children and families to support, often find that their choice of partners is limited. Because most people are married, relationships with married men are common for single, divorced and widowed women. Exchanging sex for money, housing, food and other material goods may be the only way women can meet their own and their families' needs. Women in these situations do not consider themselves to be sex workers nor does society see them that way.

Bisexual and homosexual relationships

Thanks to gay and lesbian movements in the past two decades, more people feel able to be open about same-sex relationships, and bisexuality is more openly acknowledged as well. But many people have experienced relationships with both sexes and never told

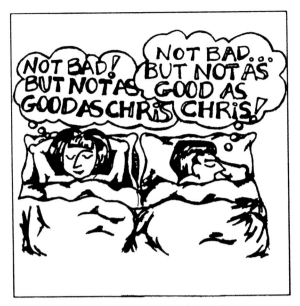

Queensland Dept of Health and AIDS Council, Australia

anyone. They may also have partners who have done so.

Homosexual women and men may get married or have sexual relationships with the opposite sex because they are bisexual by preference, in order to have children, because it is socially expected, and/or in order to hide their same-sex relationships. Where same-sex relationships must be kept hidden, any risk of HIV infection for partners must be kept hidden as well. Many women do not know that their husbands or male partners have relationships with other men.

Male sex workers may sell sexual services to other men because that may be the only way to find these relationships. Others do it for the money. Men in this situation often have women partners.[58]

In Africa, homosexuality is still mostly condemned and denied, although its existence in institutions such as the army, prisons and single-sex schools is tacitly acknowledged.[3]

In countries with strong Arabic and Islamic influence, homosexuality is acknowledged, sometimes accompanied by the belief that it leads to wealth, since it used to be practised by feudal aristocracies. In Nigeria, homosexual relationships among the Hausa were publicly acknowledged in the late 1980s as a consequence of publicity about AIDS among gay men in the West. Lesbian relationships in Nigeria among urban, educated women, married and unmarried, are also being acknowledged.[3]

In Denmark, where people are relatively open about homosexuality and bisexuality, about 10 per cent of gay men in one survey said they had had sex with a woman in the previous year. One-third of women with HIV in Copenhagen had bisexual partners with HIV.[59, 60]

In Honduras, Guatemala and Costa Rica, HIV rates in the population have been increasing rapidly and there are a large number of HIV-positive bisexual men. Fifteen per cent of patients at an HIV clinic in Rio de Janeiro and 33 per cent of those attending an HIV clinic in Belo Horizonte in Brazil said they were bisexual.[43]

In Mexico, the proportion of AIDS cases among gay men decreased between 1981 and 1990, while the proportion among bisexual men rose. In 15 per cent of cases of pregnancy-related HIV in infants, the mother was the partner of a bisexual man.[43] Bisexuality remains highly stigmatized in Latin America, but a growing gay movement and studies on male sexuality are bringing the issue out into the open. Hopefully, this will help to reduce HIV infection among men and their partners.

The project *Mano a Mano* for Latino men in San Francisco is doing outreach to bisexual men in bars, prisons, among gangs and in the streets. The men often act tough and insist that they are not gay. They are told: 'I don't care what you call yourself, your behaviour is high risk and you'd better learn to protect yourself.'[61] A group called *Pegação* in Rio de Janeiro encourages bisexual men to accept their own sexuality, as well as to protect themselves and their partners from HIV.[58]

Bisexual men and women are not part of supportive communities, groups and movements to the same extent as gay men and lesbians may be. Bisexuality may be the most stigmatized form of sexuality; belonging to two camps, as it is perceived, may mean not belonging to either. Bisexual men and women may describe and consider themselves as heterosexual, because that is more socially acceptable. More campaigns by and for bisexual women and men are needed.

Women need to be made more aware of the fact that their partners may be bisexual and of the potential risks of HIV infection that may arise.

Mixing sex, drink and drugs

Combining sex with money and/or drugs of any kind makes people more willing to take risks of all kinds and increases the risk of HIV infection.

Among more than 200 adolescent crack cocaine users in California in the USA, 55 per cent of girls and 34 per cent of boys reported a history of an STD. If they combined the use of crack cocaine, which is known to stimulate sexual desire, with sex, the rate was higher than if they had not. Additional risk behaviours reported by these young people were failure to use condoms in their most recent sexual encounter, exchanging sex for drugs or money, and having five or more sexual partners a year.[62]

Any mind-altering drug, legal or illegal, will affect the ability to make decisions, and may make people more likely to have unprotected sex than otherwise.[63] In Zimbabwe, one study found that 80 per cent of men sought a sex worker in bars and 60 per cent were drunk the last time they had sex with a sex worker. In Rwanda, wives of men who drank regularly had a high rate of HIV infection.[64]

Any woman who regularly uses drugs to the point where she is dependent on them is very vulnerable. She will eventually have pressure put upon her sexually, whether from drug dealers, police wanting a pay-off for not arresting her, or financial desperation. Drug use can push women into selling sex.[63]

On the other hand, drug dealers or the embarrassment of selling sex may push sex workers into drug use. In the Philippines, drug use among sex workers is not uncommon, to get over the shame of the work, perform vaginal tricks, dance naked on stage, or overcome shyness about approaching customers. Marijuana, valium with beer, and cough syrup are most commonly used.[65]

Users of illegal drugs are getting younger, and the risk of HIV from combining drug use and sex is more likely to endanger younger women who are less experienced and less confident about laying down limits, do not have the businesslike attitude or take the same protective measures as experienced sex workers would do.[63]

Casual sex

Many people have sexual encounters without any intention of forming a relationship. They may meet someone in a bar, at a party or other social gathering, spend the night with them and perhaps never see them again. Few studies indicate the extent of these encounters, except among gay men and people who travel.

Studies in Britain, Switzerland, Denmark and Sweden have all found that travellers, especially men travelling without partners and young people of both sexes, regularly have sex in the places they visit. Many professionals travel and migrate for international politics, diplomacy, business and trade, relief and development projects and war, as well as holidays. Although the sexual behaviour of these groups while travelling has not been well studied, earlier studies have shown high STD rates among business travellers and their contacts.

Among a group of British men aged 16–25 travelling without a partner, 26 per cent reported sexual intercourse while away. Among 1,229 guests in a youth hostel in Copenhagen, 13 per cent of men and 9 per cent of women had sexual contacts. And among a group of male Swedish travellers aged 19–21, of those who had sex while travelling, more or less one-third had casual contacts with fellow Swedish women travellers, one-third with women tourists from another country, and one-third with girls living in the country they were visiting.[66]

Sex tourism

Sex tourism, an offshoot of the rapidly growing tourist industry, has also become highly organized and profitable in many countries. Many agencies offer jobs abroad in the tourist industry and 'entertainment'. When the sex tourist industry is more developed or pays better in one country than in those of its neighbours, women are crossing borders and even continents to provide sexual services, e.g. Burmese and Laotian women and girls travel into Thailand.[67]

A much higher rate of HIV infection was found among women from the Dominican Republic who had done sex work abroad than at home. Eighty women from the Dominican Republic who asked for HIV tests at home in 1988 had been sex workers in 27 countries, including the Americas, Europe and North Africa. When found to be HIV-positive, these women found they had few or no rights and were often deported.[68]

Women are thought to comprise ten per cent of European sex tourists, with a slight preference for Kenya and Haiti.[66,69] Among male European sex tourists, favourite destinations are Thailand, the Philippines, Indonesia, South Korea, Goa/India, Kenya, Ghana, the Dominican Republic and Brazil.

Eighty per cent of all incoming male travellers to Thailand in one study arrived with the intention of finding sex.[69] US, Japanese, Korean and Singaporean men also travel for sex in large numbers. As many as 250,000 Malaysian men, mostly businessmen, cross the border into Thailand for sex each year, in spite of a sizeable but smaller sex industry in Malaysia.[47,67]

Because of AIDS, some men are being offered very young sexual partners on these trips, often adolescents and children, whom they are told are 'unspoiled'.[3,66]

Of 152 German male sex tourists (not all of whom described themselves as such), nearly half never used condoms while on tour, 20 per cent used them sometimes and 30 per cent always. The men least likely to use condoms were older and had a partner in Germany.[70]

AIDS education campaigns are targeting travellers in some countries. While people travelling can contribute to the spread of AIDS, travellers who have taken up safer sex practices could contribute to AIDS prevention instead.

Selling and buying sex

'Terms like sex work, prostitution, the flesh trade, whoredom, the world's oldest profession are qualitative indicators of how a society treats women and what it expects from them.'[27]

For many women, selling sexual services may be the only way to earn a living, and this may never rise above day-to-day subsistence. Only for some women is it a freer choice because they like the work, prefer it to other jobs that may be open to them, or can earn more than in other available work.

A substantial minority of men, whether or not they have regular partners or wives, buy sexual services from women. In Thailand, in the rural sample described above, 22 per cent of men, both single and married, reported giving money, gifts or favours in exchange for sex in the previous 12 months.[53]

In Birmingham in the UK, at least one in twelve and as high as one in five men is a regular client of a sex worker. Clients surveyed in 1988 had begun to buy sex between the ages of 13 and 69, with the majority beginning in their 20s and 30s. They had been buying sex for as little as one day and as long as 55 years, with a mean of ten years. Almost half paid for sex to avoid emotional involvement, and this was as true of men who had other partners as of men without other partners. Lack of sexual activity, insufficient sex with other partners, inability to get other partners to engage in specific practices (mainly oral sex), shyness, and boredom with sexual relations with other partners were the next most common reasons given. Loneliness and old age were cited by only a few of the men in their 60s, though not by those in their 70s.[71]

Women often begin to sell sex when they are just starting out in their lives. In Birmingham, women's first client contact was at age 18 on average. Most women moved out of sex work in their 30s with only a few continuing beyond age 40.[71]

For most women sex workers in Kananga, Zaïre, divorce or the death of a husband and, in a few cases, the refusal to be dominated by a husband, were the reason why they had begun to exchange sex for money and support. Some were younger daughters in families with a number of girls, whose parents could not manage to pay for all of them to be married.[48]

Women with little education or training have few or no choices apart from sex work when national economic policies do not provide other paid work for women and when unemployment is high. Women may exchange sex only from time to time for extra income to overcome transitory economic hardship. Having sex with an employer or manager may be the only way to reach a better position at work. In developing countries, women's access to the cash economy is often limited by regulations on land ownership or usage, limited access to credit and through culturally restricted mobility.[72]

Although well-off men can easily afford to buy sex, they can also afford stability. Fear of AIDS may encourage them to forego sexual encounters that are pursued for pleasure rather than economic gain. Poor women, with or without partners, cannot always afford sexual stability and frequently need to seek out new partners for economic and social security.[73]

Women who sell sex want relationships like everyone else. Women servicing sailors from the US Navy bases in the Philippines often formed ongoing relationships with the men during their one-to-two year tours of duty, though most were abandoned, often with children from these relationships, afterwards.[65]

An article about AIDS in a national newspaper in Zimbabwe in 1991 carried the photographs of fifteen young women, most looking happy and smiling. All of them had recently left school and home in pursuit of employment, and found nothing except sex work. They talk about their kind boyfriends. They talk about wanting to have fun and look nice for the men they know. They talk about getting presents. They also talk about helping each other to survive:

'Those who blame us do so on full stomachs. I should feed myself and my children adequately. My children should go to school. To say that AIDS kills without giving me a well-paid job is like saying I should die of hunger. To me, that is the only way to survive.'[74]

The Women and AIDS Support Network (WASN) in Harare found that articles like this were being used to blame these young women for AIDS and for not using condoms. The men, on the other hand, were seen as victims. Women were becoming divided against each other, with the 'good' blaming the 'bad' for the epidemic. The level of blame was so deep that some women's organizations were afraid of tackling issues dealing with single women and sex workers, because this would give them problems with the 'good wives'.[75] WASN therefore started a campaign to challenge negative images of women in relation to AIDS.

Targeting sex workers distorts HIV risks for all women

'There has been a serious distortion in the understanding of the way this epidemic has affected women because of the singling out of sex workers. The majority of women are not sex workers, and the largest group of women at high risk of infection are wives.

'Recent data from Mexico indicate that only 0.8 per cent of all reported AIDS cases have been among sex workers and 9 per cent among housewives. Similar figures can be found in other countries, both developed and developing. In Senegal, 50 per cent of HIV-infected women in one hospital ward for infectious diseases had no risk factor other than being a wife.'[72]

Blaming sex workers encourages blame, stigma, and discrimination against all women. It also allows the men who infect sex workers and their own wives to deny that they are infecting others.[72] Wives too can infect their husbands, who can in turn infect sex workers.

Sex workers and their clients in many countries are not serving as a 'bridge' for HIV transmission into the rest of the population. A high use of condoms, hygienic practices before and after sex, and the fact that many clients prefer oral sex and manual masturbation are the main reasons why.[76,77,78]

Among the least empowered, however, often because of poverty or, as in developed countries, use of illegal drugs, the rate of HIV infection can be high. Clients and circumstances force women to take risks in order to earn money. In Thailand, women in the lowest-priced brothels saw many more clients in order to earn a decent living, and they had more clients who refused to use condoms than women in higher-priced brothels. There was a much higher rate of infection among both the poorer women and their clients. In lower-priced brothels, 36 per cent of the women had HIV, while in the higher-priced brothels 5 per cent had HIV.[77]

Banning HIV-positive women from sex work?

Efforts to stop sex workers with HIV from working are doomed to failure. Where economic necessity motivates selling sex, women have no alternative. Alternative employment might motivate some women to leave sex work, and no one would oppose this, as long as it were voluntary. However, continuing demand for sexual services by men would ensure that as some women leave, other women would take their places.[79]

'Women wouldn't do it if there wasn't a market. We're not saying we must stop all these men needing sex. You know, they're always saying we've got to stop these women from doing it.'[80]

In fact, removing women with HIV from sex work could actually increase the spread of infection. Clients with HIV would not stop going to sex workers. All clients would feel safer because they would think women with HIV had been removed. They would continue to demand unsafe sex with sex workers and with their own partners, and could transmit HIV to all of them. Thus, more uninfected women would become infected.[79]

The fear that sex workers spread HIV has reduced client numbers and therefore some women's incomes, e.g. in Uganda, Thailand and Brazil. Women may lower their prices to attract more clients and take greater risks with clients in order to get more money.[43,81,82,83]

Legal repression?

The illegality of drugs, sex work and homosexuality influences the risks of transmission of HIV. Negative messages from governments, policymakers and church leaders, combined with fear of AIDS, have led to increased police repression in many countries against sex workers, drug users, and gay and bisexual men. This has a detrimental effect on what AIDS campaigns are actually trying to achieve, by pushing people who may be at high risk underground even further.

Discrimination and repression are most starkly expressed when sex workers and others are detained in hospitals or prisons for having HIV, which has occurred in many countries. Sweden has created the legal power to detain in hospital known HIV-infected persons who are deemed to pose a public hazard by their behaviour. For sex workers, being seen on the street has apparently been considered proof enough of such a hazard. Of the first seven people with HIV detained under this law, five were sex workers who said they were no longer selling sex.[84] In one case in the USA, a sex worker with HIV was put under house arrest and forced to wear an electric beeper which would go off if she was more than 60 meters from her house.[85]

A group of women sex workers, in detention after having been 'rescued' from a red-light district in Bombay by police and a voluntary organization, were found to have HIV. One official said they would be held until they were 'cured'. Another said they could be released if their families would take them back, but most of their families did not know they were sex workers, and the stigma would have prevented their return home. The government said they would set up sheltered workshops where the women could be trained in self-supporting jobs, but these never appeared. Finally, a court case taken by one activist secured their release. Throughout their detention, they were told nothing about HIV and its prevention. Most probably went back into sex work.[86]

Legalize sex work?

Sex work is permitted in Brazil and India, but 'exploitation of the woman' is an offence. Ironically, the main complaint of many sex workers is extortion by the police for protection against 'exploitation'. In both countries, sex workers' associations have organized against this.[27,82,87]

Legalization that requires sex workers to register and have mandatory health checks and HIV tests creates a two-tiered system. This has

---

AIDS education by radio

The Association of Prostitutes of Rio de Janeiro decided that the best way to warn their members of the dangers of AIDS was by radio, since most of them were unable to read.

The radio station they launched is located in the oldest red-light district in Rio. It transmits music, news, interviews and advice on how to reduce the risk of STDs and AIDS.

A survey carried out in 1990 found that only half of the sex workers demanded that their clients use condoms. As a result the radio station encourages the women to come to the station where they will be given free condoms. BENFAM, the family planning association of Brazil, paid for the radio equipment and provides medical information for programmes, as well as 12,000 condoms for distribution per month. More than 300 of the 400 women working in the district signed up to receive condoms after the station opened.[82]

been shown to be a major problem in the Philippines,[65] and in Nevada in the USA,[88] as unregistered women become more vulnerable to poverty and abuse by clients, pimps and the police. In developing countries, poorer women in rural areas would be the least likely to register or have regular health checks.[80]

Thus, many sex workers' groups support full decriminalization of sex work and oppose legalization that involves registration.

Sex workers and clients need safer sex

HIV prevention programmes for sex workers have benefited many through counselling, support, services, access to condoms and assistance in adopting condom usage. Empowered sex workers are educating each other and their clients, and all women benefit as a result.

Clients are not victims of sex workers. It will never happen that a client wants to use a condom and the sex worker refuses.[25] Clients need educating. In Asia, these lessons are being ignored. Sex workers have been the only women targeted in India, Indonesia, Malaysia and the Philippines. In Indonesia the National AIDS Committee and NGOs have made no efforts to educate clients because they are considered a population too difficult to identify.[47]

Sex work involves many more people than sex workers, and supports local economies and the people who work in them, wherever it takes place. This includes the owners and staff of hotels, clubs, bars, brothels and escort agencies that employ sex workers; local shops and food sellers; and taxi drivers, pimps, police, drug dealers and criminal elements who feed off the trade. The entire sex industry can be mobilized to ensure safety. In many cases, sex workers have empowered themselves through collective action and condom-only policies in their workplaces.

Proposals for safer sex work

- Sex workers' unions associations to self-determine their conditions of work;
- access to free or low-cost quality health services, legal aid and social workers;
- minimum income and welfare for sex workers, paid through taxation of establishments;
- elimination of forced prostitution;
- minimum-age requirements for sex workers;
- banning of intoxicated and other undesirable clients;
- allowing sex workers to reject clients;
- safer sex education for all the participants in the sex industry;
- safer sex education for women that addresses but does not single out sex workers;
- safer sex education for men that addresses but does not single them out as clients;
- absolute enforcement of condom-only policies with harsh fines for sex establishments, sex workers and clients alike;
- regular and adequate supplies of condoms;
- welfare officers and inspectors, recruited from among sex workers themselves;
- educational and occupational training, and alternative employment options for sex workers. [25,79,81,89,90,91]

Achieving safer sexual relationships

Dealing with the sexual transmission of HIV is not merely a personal issue for individuals. As women struggle to reduce the imbalance of power between women and men, there seems to be a clear trend towards more partner change. Is this a positive sign of greater sexual freedom for both men and women, though not equal for each? Or is it a sign of a breakdown in the social order, with more risks than benefits, not least of which come from AIDS. Trends at a macro-level are having profound effects. It is difficult to stand back from what is happening and evaluate its import.

Condemnation and exhortations to return to lifelong monogamy may appear to be the only safe and moral stance, shadowed by negative images of the relationship between sex, AIDS and death. But this has not stopped sexual trends – or AIDS. If we, as societies and individuals affected by these trends, do not begin to take some control over them, they will continue to control us. If AIDS prevention and education campaigns do not address these issues, they will miss the mark.

Women have begun to challenge narrow definitions of sexual risk as defined by most AIDS campaigns. Safety in relationships for women can be defined as:

- The right to a self-defined sexuality, the right to choose which sexual practices to engage in and with whom, and the right to practise these safely.
- Safety from being pressured, expected or forced to have unwanted sexual relations of any kind, whether as a duty, service, tradition or through physical force.
- Safety when trying for a pregnancy.
- Safety during pregnancy, childbirth and breastfeeding.
- Safety from unwanted pregnancy, including safe contraception and abortion.
- Safety from reproductive tract infections, including HIV.
- Social, economic, legal and health service support in making these possible.

The freedom of women to express their sexuality safely in the kinds of relationships they want will take an incalculable period of time to achieve, but we are working on it.

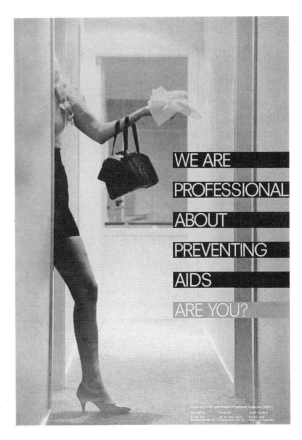

New Zealand Prostitutes Collective

Don't die of ignorance – I nearly died of embarrassment: condoms in context

by Janet Holland, Caroline Ramazanoglu, Sue Scott, Sue Sharpe and Rachel Thomson

In the official campaigns which encourage condom use and disparage complacency about the risks of spreading HIV through heterosexual intercourse, condoms are represented as a means of self-help in which the individual takes responsibility for safer sex. Campaign advertisements represent young women as well as young men as bearing a responsibility for sexual safety, and now recognize some of the problems that young women face in introducing a condom into a sexual encounter. One advertisement comments, '. . . and she's too embarrassed to ask him to use a condom . . . wouldn't it have been easier to talk about it earlier . . .' We have found that embarrassment over condoms is not simply a question of bad timing, but indicates a very complex process of negotiation.

The Women's Risk and AIDS Project [UK] currently has data from 496 young women aged 16 to 21, and qualitative data from 150 of them. These data are beginning to provide knowledge of the social situations in which condoms are used or rejected, and of the symbolic significance of condoms as young women negotiate their sexual relationships. Condoms carry symbolic meaning which can differ for each sexual partner and for individuals over time.

Our data illustrate the importance of men's power in sexual encounters and their control of sexual pleasure; women's opposition to condoms; the ways in which women can demand safer sex; the complications of love in unequal relationships; and the contradictions of asking young men to use condoms. These meanings cannot simply be swept away and replaced by public education.

The social context

The physical intimacy which can lead to orgasm, pregnancy or sexually transmitted disease is potentially an experience of both pleasure and danger, but it is also unknown social territory. Even for the sexually experienced, encounters with new sexual partners are not wholly predictable. Sexual intercourse entails entrusting our bodies, our identities, our self-respect to others and, not uncommonly, to strangers. Sexual practice in Western society is heavy with moral meanings. While the English education system may equip pupils with some knowledge of the mechanics of vaginal intercourse, much of the danger and virtually all the pleasures of sexuality are an embarrassed area of silence.

In many sexual encounters women have little choice about whether or how to engage in sexual activity with men, the options being physical injury or more subtle forms of sanction. The accounts given by the young women in our sample support Liz Kelly's conception of the continuum of sexual violence, from sexism, to mild pressure to have unwanted intercourse, to more overtly coerced sex, child abuse and rape. But women are not simply helpless victims in the face of male control of sexuality. Male power in sexual relationships is both embraced and resisted by young women in the course of negotiating sexual encounters. The same woman can negotiate very different sexual encounters with different men or at different points in her sexual career.

The social context of condom use may or may not be problematic for young women, depending on their priorities in a particular relationship, the degree of trust between partners and other factors. But condom use remains the focus of a number of social tensions. Male sexual power, the privileging of men's sexual pleasure and the dominance of men over women can be challenged by a woman's insistence on her needs for safety being met. Asking him to use a condom is embarrassing when it is a potentially subversive demand. The spontaneity of passion can be undermined by recognition of risk and responsibility. If coming to orgasm means losing control, being taken over by sensation, then condoms symbolize control and a curb on passion and spontaneity. Sexual fulfillment and sexual safety pull against each other when they are defined in terms of men's fulfilment.

There is more than one way in which men can express their masculinity. But it takes a special combination of circumstances for young women to gain sufficient control in sexual encounters to ensure both safety and their own sexual pleasure. Shere Hite concludes from her survey of predominantly well-educated American women that women are tired of 'the old mechanical pattern of sexual relations, which revolves around male erection, male penetration and male orgasm.' We have found that much, if not most, of young women's sexual experience is not particularly pleasurable. Sometimes it seems

that what is valued is the social relationship with a partner rather than the sexual activity. Young women are not without the ability to choose and to act for themselves, but they are socially heavily constrained. Young men are much better placed socially to gain sexual pleasure for themselves. When a young woman insists on the use of a condom for her own safety, she is going against the construction of sexual intercourse as men's natural pleasure, and women's natural duty.

Use of condoms – the figures

Of our 496 respondents, 16 per cent said they had used condoms without any other form of protection; 13 per cent had used condoms while they were taking the contraceptive pill; 0.5 per cent had used condoms with spermicide, and 1 per cent had used a condom and a cap at the same time. We can therefore say that 30 per cent of our sample had used condoms, but this tells us nothing about the circumstances of condom use. The fact that a young woman uses a condom on one occasion does not necessarily mean that she will be able to negotiate the continuation of this practice even if she wants to.

Power, control and pleasure

The young women's own definitions of what constitutes sexual encounter or relationship include practices which did not involve sexual intercourse. But when asked what sex meant for them, most of the young women accepted the prevailing view of sex as heterosexual sex with male penetration.

It was much more uncommon to find young women who had thought of the possibility of sexual pleasure without sexual intercourse. It also became clear that for many, vaginal intercourse was something they did not particularly enjoy, although they assumed that it was what men wanted. A number said they had never experienced orgasm through penetrative sex and that they much preferred other sexual activities in which they engaged. One felt that to stop short of intercourse would label her a tease.

Behind this definition of sex – as the need to fulfil male sexual desires in a specific way – lies the notion of men's uncontrollable sexual drive, which cannot be interrupted or diverted. This idea implies that women must take responsibility for moral standards and contraception. It can also lead to failure to use contraception, particularly condoms, where these have connotations of breaking the flow and destroying the passion.

Some women showed a limited sense of the potential for their own sexual pleasure, particularly when this was something which they had not experienced. Even where they had high expectations of sexual pleasure they were often prepared to settle for less.

'One young woman, discussing her first experience of condom use, explained that her boyfriend had been certain that the condom should be blown up first. She had strongly doubted this, but she allowed her views to be overridden on the assumption that men knew better.'

Men exercise power when they are considered to be the initiators of sex, when they threaten the loss of the relationship if the young woman will not have sex, when they refuse to use a condom even when asked, and when they destroy a young woman's reputation by describing her in sexually abusive terms. These are the framework of male power within which young women negotiate sexual encounters and relationships. In turn, women can demonstrate acceptance of male power, ambivalence towards it or resistance.

Where men did agree to use a condom, there was still the problem of how to make sexual activity pleasurable. Couples need to be relatively sexually experienced to deal with the woman's need for pace and timing.

'Unless you're quite close it does interrupt things. They [boyfriends] have got to be quite liberated themselves to use them in a way that's really good. It's frustrating because there isn't an equal amount of knowledge on how you use them.'

Women's demands for safe sex

Despite a very general perception that men dislike condoms our interviewees did not necessarily see that men's needs must always dominate a sexual encounter. Women are not without agency in protecting themselves when they define sexual safety as a priority.

When we asked young women about how they felt personally about using condoms, 26 per cent of 78 young women disliked condoms themselves, and 38 per cent reported that they had partners who disliked them. But 47 per cent of the young women liked or preferred condoms, and 32 per cent reported this for their partners. Condom use for safe sex could then be seen either as a problem or as a solution or, in a contradictory way, as both.

When women did insist on sex being safe, they were often able to get men's cooperation. Sometimes they had to assert themselves quite strongly.

'He really hates using them, so I used to say to him, 'Look, right, look, I have no intention of getting pregnant again and you have no intention to become a father, so you put one of these on.' And he starts whingeing. He goes, 'Oh, no, do I have to?' I say, 'Look, Alan, do it or you know . . .' He's all right, he knows how to do it now.'

Insistence could mean being prepared to give up the relationship.

'Some boys are just stupid, but if they don't want to wear a condom, then tough, you know, go and find someone else. That's it. But most of them don't mind.'

A very small number of young women in our sample seemed to be prepared to attempt to negotiate either non-penetrative sex or condom use in a range of different situations. These young women all seem to have a fairly strong sense of themselves, rather than being highly dependent on having a relationship with a man. They also talk about sex in terms of pleasure and their own needs, and about safe sex as more than just condoms.

'Safe sex is as pleasurable an experience as actual penetration. Oral sex, things like touching somebody else's body in a very gentle way, kissing, appreciating one another's bodies.'

A more common way for young women to counter young men's rejection of condoms is to assert their fear of pregnancy. There could be considerable embarrassment about telling a new partner that a condom is wanted for protection against possible infection, but it is allowable for protection against pregnancy.

Women's opposition to condoms

Some young women had a range of reasons for not using condoms. This generally seemed to indicate an accommodation to their own relative powerlessness in sexual encounters.

'Well, it would be nice if it was easier for girls to actually initiate things with men without feeling difficult about it. But I don't really know how it happens.

I don't really know that many blokes who I think would use a condom or are even concerned about it. I mean, they've never been concerned about getting women pregnant, have they.'

These young women also reported a wide range of negative descriptions of condom use, which seemed to reflect male perceptions. For example: 'It's like picking your nose with a rubber glove.'

Others used condoms when they were available or agreed upon, but went ahead anyway when they were not.

A further group of reasons for reluctance to use condoms came from the women's fear of upsetting men by asserting their own needs. These were partly to do with the fear of losing a boyfriend and the hope of a more committed or steady relationship, and partly a general unwillingness to hurt the man's feelings.

A clear way of avoiding control was to enter into a sexual relationship with no specific expectation that there would be sexual intercourse. Some convince themselves the man is 'safe' to avoid asking him to use anything, or believe that they themselves are invulnerable.

These types of explanations were used by young women who feared both pregnancy and HIV infection and occurred in the context of both steady and casual relationships.

Going steady and trusting to love

There is a common sense assumption that negotiations around sex are easier in the context of steady relationships, but this is not necessarily the case. Going steady implies a degree of trust which is lacking in less persistent sexual relationships. Trust then becomes a significant aspect of the context of decision-making about condoms. If love is seen to be the greatest prophylactic, then trust comes a close second.

Condoms can be seen as a strategy for occasions when it is not clear whether partners can be trusted. Some young women who were on the pill told new partners they were not, so that condoms were used as well.

A trusting relationship provides a social context in which condom use may be relatively unproblematic. In some of these young couples, both lacked sexual experience or had been going steady for some time before their first experience of intercourse. Inexperience provided a basis of trust so that they could discuss the problems of using condoms and their own embarrassment. Reaching the stage of going together to buy condoms could become a joint commitment to a deepening relationship.

Once the relationship was felt to be well established, the young woman would go on the pill. The transition from condoms with new partners to the pill with steady partners is laden with symbolic meaning. It can be used to signify the seriousness of a relationship. For the current generation of young women, the pill (despite the problems connected with its use) is closely associated with grown-up status and grown-up sex. This makes the prospect of long-term condom use highly problematic.

The question of what counts as a steady relationship is clouded by fears for loss of reputation, particularly by young women. Most young women are reluctant to describe themselves as having casual sex when the culturally approved objective is to be in a steady, preferably monogamous relationship, supported by the ideologies of romance and love. Conversely, they are likely to expect or to express the hope that relationships of short duration, including one night stands, will in fact last. Sex as leisure and pleasure tends not to be available to young heterosexual women.

The young women who described themselves as being in steady relationships tended to think of themselves as not being at risk in relation to HIV and to focus their attention on avoiding pregnancy.

Often the young women's experience of sexual pressure and physically unpleasant encounters conflicted with their desire for romance, caring, closeness and trust. There was a widespread negative perception of male sexuality.

Others insisted that if they did not trust the young man, they would not have sex, or they would not be in a relationship with him. Where there are social pressures on young women to police sexual encounters and look out for problems, particularly the risk of pregnancy, this mitigates against developing trust even when a steady relationship is wanted. Many women took risks with partners they loved but did not wholly trust.

A small number of the young women clearly stated that they had casual sex or one night stands. Some of these had taken on the idea that it is legitimate for women to be sexually active, to have their own sexual identity, but they were not necessarily any more in control of their encounters. One young woman who was very clear that she wanted to be sexually active and child-free was in fact having unprotected intercourse with partners who were potential health risks. She said that she had come to be interviewed to make her think about what she was doing.

Condom use tends to be associated with one-night stands rather than 'steady' relationships. If young women's relationships are conceived as 'steady' until proved otherwise, this makes condom use rather unpredictable.

Conclusions

The mixture of positive and negative ways in which the young women we have interviewed react to sexual safety makes it clear that young women cannot be treated as a unified category. A number of couples used condoms with few apparent problems in negotiation, particularly where couples were young and inexperienced, where women were assertive, or where men habitually used condoms with new partners for their own protection.

Public education campaigns need to be sensitive to the different ways in which young women are positioned in relation to safer sex. Our sample indicates not only a range of sexual experiences, but also variations in levels of power and autonomy in the negotiation of these sexual relationships. While most of these young women do not use condoms most of the time, they are coping with considerable and conflicting social pressures in organizing their sexual behaviour.

We found embarrassment about every stage of condom use. Young men may well be just as embarrassed in sexual encounters as young women, especially when they are inexperienced, but the meanings carried by condoms allow them to hide embarrassment by rejecting condoms. Young men can be fearful of sexual inadequacy and apprehensive about sexual encounters, but as these emotions are not defined as natural aspects of male sexuality, there is no discourse around this issue to which women have access.

Many young women who were unable to negotiate condom use recognized that what they were doing was not in their best interest. This was particularly so for those who were informed and concerned about HIV infection.

'I thought straight after, 'You stupid, stupid girl,' and immediately resolved that next time, I would, you know.'

'I would like to think that I would, I hope to death I would.'

If young heterosexuals are to be able to protect themselves against the spread of HIV, we will have to restructure the common sense of sexual relationships. The language of sexuality needs to be challenged, changed and expanded so that women and men can recognize the contradictions of their own experiences, their own responsibilities and their own agency. Women can then develop a positive language which will make public the continuum of sexual pressure, ambivalence and pleasure in sexuality. When women have self-respecting sexual identities which do not depend primarily on being attached to a man, they will be in a stronger position to promote sexual safety. The embarrassment of negotiating condom use with the one you love indicates the current contradictions of female subordination in the close encounters of heterosexual sex.

Sexual insecurity of the boys of today

by Erik Centerwall

The emotional isolation of boys

The basis for my own sex education work with teenage boys is a study that was made in a suburb of Stockholm fifteen years ago. This study showed that teenage boys had no one to talk to about matters that were sensitive, complicated, fraught with problems and causing anxiety. In fact, 80 per cent of the boys said they had no one to talk to.

Many girls also lack a confidant(e). However, there is a kind of protective network surrounding girls in Sweden. Most girls, in spite of everything, have a far greater chance of experiencing the comfort of words, talking to someone about a deep love affair, and obtaining experienced advice on sexuality and contraceptives.

Girls have a closer relationship with their mothers – they go through the same things. When a girl has her period, Mum is there, showing her what to do. Mum is involved in the girl's sex life in a more intimate way.

When a boy has his first involuntary ejaculation, Dad is hardly likely to be there cheering him on. I continue to believe that many boys can be uneasy and surprised when they first ejaculate.

A boy tends not to go to his father with his questions as their relationship does not allow this. But neither does he go to his mother. For a mother, physical sexuality is something to be kept from her and can, in fact, be experienced as something that takes a boy away from her. Boys do not find it possible to talk to their mothers about this wave of sexual experience.

Girls are often closer to their friends and they may have a best friend with whom to share their worries about love. It is possible that some boys also have a friend they can talk to about intimate matters, but it is more common for boys to be part of a gang, which leaves little scope for sensitive conversations on love and one's hopes.

The message of 'bad' male sexuality

Girls in Sweden have far more opportunities through youth clinics, school nurses, counselling on contraceptives, etc., to discuss their questions and what they wonder about with experts – most of these experts being women. Moreover, Swedish sex education follows a female tradition with an emphasis on fertility and the control of the woman's reproduction. The message communicated to boys and men in this tradition has generally been to be

considerate and not to make the girl pregnant. The message has often been that male sexuality is wicked and that men are dirty and inconsiderate.

This message may also be a male self-experience. It is a negative sexuality which makes me a man in the eyes of other men. The wicked urge becomes something that creates identity. The male urge is opposed by a female morality – my sexuality is in some way bad because it wants something which girls do not.

Do girls actually want sex? This is one of the more difficult and most concealed questions among boys in their teens.

Male educators are needed

The purpose of aiming special education at boys in their teens is to break a silence and to strengthen boys' search for identity. We would like boys to be able to recognize themselves in each others' experiences. And we would also like adult men to play a greater role in sex education work with teenage boys.

Both male and female experiences are needed, e.g. when talking about condoms. Only an adult man can talk about condoms with all the torment and problems associated with this shameful sheath. Only an adult man can talk and give feelings about the significance of wearing or not wearing one. Because we know how it feels!

Another point is that we would also like to know how women experience the condom. Many women say that it is of no significance whatsoever. Others insist that having or not having a condom makes a huge difference.

The purpose of our project has not been just to create dialogue between men and boys, but also between men and women – and ultimately between boys and girls. What we want is that boys and girls should be able to talk together, have a dialogue on what they want and feel – instead of morality forbidding this. We want to stimulate conversation. Our belief is that conversation provides better opportunities to control one's own life than moral rules established by others.

I often go into classes where I do not know the pupils, to talk about sex education. I frequently find that I have to take a deep breath before I go into the classroom. Beforehand, I try to see the boys in front of me, think about what I was like myself in such a situation and what I would have wanted to hear. Such thoughts are almost enough to make me turn round at the door and back out. As a boy I would not have wanted to hear a word, and would have thought it highly embarrassing if a grown man had come into the classroom to talk about sex in the way I talk about sexuality to boys.

The following relates to a class of boys aged 16:

- They are above all afraid of revealing themselves in front of each other: 'It must not be revealed how silly I am; how little I can do; that I have never done it; that I masturbate so often; that it's over so quickly', and so on.
- There may perhaps be a boy who is not sexually mature, and most of the boys have not had intercourse. In Sweden, girls are slightly ahead of boys. The majority of boys start sexual activity between the ages of 16 and 19, a relatively large number even in their 20s. Some boys think that girls of the same age fail them when they go with older guys.
- There may be a gang who are quite boastful about their sexual experiences. Some boys are experienced, but this need not mean that they are mature.

If girls are present, it is often very difficult to work with these misunderstandings and also to talk about such things as masturbation.

In front of girls, and also in front of adults, boys have had to learn to behave and not 'talk dirty'. The whole joy and pithiness of the language which is part of the world of boys and men is therefore often lost in the company of women. Using dirty words, deducing their meaning, talking and laughing about sexuality can often be a gateway to conversation.

If one is allowed to laugh, it is easier to be oneself. I can then talk about my sexual failures, e.g. how tricky I found it to use condoms during all these adult years. If he dares talk about it, if perhaps a boy dares to say that he does not like this business with condoms, the conversation is at once on its way from morality and idealism to the realities of existence: What it feels like to put a condom on. What it is like if an erection fails. How one has been unsuccessful in putting it on in the dark. How one feels towards a girl when pulling it out of one's pocket, etc.

This realism is part of sex education. It is the condition that has to be met for sex education to succeed.

Realism also includes conversations on the age of starting sexual activity. Boys have to know that they are not particularly late and that most boys have a sporadic sex life in their teens. Only a small number enter into a steady relationship.

They also have to know that both young boys and adult men can find that sexual intercourse can happen too quickly, that they may not have time to enjoy it themselves before it is over. It is not just the girl who feels cheated. The boy can too. As an adult man, one can also talk about what can be done about it. One can talk about what one has done oneself – when one was young and later on. In our time, we were told to think about icebergs, barbed wire or multiplication tables during intercourse – but perhaps this was not the best answer to the problem.

Learning to masturbate is an integral part of a boy's development to becoming a man. Masturbation is also a way for a boy to learn his intercourse cycle. My experience is that masturbation is far from being as great a source of anxiety today as it was in previous generations. Over the years I have been talking to boys, I have found a great many synonyms and slang words for masturbation. There is great fun about the whole topic, which suggests that the act itself is not particularly associated with shame.

There is shame about sexual fantasies and infantile aggression and dreams in relation to girls and women, something which one would never consider talking about with any other person. This is also one of the limits to conversation on sex.

There are several such limits, and they are all concerned with not exposing another person to enforced frankness. Sexuality must be respected as a deep personal urge, a way to independence and maturity, a secret world which precisely by virtue of its closed nature, gives strength and an experience of being a personality.

Love itself is nevertheless still taboo. Let the girls chat about it and the boys shout. The boys can be dirty but not tender-hearted, at any rate, not in front of their friends. It is also a fact that most boys of this age perhaps have not been in love at all, not in such an overwhelming way that it feels as though they cannot think of anything but the girl. They may perhaps have fantasized but have not had their love requited – not dared to. And the lives of many boys are marked with feelers put out, signals sent and attempts at making contact. What does one do to make contact with girls? This is one of the most important questions. The answer is found when one sits down together with a group of grown men and talks. None of these men, or perhaps one, has been particularly good at this with girls. And everyone thinks that everyone else is far better.

When one nevertheless falls in love, it is a great thing which affects oneself as a man, and sex education is then meaningless. It is for this reason that we must inform beforehand, talk beforehand, so that sense is also retained when one falls madly in love. Boys and girls need both male and female experiences on this.

We not only talk about all this when we train adult men who are to talk to teenage boys, but also about the love and sexuality we are living with right now.

Many people think they have to be good at sex to teach about sexuality, but this is not the case. What is important to pass on to boys in their teens is that we live a long life – certain periods without any partner, other periods with one. I usually show the young boys my one life-line, how I have lived during the different parts of my life. This too can show that love and sexuality are not a utopian striving for something which has to be as good as possible, but a reflection of our life and our past.

The position of women in our society

by Elvira Lutz

Women's sexuality has never been their own to experience by themselves and for themselves. So it is hardly surprising that we have to wait until the second half of the twentieth century for the first references to be made to women's right to sexual pleasure and for people to begin to talk – even if only timidly – about women's inalienable sexual rights. Inalienable rights they may be, but they are rights which are universally alienated.

Twenty-five centuries of puritan education have prevented women from developing the kind of sexual response of which they are potentially capable – and which is biologically equivalent to a man's.

Women's sexual problems are not individual but social, not biological but ideological, not a problem related to health or illness but to politics.

So-called 'female frigidity' is not an illness; it is the result of a female stereotype which is fabricated by a repressive society through two instruments that oppress and discriminate against women:

- the double standard of socially acceptable sexual behaviour, and
- the different rules on sexual morality which are used to educate girls and boys.

Years of struggle by the women's liberation movement throughout the world have opened up new areas of participation. We must not underestimate the achievements which have been made in education, employment, social affairs, economics and politics. But at a sexual level, the traditional roles remain untouched. The lack of genuine sexual freedom continues to make women second-class citizens, always pitifully dependent on men.

Genuine sexual freedom for women will only become a reality when they no longer have to provide compulsory sexual services, when sex is no longer a marital duty imposed by law, religion or society. When women can say yes or no, now, later, or never.

True liberation is not found in elitist and individualistic sex therapy that teaches us multiple orgasms. It is not found in the alienation of promiscuity as a replacement for the puritan alienation in which we were trapped.

When Latin American women assume their sexual identity, when they decide to be themselves and want to control their own sexuality, they become threatening – not just for men, but also for many women who judge them harshly as being unfeminine, pushy, too independent and over-ambitious.

It is interesting to see how even the most progressive and radical men and women are still infected by the virus of male chauvinism. Even though most of them say they want women's liberation, there is always a condition that it shouldn't go too far. And for them liberation always goes too far if it involves sexual freedom, questions traditional sexual roles or threatens to make men and women equal in erotic and sexual matters.

Even the most radical progressives still educate their children in the double standards. They still worry if their daughters start to be sexually active too early or if their sons delay their first male 'performance' too long. Deep down they don't want them to be equal, but different, so that they can adapt and be successful in a discriminatory world.

Male and female sexuality is not something which exists, but something which develops. It is created gradually through the educational models we come into contact with each day, and it is branded by the ideology of the teachers. Obviously, these models conform to the expectations of those who hold the power – men.

Paradoxically, or maybe not so paradoxically, it is women who are given the unfortunate task of passing on male chauvinist ideology to boys and girls. It is women in the role of mothers, aunts, sisters, grandmothers, neighbours, teachers and domestic servants who, as victims and accomplices of men, are responsible for passing on and strengthening male privilege and for praising girls who show traditional female virtues. They are the ones who venerate us for being 'delightfully' submissive and dependent. This is the educational influence which is passed on to us and which we pass on ourselves, convinced that we are doing our best.

It is through this unobserved, behind-the-scenes process that our private lives lay the foundations for our public and political lives. By being forced to relegate anything sexual and erotic to the sphere of personal intimacy and to the modesty of our private lives, we have been prevented from seeing sex as it really is: as an essential component in the use and abuse of power and a collective and political problem.

Women have been locked away in their intimate, private lives whereas men have grown up used to playing a leading role and taking chances. Women have been condemned to the constrictions of family routines, to looking after the children, preparing meals and serving in bed. And they still carry on preparing meals, looking after the children and serving in bed, even though their status is now apparently equal to men's educationally, professionally, scientifically, artistically and politically. They pay an exorbitant price for this 'equal status' through a double or even triple working day.

This narrow domestic and domesticizing world has made women conservative, over-protective and afraid of anything that might involve risk and adventure. It has turned us into the natural bearers of an ideology based on stability, fear of change, conformism and servitude.

If this is the case, and there is no reason for us to feel guilty, we are justified in asking: What if we were to wake up to our role as 'conscience builders' and take advantage of the power we have to change the world instead of letting it carry on as before? What would happen if we were to say 'enough!' and started to walk on our own?

Roger Garandy said that 'no one can be liberated on their own or just in their thoughts'. We become liberated with other people and by taking action.

Therefore, it is not enough for women to become gender conscious and class conscious. We will also have to learn the hard lesson of solidarity towards our own sex. Men will respect us when we begin to command respect. And we will command respect not only when we become aware, but when we unite and organize as a movement, when we have undermined rivalry through solidarity.

Translation from Spanish by
Ruth Mahnen.

Issues in women's perception of AIDS risk and risk reduction activities

by Vickie M. Mays and Susan D. Cochran

Perceiving AIDS risk

Despite the increasing attention focused on AIDS, women may not consider their own personal risks to be high for several reasons. Most women, particularly when their life reality is that of being poor, from an ethnic minority, or outside the law through drug abuse or prostitution, have always lived with risks of some kind. AIDS is simply one more risk with which to be concerned. These women have long histories of facing omnipresent dangers not often experienced by the middle class and mustering what scarce resources exist to cope with these dangers.

The key to their response to AIDS is their perception of its danger relative to the hierarchy of other risks present in their lives and the existence of resources available to act differently. Competition for these women's attention includes more immediate survival needs, such as obtaining shelter for the night, securing personal safety or safety of their children, or interfacing with the governmental system in order to obtain financial resources. For women who often, realistically, feel powerless to change the external realities of their lives – where they live, how much they earn, or the system's rules for getting financial supplements – AIDS may be of relatively low concern. In addition, even if AIDS is perceived as a relevant danger, women may not readily have the means to reduce their risk.

Encouraging risk reduction

Behavioural scientists have known for some time that people are more likely to engage in a target behaviour if the information is not presented in an overly fear-arousing manner. Rather it is important to present individuals with concrete steps that can be taken on their own behalf. This lessens the likelihood of engaging in denial, adopting a fatalistic attitude, or dismissing the information. The lesson was well learned in the educational campaigns directed at gay men. Many of these interventions, rather than insisting on abstinence, promoted lower-risk safer sex and emphasized new, substitute activities.

These same principles of specifically tailoring advice to the cultural and political realities of the target community are essential for risk reduction interventions aimed at women. Yet women are asked to engage in safer sex when they may not know or understand what safer sex is because the preventive messages have been much too complicated. For instance, women are asked to 'negotiate' safer sex contracts in relationships when some may not understand the word 'negotiate'. But women do understand male-female relationships within their own communities. Despite risk reduction advice to 'talk to their prospective partners', a rather middle-class notion, poor women may not bother to ask men about previous sexual or drug-use behaviours because they know the men will lie or discount the risk.

Women are advised to have one lifelong sexual partner, although they may live in a community with a high sex-ratio imbalance and instability of relationships. Should a woman fail at her latest relationship, is she to conclude that another involvement this year would mean that she has had multiple partners? Messages in the USA, for example, that advocate monogamy, when 65 per cent of black women, 47 per cent of Latina women and 43 per cent of white women over age 15 are not currently married, ignore the social and contextual reality of their lives.

Developers of risk-reduction messages may be taking a friendship-like model of love relationships, a model based more on power equality, and imposing it as the foundation for their advice. In friendship-based love relationships, honesty and disclosure are valued. However, there are other models of relationships, ones where past sexual behaviours or relationships are expected to be kept secret until the relationship has been well established.

It is wise to remember that poor people do not always have the luxury of honesty, which is much easier when there is sufficient money and resources to guide one's choices. When a poor, ethnic minority woman meets a man of unknown background whose current presentation appears to be that of a clean-cut, upwardly mobile man, she does not ask questions. A prior jail term, so much more common for poor and ethnic minority men, may have involved same-sex consensual activities or rape. Or there may have been drug addiction in a man's past because drug addiction is a widespread problem in the poor ethnic community.

Equally possible is that a woman may conceal her own background. In a *New York Times* article in 1987, one drug-addicted woman acknowledged that although she had her partners use condoms and practised safer sex, she had not told her current boyfriend that she had AIDS. Cognizant that this omission might cost her the relationship, her hope was that the relationship would be strong enough to continue once he became aware of her illness. Having lost an earlier prospective boyfriend after disclosing her illness, she had learned to conceal this information because, in her own words, she 'can barely imagine life without a man'. For some women, the risk of being alone and unsuccessful in relationships may seem greater than the risk of having or transmitting HIV.

However, there are other ways of structuring AIDS prevention messages that may prove more effective. This involves incorporating two dimensions into current activities. First, in targeting behaviours for change, it is important that the origins of those behaviours be understood from both an individual and socio-cultural perspective. What is the role of community norms? How will behaviour change affect economic or emotional support within relationship or family units?

Second, prevention approaches need to focus comprehensively on the individual as a responsible member of a social or familial network. Culturally-based values of co-operation and unity may be more powerful motivators of behaviour change than strict appeals to individualistic action, such as 'protect yourself'.

All of these values can readily be incorporated into AIDS risk reduction messages. For example, one model of AIDS education that appears effective in changing attitudes and behaviours in some communities is an appeal based on responsibility to others in the community. Men are asked to practise safer sex in order to survive as a needed father or support for their parents. Women are asked to be more assertive regarding condom use in order to stay alive to take care of their parents and children. Possibly men and women could be encouraged to practise risk reduction in order to ensure the existence of the community and to build a future for others. This approach is based on a model of social responsibility rather than individualistic preservation.

Involving the community

Community and normative pressures on individuals' sexual and drug-related behaviours may be seen initially as problematic. For example, conservative religious beliefs and important church affiliations can be viewed by AIDS educators as impediments to AIDS-related education and risk reduction activities.

This is because some risk reduction messages clash with the theology of particular denominations. An often used AIDS risk reduction message is that of 'Play it safe'. The assumption here is that sex is play, fun, or a leisure activity. However, within most religions, sex is viewed as behaviour sanctioned by God for procreation. Religious beliefs that reject the use of condoms on the grounds that the purpose of sex is not recreation may frustrate some AIDS educators.

To some extent, though, this frustration may stem from an overdependency on using churches as the major site for programmes and a failure to plan multilevel interventions. Those churchgoers who cannot learn about condoms within the context of church-sponsored AIDS education should, none the less, be able to receive this information from their local pharmacist, through television and radio public service announcements, or from community outreach workers in, for example, the local beauty shop. It is important to work within the natural context of the community.

Churches can still provide needed supports for both those who are attempting to reduce their risk of getting AIDS and others who are directly affected by the HIV epidemic, including caretakers, orphaned children, and the sick. Among terminal illnesses, AIDS is a particularly treacherous and stressful one. The emotional and tangible resources of the community of churchgoers may assume increasing importance as the epidemic spreads in ethnic minority communities.

Recommendations

It is necessary that public-health officials interpret the risk of AIDS to women in a manner that is understandable, relevant, and effective. AIDS messages may best be delivered by individuals with whom women can identify. Although most women view health care professionals as credible sources, they may dismiss, not the facts of their messages, but the personal relevance. Health care professionals have long been associated with other risk messages (e.g. smoking, obesity, cardiovascular diseases) that carry warnings of death.

Results from smoking cessation research provide some evidence for the effectiveness of messages when they are delivered by a credible source, targeted at a specific audience, and combined with community and peer support. Although AIDS risk behaviours differ, the same principles appear to be effective in campaigns aimed at gay men. For drug users, the effective message carriers appear to be other users or ex-users; for sex workers, it may be other sex workers or ex-sex workers.

Condoms, yes, but why?

by Susan D. Cochran

A working-class black woman in her late 30s, whom I was seeing for therapy began a dating relationship with a black man in his early 50s. As a single mother with many pressing financial debts, she currently views her relationships with men as falling into one of two camps. The first is a romantic, idealized relationship where she is sexually and emotionally attracted to the man and seeks permanency of the relationship for these emotional reasons. The second type of relationship, more commonly experienced by her, is simply pragmatic. In the latter relationship, she generally is not especially attracted to the man himself but feels that he will spend money on her, perhaps give her money to spend on herself, or provide assistance in raising her young daughter. Her desires for financial support include help in paying for extensive car repairs, long-standing credit-card debts, and the monthly rent on her apartment. These are in addition to expenses associated with dating, such as dinners out and movies.

Over the past eight months she has had several brief relationships of mostly the pragmatic kind and is grateful when her partner suggests using a condom, although often he will do so in a way that makes her feel accused of being diseased or someone he does not care about very much. Her interests in condom use are more for contraception than HIV prevention, although she acknowledges that it is probably good to prevent catching something she does not need to be bothered with. But she does not insist on condom use

for two reasons. She feels it is the man's responsibility, and she is concerned that he may have a negative reaction if she suggests using condoms. From her perspective, there is no possibility that she has HIV. Her only concern is that the romantically exciting men she dates are infected.

Her relationship with this new man fell into the second category of pragmatic dating. She very quickly reassured herself that he was not HIV infected by bringing up the general topic of homosexuality and watching his reaction to it. He displayed no interest either way, saying whatever those people do is their own business. His strategy with her was also indirect, although more awkward. Soon after they began going out, he handed her a letter. In the letter, he brought up the issue of AIDS and sexual histories, and closed by citing the US Surgeon General's advice that it never hurts to ask. The letter itself was fairly inarticulate and angered her because it demonstrated his ineptitude in dating. She told him if he wanted to use a condom then he should, much to his apparent relief.

The story, however does not end there. After a couple of months of getting to know her better as a person, he decided that she was safe and asked to have unprotected intercourse. At the time, she was coming to see that his financial help was going to be more tenuous than she had hoped for, while his demands on her for emotional support were more than she wanted to give. She refused, in punishment for his earlier letter. Thus, for the time being, at least, these two individuals continue to practice safer sex although not for reasons motivated by prevention concerns.

One is left to contemplate what this man will do with his next sexual partner. The odds are slim that he will write another letter and face the wrath of his partner. He may also choose not to talk about safer sex, to avoid committing himself to perpetual condom use if he changes his mind later in the dating relationship.

Black women and AIDS prevention: a view towards understanding the gender rules

by Mindy Thompson Fullilove, Robert E. Fullilove, Katherine Hayes and Shirley Gross

Despite the complex issues surrounding sexuality, the research examining the sex lives of black women [in the USA] has been confined largely to the study of the sexual activity and contraceptive use of teenage girls. For example, of 191 articles devoted to an examination of black sexuality and published between 1964 and 1989, only 22 per cent were concerned with adults; 42 per cent with pre-teens and teenagers, and an additional 28 per cent with both. One-third of the articles examined issues of contraception.

This rather narrowly focused research effort has established that:
- black heterosexual teenagers initiate sexual intercourse at an earlier age than white teenagers,
- they are less likely to know about and use contraception than white teenagers, and
- they wait for a longer period of time between initiating sex and initiating contraception.

This literature describes significant gender differences in attitudes toward sexual behaviour and sexual activity. Black boys and men have attitudes toward sexuality that differ sharply from those of black girls and women. Men are more 'permissive', that is, they are more likely to endorse pre-marital sexual relations than women are. Men are more oriented toward the erotic, the enjoyment of the physical aspects of sex, while women are more oriented toward the romantic, that is, sex as part of love and marriage. The sexual behaviours of the genders also differ: black men have more sexual partners and are more likely to have sex outside of marriage than women.

Information is lacking, however, about such basic issues as: What sexual practices are engaged in and preferred by black women at various phases of the life cycle? How do black couples negotiate meeting potential sexual partners and initiating sexual relations? What is the impact of drug use on a woman's sexual behaviour?

Open discussion of sexuality is common in the black community. This is evidenced in the music – traditional blues, jazz as well as contemporary rap music – and in the literature. In community settings such as barbershops, beauty parlours and bars, sex is a frequent topic of conversation. The common profane language in the black community is concerned with sexual activity. Talking about sex is important and commonplace. This rich source of information about sexuality has particular relevance for AIDS prevention and education because the dialogue about AIDS must be incorporated into these natural conversations about sex.

We asked working-class and lower-income black women and teenage girls to participate in group discussions of sexuality. The conversations contained vivid descriptions of sex and its meaning for black women. Our major focus was an examination of the rules defining gender behaviour, that is, the rules that define 'what a woman does' (both in terms of sexual and non-sexual behaviour) as opposed to 'what a man does', information that is critical to the development of effective AIDS prevention for black women.

Six groups met for two hours each on one occasion. Nine adult women and nineteen teenage girls participated. The groups ranged in size from two to eight women.

Sexual roles and their impact on behaviour

Participants described two sexual roles for women. The 'good girl/madonna' role was consistent with serial monogamy. The 'bad girl/whore' role was characterized by simultaneous multiple sexual relationships. Though similar to stereotypes described in many cultures, the definition of the 'bad girl/whore' did not include participation in pre-marital sex, an activity that was ubiquitous among respondents. Rather, the following criteria defined a 'bad girl':

- sexual aggression;
- giving sex in a casual manner without regard

for who the partner was or requiring anything of the relationship;
- giving sex in exchange for money or drugs.

Gender roles appeared to be closely related to sexual practices. For example, one woman said that in an earlier historical period, only 'bad' girls were expected to enjoy sex. In contrast, the women made it clear that taking pleasure was no longer taboo, but taboos as a method of defining sex roles had not disappeared. One woman related that her sexual overtures made her husband uncomfortable because he felt that a man should initiate it, but then they talked and decided it was no problem. Another said a lot of black men have that problem.

The definition of 'respectable' is critical to these sexual roles. Teenage girls maintained their own respectability by being faithful to a teenage boy in spite of his unfaithfulness to her. In that situation, her respectability was not threatened by his infidelity: the behaviour of each was sanctioned by the double standard. For others, working from a monogamous norm, the acceptance of a male partner's infidelity was looked upon with scorn.

It was clear that women, as well as teenagers, differed in their willingness to accept a sexual double standard.

A woman who is abused by her lover(s) is not respected. But, the loss of respect does not imply that the woman is 'bad' or 'wild' but rather that she is pitiful or to be pitied.

The ultimate loss of respect for self and from others appeared to be related to addiction to crack, a smokable form of cocaine. One teenage girl described girls she had seen who would do anything for drugs.

The teenage girls used the term 'tossup' to describe this exchange of sex for drugs, though the term could also be used to refer to a person who moved casually from partner to partner.

The easy availability to men of these alternative partners was a constant source of tension for women and for teenage girls. The tossup, though outside the woman's sphere of influence or control, is clearly a part of her life: even some of the more stable relationships were affected by the outside sexual activities of the male partner. Two young pregnant teenage girls, recently diagnosed with gonorrhoea, bemoaned that their partners had not even worried about 'bringing disease home to the baby'.

These stereotyped roles also affected sexual practices. 'Whores/tossups' were expected to participate in the more taboo sexual practices. This was expressed by the teenagers as 'things you don't do with your steady partner, just with a tossup'. For women and teenage girls in this study – none of whom admitted to 'tossing' – vaginal sex with the man on top was by far the dominant mode of sexual expression. Participants referred to this practice as 'normal sex'. Many had participated in cunnilingus and fellatio, but a much smaller number reported enjoying these practices. One woman described:

'I have a real problem with just the thought of putting my mouth on a man's penis knowing that the penis was in somebody else's vagina. So I would probably have to have a very, very, very close relationship. With love, you can do a lot of things that you wouldn't be able to do.'

Study staff knew participants in other contexts and were aware that they actually had participated in 'tossing'. The fact that the participants could not say this in public reflects the public scorn for this activity.

Masturbation was reported commonly, though again, hesitation was noted in some of the descriptions. In particular, women noted that having an orgasm felt incomplete if it took place out of the context of sexual communication with another person. None of the respondents reported anal sex, group sex, or same-sex sexual activity.

What was perhaps most striking was the extent to which participants of all ages saw sex as the consummation of a relationship, not as an isolated pleasure-giving act.

Sexual knowledge and communication

Sexual knowledge was acquired through family, friends, and school-based education. The participants varied in their mastery of the subject matter. Some of the confusion about STDs and AIDS is created by the unclear manner in which the material is presented. One woman told a story about trying to learn how you get pregnant.

'I know when we started having sex education I was in junior high school and we had to watch this cartoon. OK. I had more questions after I watched the movie than I had before. It was like, OK, if a girl has her period, OK, but how does she actually get pregnant? When I went home, my mother pulled out this big old book, dated 1958. OK. And she showed me a picture of a uterus. OK, fine, I saw that in the movie. But how do you get pregnant?'

The failure of school and parents to provide clear communication appears to be closely linked to the fear that clear communication will violate social taboos.

Condom use is an important behaviour for examining communication patterns. Condoms are only indirectly used by a woman. Rather, what women do is request that a man use a condom in the sexual encounter. Communication with the sexual partner emerged as central to the woman's ability to protect herself from infection, but the ability to negotiate the finer points of sex varied considerably.

Some women were remarkably poised. One teenage girl said:

'Before I'm in a relationship, you gotta tell

me your life story. I gotta see what I feel about you and then it's up to me . . . But we gotta talk. We just can't rush into things . . . Because that's where you get the most pain and catch a lot of stuff, if you rush into things.'

But for most, the communication was complicated by planning, trust and fear. Where there was deep trust, women were willing to 'take a chance'. Where the trust was not established or had been eroded, women tended to ask – however ambivalently – for condoms to be used. One woman demanded condom use when she wanted to punish her husband for coming home late.

Planning was important in condom use. One woman – one of the few who always used condoms – said that they were like her credit card, she didn't leave home without one in her bag. A teenage girl, in describing why teens do not use condoms, suggested, 'Sometimes you'll be in the mood and a condom won't be right there and you think, so what. I guess that's it.' The teens also suggested that lowering the price would make it easier to have condoms around.

None of the participants expressed a fear of raising the question of condom use with a man, though this does not imply that fear did not exist. An indirect indicator of fear was the women's awareness of date and marital rape. One woman described, 'Just having an encounter with someone and I'm saying no and they're persisting, it's just devastating.' Another woman added, 'It's not uncommon, I believe, it probably happens in 90 per cent of marriages and relationships where women live alone. I know it's very common for a husband to force his wife to have sex and think nothing of it.'

Several factors were noted to be related to power in sexual communication. The older women were clear that their ability to communicate with men had changed as they had matured. With experience, they had become clearer about what was acceptable and what was not. One woman noted:

'I would say for most, almost exclusively, of the years that I was sexually active, I more or less would just go along. I always felt cheated. The last couple of years, the person I'm with now, I talk about up, down, in and out, everything. So, it's not a problem. And I have noticed a big change when you can do that. Especially when they respond and start satisfying you.'

None of the participants in any of these groups discussed the relationship between physical beauty and sexual power. But it is perhaps relevant that those most confident about making demands on men were also pretty. By contrast, the most helpless girl, who had got gonorrhoea from her boyfriend five times, was overweight and appeared depressed. Throughout the group, this young woman looked at the floor, gave monosyllabic answers to questions, and had a sad look on her face. At the end of the session she finally made eye contact with the leader of the group and said that she always found it hard to talk.

This was an important call for help. She acknowledged her helplessness and her despair to others. The leader and another participant responded to her need. This exchange, however fleeting and tentative, carries the most important AIDS prevention message we found: in the group process a high-risk participant was able to address her vulnerability.

Changing times

The teenage girls had a sharp awareness of the epidemic levels of drugs in their neighbourhoods. They all knew friends who had 'gotten into trouble' with drugs: all expressed the sense that drugs were 'everywhere'. Several girls had friends who had been pregnant at young ages but had their babies taken away by children's protective services because they were addicted to crack. The absence of drugs as part of the teenage experience of the older women was in stark contrast to the central role drugs were playing in the lives of the teenage girls, and has marked implications for the spread of AIDS.

Discussion

As we promote AIDS prevention for black women, AIDS educators are proceeding from a model of ideal attitudes and behaviours. In this model, a woman who was able to protect herself from infection would:

• insist on condom use with her partners,
• reject the double standard as applied to herself or other women, and communicate clearly about sexual issues.

In addition, others around her would also practise ideal behaviours such as:

• teachers and parents would provide explicit information about sexuality;
• men would not base their behaviour on the double standard;
• female-controlled barrier protection would be introduced, and
• condom/barrier-protection use would be adopted as a community standard.

There is a broad gap between these hypothesized ideals and many of the real experiences related in the groups. A key issue emerges here: to what extent are women responsible for their own plight? Women in the groups underscored that some women 'have to have a man' and will accept a relationship at any price. While the inability to 'just say no' contributes to the maintenance of the imbalance in male-female relationships, this female powerlessness is best understood in the larger context of change in the black community.

As participants noted, there have been dramatic changes in the black community in the past decade. What one participant noted as 'respect that used to exist for black women does not exist any more' is a poignant expression of a complex reality. The very dramatic increase in male unemployment is closely tied to increasing imbalance between the number of marriageable men – that is, men who are heterosexual, employed, and not incarcerated – to marriageable women. The decline in the stability of adult relationships – as measured by out-of-wedlock births, divorces, families headed by one parent, or other markers – implies a concomitant instability in adult sexual relationships, with people establishing and re-establishing sexual partnerships. The increased pace of entry and exit from the 'available partner pool' has obvious implications for the spread of sexually transmitted disease. What is less obvious, but equally important, is the extent to which gender-based behaviour will regulate risk for infection.

Two suggestions emerge as critical rate-limiting factors in the spread of infection. First, although the black community has a vital public dialogue about sex, the private, intimate conversations between an individual man and an individual woman may be less open and less forthright. Negotiating condom use, for example, is highly emotionally charged for casual as well as stable partners. Second, women and men enter into these negotiations from distinctly different power bases. Recent changes have undermined the economic standing of black men but, paradoxically, have increased their power in relationships with women. Men, oriented towards erotic fulfilment, are more able to satisfy themselves. Women, oriented towards romantic attachment, are less able to attach to a man who can meet that need.

This analysis suggests that women and men are acting/reacting in a context of community disintegration, in which men have been empowered to have greater sexual freedom, but women have lost ground in their ability to insist on protection from infection. The deeply challenging problem of intimate, sexual communication is heightened by these imbalances in gender-based power. This has several implications.

First, AIDS prevention cannot be left to 'messages', however cleverly designed. The issue is not the development of a mutually acknowledged message (e.g. 'just say no') but rather of a means of communicating that will empower women to negotiate with men how, and under what circumstances, sexual activity and relationships will be conducted. It is person-to-person and group-to-group contact that offers the best hope for change in power-related communication behaviours. Individuals, in conversation with others, must begin to acknowledge the choices they are making and critically examine their strategies for survival. At the heart of such preventions is the development of explicit communication, free of jargon and ambivalence, set in a context in which black women are again restored to a position of respect.

Is AIDS prevention unrealistic? We think not. In fact, there are many such efforts in evidence around the country. For example, at Montefiore Hospital [in New York], a group of women drug users have met in a drop-in group which has given them a place to discuss AIDS prevention and other life problems. In San Francisco, outreach workers take AIDS-prevention messages to the streets in an effort to reach out-of-treatment populations. In Cincinnati, health educators and community leaders have begun to train teenagers to become peer counsellors and AIDS educators in their own communities.

What is critical about these programmes is not the content of the information but the use of social organizations to intervene, to recreate human contact in the face of community disintegration. The re-knitting of community connections renews the power base that women must have in order to build equitable, protective relationships with men.

Sex work and personal life

by Sophie Day and Helen Ward

This study consisted of unstructured, informal interviews with 148 sex workers who attended the Praed Street Clinic at St Mary's Hospital in London for screening and treatment of STDs from 1986 to 1988. They ranged in age from 16 to 55 years. Injection drugs were used by 7.4 per cent. They had worked as sex workers for 1 month to 27 years and in the week before their first visit to the clinic had seen from none to 70 clients each.

The women described themselves as 'business girls' or 'working girls' and invariably stressed that the exchange of sex for money was 'work'. Many stressed the service aspect of their work, suggesting that they stopped men from raping other women or kept marriages intact. Some, usually those who worked as escorts, described themselves primarily as companions or hostesses. Others presented themselves as counsellors, social workers and sex therapists. Such arguments do not seek only to establish sex work as work but as an essential service.

The women originated from eleven different countries and a wide range of work places and socio-economic backgrounds. They rarely worked together. Indeed, one of the more important aspects of sex work in London is an enforced isolation at the work place.

Condoms were associated with 'work' among this group. Certain sexual activities were distinguished by means of condom use and turned into 'work' that had no relationship with a personal or private sex life. One young woman's comments about her work on the street were typical: 'I always use a sheath. I'd commit suicide if I didn't. But I don't use anything else, I couldn't prevent nature.' Other women mentioned a range of protective devices, including at times, a diaphragm, spermicides, and the oral contraceptive pill as well as a condom. One woman reported that she always put two condoms on her clients, and that they 'never noticed'. She was currently seriously considering using three condoms during each client contact in order to protect herself from AIDS.

The women often stated that they regarded semen as 'dirty'. Both semen and any organisms it might carry were rejected. However, it was only clients who had 'dirty semen' and it was substances associated with work that must be kept outside their bodies.

A number of women said that condoms protected them from STDs in general and not just HIV infection. They were particularly worried about infections that might cause infertility. More generally, however, condoms provide a means of keeping clients at a distance and making sex at work distinct from sex outside work.

If condom use with clients makes sex into work, it is the absence of condom use with boyfriends that makes this kind of sex a private affair. Little condom use was reported with boyfriends, except when related to changes of partner and concerns about possible infections. Condoms were also used for contraception. High and increasing rates of condom use at work contrast with little or no use outside work. Eighty-two per cent reported no condom use at all in their private lives.

Many women were horrified at the thought of using condoms with their private (non-paying) partners. Most said that their relationships would be finished:

'We have a very good sex life. It would be spoilt if he wore a sheath. We would be finished.'

'I don't want strangers' semen inside. I only drop the barrier with someone I really love.'

'How could I? He would be like a client. It's different for people who don't work.'

Much research with female sex workers has focused only on the domain of work. However, women's private lives are equally important. It may be more relevant to consider sex workers' non-working lives, which are not associated with high rates of partner change or directly with the sale of sex, but which commonly involve unprotected sex. Many women attending the clinic with infections immediately attributed them to their private partners. Approximately half of the women with boyfriends reported that they knew these men had other sexual partners with whom, it was suspected, condoms were not used.

One woman had moved from soliciting on streets to advertising and working in a flat because it was safer. She currently uses two condoms each time for penetrative sex and one for 'hand relief' (masturbation of the man). She engaged only in safer sex with her clients. She commented:

'It's all right for you [the interviewer]. You don't work with a hundred condoms by the bed, six days a week. How could I use condoms outside work? . . . The mere thought of putting a condom on a boyfriend or watching him put it on leaves me cold. I'd rather not have sex.'

In fact this woman later left her boyfriend because he had other sexual partners. She had not had a sexual relationship outside work in the previous four months. Celibacy proved a more palatable alternative than the use of condoms outside work.

There is a third type of sexual partner, in between the casual or new client and the private partner. This is the 'regular client' who pays to see the same woman repeatedly. Regular clients play a central role in a sex worker's career. With 'regulars', women are assured of an income. Moreover, they can begin to establish themselves as self-employed businesswomen rather than employees. Money is frequently evaluated in a very different way from the transactions that occur with casual or new clients. Sometimes, regulars do not pay. On other occasions, they agree to meet expenses such as rent, private medical bills, or school fees.

Regular clients may also be involved in women's personal lives. Indeed, a small number of women have turned regular clients into private partners. One is now married to an ex-client. In such relationships, women do not see themselves as sex workers.

It is possible that the development of alternative distinctions between different types of sexual activity might make it easier for women to introduce condoms into non-working relationships. Some women did not sell penetrative sex but instead catered for a variety of fantasies, domination, and masturbation. Most women restricted the types of sex which they sold at work. Thus no one in the cohort was currently selling passive anal sex at the end of 1988. If these other distinctions were developed, condoms might become less central to the demarcation between work and the rest of life. It is possible also that different types of condoms might come to stand for different relationships.

Empowerment through risk reduction workshops

by Brooke Grundfest Schoepf, with Walu Engundu, Rukarangira wa Nkera, Payanzo Ntsomo and Claude Schoepf

CONNAISSIDA Zaïre's action-research workshops engaged women residents of a low-income community, with little or no literacy, in a problem-solving approach to risk reduction. The workshop design uses active learning methods, including role plays, simple posters, small group discussions and structured group 'processing' to demonstrate to participants their own ability to reduce their risk of AIDS. Didactic presentations are kept to a minimum.

The workshop leaders (or trainers) do not give advice. Instead, they promote the search for solutions appropriate to the participants' lifestyles.

Grounded in principles of group dynamics, experiential training begins with the principle that people already know a great deal about their situation. Group leaders assist people to develop a 'critical consciousness' leading to cooperative social action and self-reliance. While some risk reduction strategies, including individual counselling, tend to stress 'responsibilization' of individuals at high risk, the training strategy aims to develop participants personal power. In this case, power is defined as the capacity to control risky situations.

In the case of women, and especially in the case of sex workers who have experienced social stigma, feelings of powerlessness, and low self-worth, telling people how they 'should' act is tantamount to blaming them for their predicament. Instead of focusing on behaviour that cannot be altered in present circumstances, experiential training helps people to discover what they can do to make their situation somewhat better in the short term. While the method concentrates on self-empowerment, it also can be used to initiate and sustain other types of socially transformative change. The need to increase feelings of personal competence and to minimize anxiety and guilt, with their resulting denial, blame-casting and avoidance, was identified from data contributed by women with multiple partners and others.

The first workshops were conducted with a network of fifteen sex workers. The women report serving between five and forty clients per working week. They charge very low fees and have had recurrent bouts of STDs. In July 1987, most recognized that their activities place them at high risk for AIDS. However, with no other way to support themselves and their dependents, their attitudes included apathy, fatalism and denial. By October 1987, their awareness of AIDS had grown, partly as a result of the national mass media campaign. Their existential dilemma could no longer be denied. As the national campaign against AIDS became more visible the women reported that neighbours had begun pointing hostilely at them as 'disease distributors'. The leader of the network asked CONNAISSIDA to provide the group with information on AIDS prevention. We held the sessions in a private garden, some 500 yards from their homes. Four morning workshops were held in late October and early November.

An initial role play served as an 'ice-breaker'. It portrays a male visitor who fails to recognize that the woman who welcomes him to her village is a chief. The women immediately saw the visitor's problem and laughed at him. Participants were asked to describe what they had seen, heard and felt. They remarked that women's responsibilities often go unrecognized. Applying this insight to AIDS, they concluded that they must take care not to become infected because AIDS is fatal and others, including children, siblings and elderly parents, depend on them for support.

Other exercises show how HIV progressively attacks the body's defences against disease. Role plays demonstrate transmission routes and social situations that involve risk. A dramatization of pregnancy-related transmission elicited strong emotional reaction.

AIDS prevention was addressed in a broader community-health context, which helps to remove some of the stigma and guilt associated with sexual transmission. For example, we include ways to prevent malaria, as one means to reduce the need for blood transfusions among anaemic children. Sterilization of needles and syringes also is addressed, since poor people cannot afford to purchase disposables for each injection. Role playing helps women to check on hygiene standards in local dispensaries. The experience is empowering and will help to reduce risk of other infections.

An entire session was devoted to familiarization with condoms, demystifying what is to most an unfamiliar, uncongenial, unnatural, unwanted foreign technology. The group consumes soft drinks together. A trainer produces a box of condoms and irreverently displays one on her forearm. The condoms are passed around and each participant rolls one over her empty soft-drink bottle. Some break, giving rise to jokes which provide opportunities for further teaching. In the ensuing role play, a sex worker shows a reluctant client how to use a condom, using her powers of seduction to eroticize the situation and overcome his resistance. The women take home condoms to try before the next workshop, during which they share their experiences with trainers and the group.

When a local Protestant Mothers' Club learned of CONNAISSIDA's workshops for sex workers, they requested that we come to their church to hold workshops, which we did. In this group we began by exploring the wider health context and then took up sexual transmission. We added a role play to help wives persuade husbands to remain at home instead of accompanying their friends to bars where they buy beer and sexual adventures. The drama enacted by participants showed how male peer-group pressures work to prevent behaviour change. This role play has proved useful in all-male and mixed-sex groups as well. Participants decided that although married women are definitely subordinate within the household, the wife-and-mother role also provides some opportunities to cajole husbands into dialogue about the need for protecting parents and children. The workshops provided a forum in which to practise communication skills and to develop confidence in parrying male resistance.

The 'condom seduction' was expertly performed by two volunteers: a grandmother who was formerly a professional sex worker acted the reluctant husband. A young sex worker who is a member of the congregation acted the cajoling wife. Their inclusion in the church group taught the research team that categorization of women in mutually exclusive social/sexual status pigeonholes such as 'prostitutes', 'mothers', or 'church members' can be misleading and counter-productive. Negative value judgements and reluctance to be associated with stigmatized social categories hinders people from examining their behaviour and making realistic risk assessments.

In fact, sexual relationships vary according to the circumstances in which women find themselves at different moments in their life careers. Several divorced, abandoned or widowed mothers and their children were receiving alms from the congregation. The Mothers' Club president stressed that dire poverty and lack of economic alternatives made it likely that such women would soon become sex workers. Former sex workers who had attempted to find other means of support also feared that they would be obliged to resume this high-risk occupation. Working with the two groups simultaneously reinforced our conviction that for many poor women, sex work is not a profession but merely a survival strategy resorted to when other strategies fail.

Evaluation

User-focused evaluation meetings held at three and eight months following the risk-reduction workshops sought to discover participants' reactions to the interventions. We asked what changes, if any, had been tried and sustained. At the end of three months, all but one of the sex workers reported using condoms regularly, both those supplied without charge by the project and purchased at the local pharmacy. The non-user reported that a genital ulcer made condom use painful, so we drove her to the hospital, as local dispensaries are without testing facilities. Client acceptance of condoms was reported high. Two women said that they had turned away men who refused condom protection. Their colleagues agreed that this was a wise practice, but that sometimes they needed immediate cash and had no other clients waiting.

Knowledge of condom protection apparently raised the sex workers' status among clients and community residents. Clients were surprised to discover that the women knew about the value of condoms for AIDS prevention. The women felt somewhat less threatened by neighbours. Participants said that they would like the government to provide regular health examinations and testing for HIV infection, so that they might be issued health cards, as had been the case formerly with syphilis and other treatable STDs. They had not grasped the significance of the long latency period of AIDS and the continuing risk of an almost certainly fatal infection. These make such procedures illusory as protective measures in the case of AIDS.

The training was perceived as valuable. Participants asked: 'Can you teach us to do what you do, so that we can inform our colleagues?' Following a practice session the sex workers demonstrated the method to friends. Considerable knowledge about AIDS had been retained. Condoms were made available on a continuing basis and the participants were encouraged to share their knowledge and supplies with others.

At eight months' post-intervention, however, participants reported that condom use had declined from 'almost always' to 'sometimes'. Their confidence in condom protection had waned. Two women said that student clients had told them that the condoms we supplied were outdated. They wanted us to provide a more attractive product called 'Prudence', which had become synonymous with 'condom' among university students.

Still more serious, the sex workers' felt need to use condoms with their multiple partners was undermined. The reasons are complex and indicate the permeability of the local social field to wider influences. The neighbourhood in which the women live and work is situated near the university. Student clients are highly regarded by these poor women, who were born in the interior and have had little or no formal primary education. Studies of knowledge, attitudes and practices among students conducted in May and July 1987 discovered that, like others, they held numerous misconceptions about condoms and that despite knowledge of AIDS as a fatal disease, few had begun to change their behaviour. One year later, some students reported that they avoided sex workers and used condoms with other women. Nevertheless, these students appear to have been a minority.

Like other members of the elite, many university students had read or heard about the April 1988 issue of *Paris-Match* which carried an interview with US sex researcher Jonathan Kolodney. He was quoted as saying that condoms provide incomplete protection from HIV infection. In Kinshasa, this was translated to mean that condoms are useless. A television appearance that same week by the Public Health Department's AIDS coordinator, promoting condom protection, had not prevailed over the authority imputed to the international news media.

The sex workers, in turn, had been misinformed by the students. Like most poor and working-class inhabitants of Kinshasa, they do not own radios or have access to television on a regular basis. The women could not remember having heard anything about AIDS from these sources during the three previous months. Nor can they read newspapers or handbills. Thus, apart from *SIDA*, a record of advice set to music, issued by the popular singer Luambo in May 1987, and the CONNAISSIDA workshops, the grapevine was their principal source of AIDS information. The students were saying: 'No need to use those things!' and the women acted upon this incorrect advice, for they were not ready to lose their preferred clients. This is testimony to the influence of social status as a determinant of popular knowledge.

Sex workers are considered as the major reservoir of AIDS as of other STDs in Africa, as in other parts of the world. Viewed from a different perspective, however, poor sex workers are at higher risk than their student clients. The women serve between 250 and 1,000 clients annually, whereas the students use their services once or twice a month. Condoms are commonly perceived as offering protection for men against women. This stigmatizing gendered perception is involved in many women's refusal of condoms, as we discovered from interviews in many different settings. The young men's disparagement of condoms and the sex workers' acceptance of their authority increases the women's risk. It also underscores the need for activities which can effectively increase their sense of self-worth and over the long term, lead to empowerment.

A third evaluation in early 1990 found that two women in the network had died, reportedly from AIDS. All the survivors reported using condoms in all encounters. They all carried condoms, which they supply if the client does not have his own, or if a second episode takes place during the encounter. They expressed gratitude for CONNAISSIDA's effort, which had enabled them to become aware of HIV risk earlier than most of their colleagues, for whom they had served as sources of information and support.

Empowerment is an issue for the churchwomen as well. One-third of sixty participants reported that their husbands utterly refused to consider using condoms or even to discuss the risks the couple might face.

Some of these were older men. Their wives believed they no longer sought extra-marital sex. Some husbands known to have multiple partners were reported to have responded with anger and hostile threats. For example, one woman said that her spouse refused to give her the monthly housekeeping allowance, telling her to go out and hustle for it.

Another third of the participants reported that they had been able to open a dialogue, but that their husbands had persuaded them that their risks were negligible. Both partners affirmed that they had had no other partners since marriage, or at least not in the past few years. Most of the women in this age group said that they had married in early adolescence and had never had another partner. The final one-third of women said that dialogue had succeeded and their husbands agreed in principle to use condoms. We do not know how many of these couples continued using condoms. Couples in both the second and third groups agreed that their older children needed to be informed and some mothers requested condoms for them.

At the third evaluation in 1990, women whose husbands had refused dialogue earlier continued to do so. However, women with older children had overcome their reluctance to discuss the subject. The workshops and continuing discussions of AIDS among the group had strengthened the mothers' resolve. The husbands did not object.

The churchwomen requested that workshops be organized for husbands, adolescents and young adults living in their households. Several mothers said that they could talk to their sexually active children about AIDS and actually began to supply them with condoms. Most felt constrained by traditional taboos against sharing intimate knowledge between parents and children. This does not mean that there is a blanket taboo across generations. Aunts, uncles and grandparents are considered appropriate instructors by many. However, these relatives may not be present or possess the necessary information. This was the case in elite homes as well, where parents requested that CONNAISSIDA hold workshops for their children and other young people living with them. Family-centred approaches offer ways to teach sexually active adolescents who are neither in school nor regularly employed.

When a new cohort of mothers attended a workshop, the first group taught what they had learned. Role plays and mini-lectures were enacted by the first set of participants with great success. It was apparent that the performers' knowledge had increased and some misinformation had been dispelled. However, both groups will need training to enhance their ability to stimulate active learning. This will be remedied by special training-of-trainers workshops.

Designs were adapted to suit the needs of several other groups and networks which requested workshops. Local officials also requested training. They were convinced that effective AIDS prevention requires community-based interventions outside the official and religious health-care systems. They subsequently asked CONNAISSIDA to work with their staffs and local influentials to develop a community-wide mobilization.

Numerous other requests for workshops came from other community groups, schools and colleges. More recently we have conducted workshops with leaders of the Traditional Healers' Association. This could vastly enlarge the networks of people who obtain AIDS information, including positive information about condoms.

Sex workers pointed to the need for accessible and affordable treatment for STDs. Several women in the church group requested money for fees and transportation in order to obtain effective care for relief of persistent abdominal pain, which was unavailable in their neighbourhood. Not only are new services needed, but they must be free services, accessible to poor women in the peripheral as well as central neighbourhoods. Since STD treatment is laden with cultural meaning and misperceptions, health workers will need assistance to provide sensitive, effective care.

The most pressing need identified by both women's groups is for income-generating activities so that women who cannot depend upon men to support them and their children can survive without providing sexual services to multiple partners. Both sex workers and churchwomen reported trying numerous other ways to enlarge family resources. Most have had scant success. Both groups drew up lists of needs and possibilities, without arriving at a realistic plan of cooperative action that might be sustainable in the medium or long term, even with initial support from a funding agency.

One month after their evaluation, the church Mothers' Club organized a festive meal for participants and trainers. Closing the proceedings, the minister advised the assembly that since AIDS is a divine retribution for sins, the righteous need not fear infection. A similar message had been broadcast by the Protestant Bishop some days earlier. Further evaluation will show which of the competing messages, the moralistic one with its avoidance of realistic risk assessment, or those developed by the group in collaboration with CONNAISSIDA, prevails.

While, at some levels, gender relations are subject to negotiation, women's struggle takes place in conditions not of their own making. More than empowerment training is needed to halt the spread of HIV.

Sex work, AIDS and preventive health behaviour

by Carole A. Campbell

Sex work is illegal everywhere in the United States except in brothels in rural counties in Nevada. Street work is the most visible form of sex work, although it represents only about 20 per cent of all forms of sex work in the United States. Street work, primarily an urban phenomenon, is the form of sex work most often associated with injection drug use. Street work is the type of sex work most likely to result in arrest since it is the most visible.

Legalized sex work in Nevada

Currently there are 37 legal brothels and about 350 licensed sex workers in Nevada. A brothel is licensed to operate within a specific geographical area. A sex worker must apply for a work card which is good for a specified time, usually around 90 days, which allows her to work only in a licensed brothel.

The Nevada Board of Health requires that sex workers in licensed brothels be tested weekly for gonorrhoea and monthly for syphilis. If found to be infected, sex workers are not permitted to work until the appropriate time after treatment when follow-up tests indicate a negative status. Since 1986, sex workers are also required to be tested for HIV antibody as a condition for employment, and once employed, monthly thereafter. If a woman tests positive, she is denied employment as a sex worker. She then receives an education programme on self-imposed restrictions from medical personnel. Since 1986, 13 job applicants have tested positive during pre-employment tests, but none of the women employed at any brothel, out of 14,000 cumulative tests.

In 1987, legislation aimed mostly at unlicensed sex workers was passed in Nevada. Anyone arrested for sex work or solicitation must submit to a test for HIV. If convicted, she must pay $100 for the cost of the test. The arresting officer is notified of a positive test result and then must inform the person tested in writing. A person convicted of unlicensed sex work who tests positive and continues to engage in sex work can be guilty of a felony and subject to imprisonment of up to 20 years, or by a fine of at least $10,000, or both. A licensed sex worker is subject to the same penalties. An operator of a legal brothel who knowingly employs a sex worker who has tested positive for HIV is liable for felony charges.

Since 1988, the Nevada Board of Health has required that condoms be used at all licensed brothels. Prior to that time, an informal survey found that 90 per cent of brothels had complied on a voluntary basis. In the brothel described below, an all-condom policy was adopted in 1985. All sex acts, including oral sex, are performed with a condom. This policy was actually brought about through pressure placed on the owner by the sex workers, who felt that unprotected sex was simply too risky and who threatened to quit unless the brothel adopted an all-condom policy. Regular medical examinations are an established routine for women in licensed brothels and this contact allows the women to get clarification on any health concerns they may have. In addition, brothels have on-site AIDS prevention education.

The work lives of licensed sex workers in one brothel

In order for a sex worker to be hired at the brothel, she goes through a formal interview process. The owner wants neither employees who use drugs nor the various problems associated with drug usage. Evidence of drug use is grounds for immediate dismissal.

The brothel is surrounded by a large security fence and its door has a chain and a small see-through opening. A visitor must ring a bell at the gate of the fence before he is admitted into the parlour. The owner is usually around and there are several employees besides the sex workers, including a hostess, bartender and cook. The hostess screens the customers carefully and at night a security guard is on duty.

Before a sex worker agrees to a customer's specific sexual request, she inspects his genitals carefully for any signs of old or active venereal disease. She looks for lesions, cuts or open sores. A newly employed sex worker goes through a formal training period, supervised by a veteran sex worker when she conducts inspections on customers. She must complete this training successfully before she is allowed to conduct inspections by herself. In the event that a sex worker sees something questionable, she then calls in another sex worker for a second opinion. If the second sex worker agrees that the customer is a risk, he is rejected. If he is accepted, he then is instructed to wash his genitals with an antiseptic solution, with warm water, and to put on a condom.

Brothel policy places sex workers in a strong position to reject a customer and to enforce condom use. Sex workers have some control over the types of sex acts in which they agree to participate and assured physical safety from the staff and legal system, though they are still vulnerable.

Sex workers work full-time for three weeks and live at the brothel during that time. Although they are voluntary workers, they do face a number of restrictions on their freedom. They are not able to leave without a chaperone and there are restrictions on where they can go. During their week off, they leave the brothel.

The main work benefit that legalization provides is freedom to work without fear of arrest. There are several disadvantages. The women must pay a substantial amount of their earnings, as much as 40 per cent plus room and board, to the owner of the brothel. They must also pay for the costs of their HIV antibody tests out of their salaries ($25 to $100). Sex workers work without benefits such as sick leave, health insurance, social security, disability insurance or workers' compensation. They are immediately terminated in the event that they test positive for HIV.

The legalized system does not provide any type of assistance to seropositive sex workers. Although they can no longer work legally, a positive test will most likely not end their working careers and they will probably continue to work clandestinely.

Illegal sex work

The work of illegal street sex workers requires a strict separation between their work and home lives. Sex among street workers and their customers usually takes place very close to the street on which the women work. Often it takes place in customers' cars. The interaction is usually quick since it is illegal and the woman must return to the street to transact more business. Street workers do not always have a warm, private place in which to conduct their work or an appropriate physical setting in which to engage in hygienic practices with customers. Street workers are usually approached by men who want quick sex at cheap prices.

Street workers are more physically vulnerable than licensed sex workers. Because of their illegal status, they have a different relationship with the police and are usually unable to seek help if they find themselves in physical jeopardy. Their contact with the health care system is also different since it is very much tied to their contact with the legal system, often the result of arrest and conviction for working.

Anecdotal evidence suggests that the relatively low incidence of heterosexual AIDS cases among males has served to undermine the women's health by providing some men with a reason to freely engage in unprotected sex without concern about the risk of HIV infection. In addition, customers of sex workers are reported to be offering more money for higher risk sex. The drug crack has also undermined sex work since some women are willing to engage in high-risk sex in exchange for small amounts of crack, worth much less than the amount of money ordinarily requested by other sex workers. If money is requested, it is usually a very low amount, as low as $3 for vaginal sex. According to reports from some sex workers, this new crack-related sex trade has deflated the price that they are able to command for sex.

Anecdotal accounts from sex workers indicate that they are getting more requests from customers for oral sex, because of its relatively low risk. The price for oral sex has apparently decreased while the price for higher risk sex has increased. Some sex workers report that they surreptitiously use condoms on customers who are resistant to using them. And some express a reluctance to carry condoms, especially large quantities of them, for fear that the condoms will be confiscated as evidence by the police.

AIDS prevention policy issues

Most of the AIDS policies involving sex workers are designed to protect the public from the potential threat of AIDS that sex workers pose. However, epidemiologic data indicate that sex workers face a very real risk of infection.

A number of studies have indicated that injection drug use rather than sexual practice is the main risk of HIV infection for US and European sex workers. Sex workers who use injection drugs comprise only an estimated 5–10 per cent of all sex workers in the USA. Although they would appear to be the main health concern, AIDS policy has not directly addressed this group.

A multicentre study in the USA found that the most likely source of HIV infection for sex workers was their non-paying rather than their paying partners. More than 80 per cent of the sex workers reported at least occasional use of condoms – 78 per cent with paying partners, as compared to only 16 per cent with non-paying partners. Other studies in Jamaica, Australia, the Netherlands and the USA also found that sex workers are more likely to use condoms in professional rather than personal contexts.

It is often assumed that sex workers know how to use condoms but this thinking may be fallacious. One study that assessed condom skills of 91 sex workers through the use of a plastic model of a penis found that fewer than 20 per cent of the women put condoms on the model correctly and 7 per cent of the condoms broke because of mistakes in use.

Examples of AIDS prevention programmes for and by sex workers

A programme in Mexico learned from focus group discussion and in-depth interviews that sex workers were concerned about how their children would be cared for if they themselves became ill and died. The programme designed a campaign that used posters and photo-novels. Women were encouraged to stay healthy for their children through key messages that stressed avoiding sexual transmission of HIV and using condoms in order to prevent perinatal transmission and in order to be responsible mothers. After the campaign had been in effect for six months, condom use increased by 66 per cent.

Several AIDS outreach programmes for injection drug users have involved ex-users in distributing bleach and condoms to users and have resulted in positive changes among users. Drug users' groups have organized in Amsterdam, New York City, and Sydney and often provide information about AIDS, bleach, needles and syringes, and condoms, as well as social support.

An AIDS intervention programme for Latina sex workers in Orange County, California used sex workers who had been released from jail to teach other sex workers about the risk of sharing needles and unsafe sex. This programme also used photo-novels to communicate the risk of unsafe sex to the clients of sex workers.

The California Prostitutes Education Project (CAL-PEP) AIDS Prevention Project was designed and is implemented by sex workers, ex-sex workers and sex workers' rights advocates to help sex workers protect themselves and their partners. Utilizing a peer educator approach, they have trained sex workers as AIDS educators to conduct outreach to other sex workers and to customers. Initially, sex workers are trained as volunteers, but upon successful completion of training are given paid positions when such positions become available.

CAL-PEP outreach workers conduct a safe-sex contest which consists of a quiz that sex workers complete and return. Drawings are then held with the first prize being $100 and the second prize being 100 condoms. The contest allows CAL-PEP to assess the sex workers' knowledge in order to determine the best focus in educational programmes and allows sex workers to assess their own knowledge in a fun and entertaining way that encourages participation and involvement.

In Australia, sex workers are working as safe sex educators and in the Dominican Republic, sex workers who have been elected by their peers work as educators. In the Netherlands, clients of sex workers organized and distributed condoms to other clients.

One intervention programme designed by Family Health International and established in Cameroon, Ghana and Mali, trained small groups of sex workers (6–10) as peer health educators. Each woman was responsible for educating and distributing condoms to a small group (10–15) of her colleagues. Preliminary results from the Cameroon project found that after the programme had been in place for a year, 72 per cent of the women reported using condoms at least half the time, compared to 28 per cent at the beginning. The women in Ghana also encouraged clients to use condoms at home.

In the Nevada brothel described above, the women spent a considerable amount of time on what might be called 'self-care', which included a range of activities intended to promote or restore their health. AIDS programmes could take up and promote this concept, including the use of condoms and birth control. This approach, which can, also include the concept of client-care, does not focus specifically on AIDS and other STDs, but instead provides a positive rubric for a number of preventive health practices and may offer an appropriate strategy for education of and by sex workers.

Testing, screening and counselling women for HIV/AIDS

Testing and screening

Being able to have an HIV test is important for anyone who wants to know whether they are infected. Testing is also important for public health and community reasons. The results of tests for individuals are used to:

- provide information to and teach people who have tested negative how to avoid becoming infected;
- provide information to and arrange care and support for people who have tested positive;
- teach people who have tested positive how to avoid infecting others;
- record and make use of epidemiological information in public health campaigns and for providing services.

If a person tests negative, but there is reason to think they have been infected recently, they will be advised to return for another test in three to six months' time, and to protect themselves and others in the interim.

International policymakers strongly recommend that individual testing is done anonymously or confidentially.

With anonymous testing, a person's name must be unknown, false, or kept separate from their blood sample, so that the two cannot be linked. If testing is confidential, people give their real names to the test provider, who is not supposed to reveal the results without consent to anyone except the person being tested. The results may or may not be put into the person's medical records. The person depends on the test provider not to reveal the results to anyone else.[1]

Screening is the testing of particular groups of people for epidemiological and public-health reasons.

The World Health Organization recommends that screening should always be anonymous and not linked to people's names. It can be done: without obtaining permission, using blood that has been taken for other reasons; or after obtaining permission, especially if blood is taken for this reason only.[2,3]

HIV screening is done:

- on blood, tissue and organ donors, to prevent infection being transmitted through donated blood, blood products, semen, breastmilk, or organs;
- among specific population groups, to find out the number of new cases of infection in those groups in a given period of time (incidence studies);
- among random samples of a population to learn trends and estimate the long term

burden of the disease (prevalence studies). Not everyone needs to be tested. Prevalence studies among random samples of well-defined and accessible groups, e.g. hospital patients or pregnant women at antenatal clinics, give a good indication of the rate of infection in the general population (sentinel surveys).[4]

HIV tests: what is available

All HIV tests currently available for public use are tests for antibodies to HIV in the blood. The ELISA is currently the best test for individual and screening purposes. A Western blot test or a second ELISA test can be used to confirm an ELISA result for individuals. Both of these tests are highly accurate, i.e. they have a very low rate of false-positive and false-negative results.

Both tests require trained staff and laboratory facilities. Test kits are expensive and have to be imported by most countries. In some countries, due to costs, diagnosis is made on clinical grounds without a blood test. Blood tests are preferable because they are more accurate.

A number of organizations are trying to develop accurate, quick and less expensive test kits, e.g. using dipsticks, which more countries could produce locally, so that testing becomes universally feasible.[5,6]

Blood tests for detecting the HIV virus itself exist but are only used for research purposes because they are even more expensive.

Antibody tests done for screening may not be confirmed, in order to keep the costs down. Less expensive tests are available for screening, especially for blood donations. These tests have a very low rate of false-negative results, comparable to the ELISA, but their false-positive rate is higher than acceptable for testing individuals. As long as people are not told the results when they donate blood, a false-positive result would not matter because the blood is just discarded.

In high HIV-prevalence areas in some developing countries, many more people are wanting to be tested than there are test kits and facilities available. As a result, less expensive tests are being used and some people may be getting false-positive results.[7]

People with no other access to testing are offering to donate blood in order to be tested. If they are at risk of HIV, they may interpret a refusal to accept a donation from them as a sign that they have HIV, when it is not. If their blood is taken, they will want the test result. Health workers will be forced to refuse, causing bad feeling, or will have to confirm the initial result, thereby reducing the number of test kits available to test blood from others.[8]

On the other hand, if people who donate blood want their test result and cannot get it at the blood-donation site, they will seek testing elsewhere. Thus three or four kits may be used to test the same person. If blood donors could learn their results, with counselling on site, this would not happen, and the tests of those who did not want their results would not have to be confirmed. In the long run, this might not only save test kits, it might increase the number of blood donors.

Policy issues

In every country, ethical and policy decisions on where, why, how and whom to test and screen have been a matter of heated debate. While policies made without debate have tended to be more coercive, the lack of clear policy guidelines adversely affects prevention work and services. Policies may be ignored or differ from one hospital or locale to another. The following issues have emerged.

Distinguishing between testing and screening

The purposes of testing and screening overlap and can be confused with each other, sometimes with negative consequences.

Letting people refuse to be screened biases the results. The more people who refuse, the more inaccurate and eventually useless the results would be.[2,4] To avoid this, it is better not to inform people they are being screened. To avoid ethical problems of taking blood only for HIV screening without permission, it is better to screen those whose blood is taken for other purposes. However, only a limited number of groups can then be screened, e.g. hospital patients, army recruits, pregnant women attending antenatal clinics, or newborn babies.

If screening is not linked to people's names, no individual follow-up can be done if positive test results are found. Those who have HIV may not get the help they may need. Voluntary testing has to be available and public education has to encourage those at risk to come forward.

The alternative is to carry out screening with results linked to people's names. Permission would be needed, but people could be given their results if they wanted. Those who were negative would be reassured; those who were positive might learn it earlier than otherwise and have access to help more quickly. It would be cheaper to give people their results than encourage everyone to be tested again voluntarily.

However, positive test results obtained through screening may be used to quarantine and/or discriminate against people with HIV/AIDS. In some countries this has emerged as the real purpose of large-scale screening. The human rights implications are serious enough that the World Health Organization and most professionals recommend unlinked, anonymous screening.[2]

Public health considerations must be weighed against protection of individual rights. Screening may be seen as a substitute for prevention work. The amount of choice people are given about being tested hangs in a difficult balance.

Individual rights and testing

People should always have the right to decide whether to be tested individually and told the results of their tests.

In places where HIV is not prevalent in women, it is not unusual for women to be told they do not need a test. Some women have found they cannot get tested even when they are sure they need it.

In many developed countries, consent is required. In practice, this is not always obtained. One Canadian woman reported: 'I was first tested for the HIV virus in October 1985, after the death of my daughter from pneumonia. Unfortunately, the doctor didn't explain what he was looking for, and didn't inform me of the results once they came back. When I went in for the birth of my second child in February 1988, I was informed that the medical records showed I was HIV-positive.'[9]

In Zambia, every patient who receives a medical registration card automatically gives consent to medical examinations. This allows practitioners to do tests without consent or even knowledge.[10] This is probably the case in many other countries.

Given the stigma, discrimination and sense of hopelessness that may follow from a positive test result, being tested is not always helpful or wanted. Advice about whether to be tested – or told the result – must take into account the person's situation if it is to be in their best interests.

With individual testing, people have the right to know their results. Again, this does not always happen in practice.

A doctor in the Congo told a researcher that he did not inform one male patient he might have AIDS because he had only an unconfirmed ELISA test and clinical diagnosis to go on. He said he would not tell the patient even if the result could be confirmed, since there was nothing the man would be able to do: he could not protect his wife sexually because they were Roman Catholic and would not use condoms.[11] Does a doctor have the right to determine this for a patient? There are arguments on both sides.

People also have the right to refuse to know their results. They may decide they do not want to know once they have actually been tested, especially if they were put under pressure to do it. However, they may return at a later date to ask for the results, and these should be kept available for them.

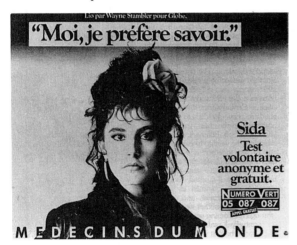

'Me, I prefer to know'

World Health Organization

Confidentiality and anonymity

Confidentiality and anonymity are among the most problematic issues in both screening and testing. An individual's test result should always be private. In practice, especially in a small town or village where everyone knows everyone, this may be impossible to guarantee.[12]

In most countries, reliance cannot be placed on the law to protect against breaches of confidentiality. Too much in the law compels, justifies and excuses the disclosure of information if it can be argued that it is for the good of others or the protection of public health. One legal expert has concluded that it is better to use the law to minimize discrimination and stigmatization than to make new laws to protect the confidentiality of people with HIV/AIDS.[13]

In Canada, a medical officer of health attempted to release the name of an HIV-positive woman in her local community on the grounds that she was either unwilling or unable to practise safer sex. He thought it might also encourage her previous partners, whom she had not named, to come forward for testing. Lawyers acting for the woman argued that no one would come forward if they saw how confidentiality had been breached in her case. They were also concerned for her safety in the community. Although the situation was resolved without her name being released, she left the area. Conditions were made if she returned, including having to tell any partners of her status and report to a hospital daily.[14]

Partner notification

Partner notification is a breach of confidentiality, but it may protect partners from HIV infection. The law often permits or requires sexual contacts to be informed that they are at risk if a person has any sexually transmitted disease, including HIV. People may or may not have the right to refuse to name those contacts, though they cannot be forced. Clinic staff can often convince them to cooperate, in the interests of their contacts. People may be given the choice to inform contacts themselves or let the clinic do it.

A survey among HIV-positive patients in Vancouver found that most would agree to partner notification if it were required.[15] A clinic in Mexico compared rate of infection and

Woman knows partner has HIV	Yes %	No %
Woman also HIV-positive	53.3	78.9
Modified sexual behaviour	88.8	27.2
Believes condoms should be used	81.8	27.2
Condom use	30.5	38.7
Avoids intercourse	86.9	50.0

behaviour in women who had or had not been told that their male partner had HIV. As the table above shows, notification had a beneficial effect for the women.[16]

Partner notification needs more gender-specific study. What may be beneficial for women if women are informed, may be dangerous for women if men are informed. Notification of male partners can lead to blame for infection, abandonment and violence against a woman. Women in many situations have given this as a reason why they would be unwilling for partners to be notified.[17,18]

One solution would be for women and their partners to be tested and to receive their results together.[19] Where this is not possible, women's concerns must be taken into account no matter what the law.

Some developing countries are considering notification programmes, but there are many medical, legal, ethical and logistic issues to confront, including how many partners to notify, how they will be notified and counselled, and what services will be available for them. Without caution, individual and social harm can be done and can detract from other AIDS prevention and control activities.[20]

Routine testing

Routine testing has been defined as the systematic testing of all individuals who meet specific criteria. Such testing can be voluntary or mandatory, though the difference can sometimes be unclear. Four types of routine testing may be found:

- Testing may be available to people who want it. For example, a family planning clinic can put up a notice saying that testing is available on request. Or an HIV-test site can be opened and people would only go if they want to be tested.
- Clinics may offer or suggest testing to people they think are at risk or to everyone who attends the clinic, but people decide for themselves whether to be tested. Antenatal clinics, drug-treatment programmes and STD clinics are all examples.
- All members of a specific population group may be tested. They may or may not be informed in advance. They may or may not be given the opportunity to refuse or to decide whether they want to be told the results. In a few countries, antenatal clinics operate this policy. All registered sex workers and all prisoners entering prison are more common examples.
- People may be required to have a test as a condition for something else and given no choice about learning the results, e.g. for studying or getting a residence visa in another country, for a particular job, or to join the military.[2] Many insurance companies require applicants to reveal whether they are at risk or have been tested, and any test results.

Routine testing for HIV is one of the most difficult areas of debate, especially when it edges towards being mandatory. Routine testing can be of value. Each case needs to be judged on its own merits.

Routine testing of individuals should not be confused with screening, though it may be. Routine testing of newborn infants might make good sense if tests were accurate for the infants just after birth. In current circumstances, routine testing of infants only provides accurate information about the mother's HIV status. At least until this changes, these tests should be voluntary unless done anonymously for screening purposes.

Routine testing has been rejected by most experts as unnecessary for either health workers or patients, because universal precautions are much more effective.[21] However, if one or other has been put at risk, e.g. by a needlestick injury or blood splash, professional bodies may recommend testing of the health worker and the patient, with or without consent.[22]

Mandatory testing

Mandatory testing raises many ethical questions and is difficult to justify. Some say people in high-risk situations or with high-risk behaviours ought to be tested if they are in a position to infect other people. But knowledge of HIV status is not protection in itself. People still have to protect others voluntarily.

Prisoners are often singled out for mandatory testing, including women arrested for sex work or injection drug use. In Belgium and Greece an HIV test is mandatory for prison inmates, while in Austria, France, Germany, Norway and Spain, all drug users in prison are offered an HIV test, and condoms are available to male inmates free of charge.[23]

Sex workers are often subjected to mandatory testing at regular intervals. Yet no one has proposed mandatory testing of sex workers' clients or men with multiple sexual partners, nor even of all injection drug users. The human rights of sex workers seem to be more easily violated than the rights of others, even other stigmatized groups. It is policy in many countries to ban sex workers from working if they are found to be HIV-positive. Women whose only livelihood is threatened by mandatory testing will try to avoid being tested. Those found to have HIV will often move to an area where no one knows them.

Testing for sex workers can have positive consequences if carried out in a programme that supports women's own interests. In the mid-1980s a hospital-based AIDS centre in Athens set up an AIDS education programme for 350 registered sex workers. The women were already required to report once a week to a special STD clinic, as a condition of registration, though it would appear that this was not strictly enforced. In 1985, the women were tested for HIV and other STDs. Since then, they have been tested every three months. At each visit, they are interviewed, counselled and clinically examined. Educational material is given about all STD prevention as well as AIDS. Their work has been protected, their health has improved and the risk of HIV has been reduced.[24] The women have clearly benefited, as shown in the table below.

Changes in (%)	1985	1987	1988	1989
Use of condoms	66.0	97.9	96.5	98.5
Incidence of syphilis	17.1	3.2	2.9	2.0
Incidence of gonorrhoea	14.0	0.0	1.2	1.2
Incidence of new HIV infection	3.4	0.0	0.4	0.4

However, the question of whether more women would have access to help if testing were voluntary, remains.

Voluntary testing

In most European countries an HIV test is offered to all drug users who contact a caring agency. The uptake in this group is much higher than in many others, yet it is voluntary.[23] This is the best evidence available that voluntary testing works when people are aware they are at risk and something can be done to help them.

The disadvantage is that not everyone will be aware or convinced they are at risk, and therefore will not be reached. Even those who know they are at risk may not choose testing when it is voluntary.

Men and women (100 each) attending an STD clinic in London were asked why they did not request an HIV test; 64 per cent of the men and 40 per cent of the women said the issue was very much on their minds. The most common reason given by the men was concern about confidentiality. The most common reason among the women was that they were afraid the result would be positive and they could not cope with it.[25] While these fears might be overcome with counselling and support, they are valid reasons not to be tested.

Testing following rape, sexual assault or abuse

If a man on trial for rape or sexual abuse has been tested for HIV, found to be positive and knew his status prior to the crime, the charges against him and his sentence may be increased, even to include attempted murder in some countries.

Many people think that mandatory testing should be done on rapists and child abusers. In the USA, mandatory testing of convicted rapists has become law in many states since 1990. Yet, testing of rapists does not actually help women who have been raped.

Only an estimated ten per cent of rapes and sexual assaults are ever reported in the USA, and the figure is unlikely to be higher in other countries. The great majority of rapists are never charged for their crime, and if charged, are usually not convicted. In the USA, fewer than 40 per cent of reported rapes result in charges, and only three per cent of these result in a conviction. On this basis, only 12 out of every 10,000 alleged rapists could be tested for HIV in the USA, and a conviction may not be reached for up to three years. The woman or child would still need to be tested three to six months after the attack, whether the rapist is tested or not.[26]

Anecdotal reports indicate that doctors may dismiss women's fears of HIV risk after a rape and tell them an HIV test is unnecessary. But coping with that fear has become part of the whole experience of rape and sexual assault for many women.[26] One STD clinic in London has found that fear of HIV infection is a principal reason why women who have been raped attend. Although the women are often not explicit about this, they often appear immensely relieved when the clinic initiates this discussion with them. Hence HIV testing and counselling is always offered.[27]

Testing pregnant women

Testing and/or screening of pregnant women for HIV, either routinely or selectively, has three main aims:

- to find out the prevalence of HIV infection in pregnant women and estimate how many infants will be born with HIV;

- to inform women of their HIV status and of the risks to themselves and their infants if they are HIV-positive and continue the pregnancy to term;
- to give HIV-positive women the option of abortion to avoid possible HIV infection in the infant.

In countries where clinicians cannot legally offer abortion, it has often been considered pointless to test pregnant women for the third reason.

Antenatal screening of pregnant women for HIV, and even more so screening of all newborn babies, is widely accepted in the USA, Canada and Britain as the best single source of data on prevalence of HIV among women.[28] It is common in most, if not all, developed countries. Since blood is taken for other tests in both instances, an HIV test is merely added to these.

However, this form of screening does not give a good enough indication of HIV prevalence in women generally. A four-week exhaustive study in Paris, reported in 1991, was done anonymously in all pregnant women attending medical settings and involved 2,753 deliveries, 249 miscarriages, 956 abortions and 42 ectopic pregnancies. It was found that 9 of the women delivering, 2 miscarrying, 7 having an abortion and 2 with ectopic pregnancies were HIV-positive.[29] As few as 45 per cent of the HIV-positive women may have been tested if women attending only antenatal clinics, rather than this range of medical settings, had been included.

Even this information is incomplete. Much more complete information about prevalence in women of childbearing age would have been obtained if non-pregnant women attending infertility, STD and family planning clinics had also been included. The fact that only pregnant women are usually screened strongly suggests that this screening is for the sake of the infants, not the women.

Contradictions in antenatal policy

Among and within developed countries, antenatal testing policy is very uneven. Although there is a major difference between screening for prevalence information and individual testing, antenatal policies and practice do not always reflect this.

The policy in both Norway and Sweden since 1987 has been to offer an HIV test to all pregnant women attending antenatal clinics and give women the results. Less than one in a thousand refuse testing in Norway. In Sweden, between one and four per cent of women refuse; they are tested without their knowledge anyway.

By the end of 1990, 324,256 antenatal HIV tests had been done in Sweden, finding 31 HIV-positive women. Eighteen of these could have been identified as at risk through counselling. In the same period, 276,852 antenatal HIV tests had been done in Norway, finding 23 HIV-positive women. Ten of these already knew they were HIV-positive.[30,31] The cost of this exercise must have been enormous. What about its value? Neither study questioned the need for a mass screening policy, nor one which links women's results to their names.

In Milan, in contrast, during 1988–9 all pregnant women (273) in three health districts of the city, whose blood was being tested for other purposes, were screened for HIV anonymously. Extrapolation from the results to the total population of Milan suggested that about 72 pregnant women in Milan were HIV-positive and had had about 29 infected infants.[32] Thus, with few tests, comparable prevalence information was gained in Milan as in Sweden and Norway. The difference is that the HIV-positive women in Milan could not be informed.

Where antenatal testing is routine, it is almost always described as being voluntary. This is not always the case in practice. Midwives attached to one obstetric unit in Geneva are instructed to test only with informed consent. Among a sample group of 112 women delivering in that unit, 105 had been tested for HIV antenatally. At the end of pregnancy, only 58 per cent said they had been told they were being tested. Five said they would have refused the test if they had been asked. Only 56 per cent were given their results. [33]

In the first of two postal surveys in Belgium, reported in 1990, half of the 237 gynae-cologists responding said they did not inform women before they tested them antenatally. [34]

Some countries and practitioners offer an HIV test to all pregnant women. Others only test women identified as at risk. Lower or higher levels of prevalence of HIV infection among women are not always the key to who or how many will be tested.

In the second postal survey in Belgium, of 446 gynaecologists, 80 per cent had never had to deal with HIV in a pregnant woman. Forty-nine per cent offered HIV testing to all pregnant women, 42 per cent only to women with identified risks. [34]

In 1989, a survey of all the main obstetric units in Britain and Ireland found that HIV testing was available in 65 per cent, and for the most part had been available since 1987–8. In 10 per cent, testing was available on request. Fifty-two per cent offered selective testing to women at high risk of infection. The test was offered to all women in only 3 per cent of the units, most of which were also involved in prevalence studies. At the remaining 35 per cent of units, which were generally in low-prevalence areas, there was no formal policy on testing.

The authors of this study noted that 46 per cent of the women tested first learned they had HIV from an antenatal test. As clinicians, they were worried that these women would not have been tested if they had not become pregnant. They point out that selective testing does not actually identify everyone who has HIV, since not everyone is aware or admits that they are at risk. In their concern to identify as many women as possible with HIV, they suggest that testing in high-prevalence areas should be offered to all pregnant women, irrespective of identified risks. [35]

When to test in pregnancy

When in pregnancy should women be tested? Most clinicians would probably reply that it should be done along with other routine screening tests in the first trimester of pregnancy, so that laboratory tests can be done together, counselling can be done early, and women have the chance to opt for an abortion if they want it.

Many clinicians do not indicate when in pregnancy they test for HIV. In the first Belgian postal survey mentioned above, 74 per cent of respondents offered or did the test at the first antenatal consultation, 15 per cent both at the first visit and at the end of pregnancy, 9 per cent only before delivery and 1 per cent only at the end of pregnancy. [34]

A Swiss study of all children born with HIV infection to the end of 1990 found that 70 per cent of their mothers first learned they had HIV during pregnancy. Among 54 women in that group who were tested at three-monthly intervals during pregnancy, as part of a sub-study, four had initially tested negative and had seroconverted during pregnancy. [36]

This and similar data from other countries suggests that testing should be done at least two times during pregnancy or even three. This would be absurd. The timing and purpose of testing during pregnancy needs to be clarified.

Why test during pregnancy?

From women's point of view, the real question is whether pregnancy is the best time to be tested. Many studies of acceptability and uptake of antenatal HIV tests have been done in different countries. Invariably, these studies find that a large majority of women favour the test being available in antenatal clinics. Fewer women usually say they would have the test during pregnancy themselves. Where testing is actually voluntary, even fewer tend to have it, and some do not return for their results. Many women would prefer not to be tested antenatally.

At one British antenatal clinic, 82 per cent of women questioned thought HIV testing should be available antenatally, but only 48 per cent said they would take the test themselves. Fifteen per cent said they would become highly anxious if they were tested during pregnancy. In contrast, the prospect of other antenatal tests made less than four per cent anxious.[37]

With HIV testing, if there is a positive result women have only two choices – to continue or terminate the pregnancy. This is not true of other routine antenatal tests. As with genetic screening, it is always better to have the information before getting pregnant than after.[38]

On the other hand, many women are not offered HIV testing during pregnancy. And many pregnant women in developing countries and poor women in developed countries do not attend an antenatal clinic until later in pregnancy, if at all.

In a hospital in a poor area of New York City, of 80 postpartum women found to be at risk for HIV infection, 69 consented to HIV counselling for themselves and testing of their newborn babies. Almost half the women had had late or no antenatal care. Only 8 of the 69 women returned for the test results, despite repeated attempts to contact them. Sixty-two per cent had no phone and 22 per cent had supplied incorrect addresses. These women had multiple problems. The end of pregnancy was not a good time to raise the issue of HIV infection, important as it was.[39]

Half the women counselled in 1989 by the Women and AIDS Resource Network in Brooklyn, New York, said they only learned their HIV status when their babies developed AIDS. This is even worse than first learning it during pregnancy.[40]

'That is why we say the time to serve women is now, not when they are in their first trimester of pregnancy and not when their baby is born.'[40]

Where and when to test women

Antenatal HIV tests should be available, but antenatal clinics should not be the first or only place where most women have the opportunity to find out if they have HIV. Instead of assuming that more HIV-positive women will be 'found' by extending antenatal testing to all pregnant and postpartum women, we should be asking where and when women should be able to find out they have HIV when they want to find out.

The most obvious answer seems to be at women's health services of all kinds, and at special testing centres for women, whether based in hospitals, primary health care facilities, or at other sites in the community. Once again, the need for an integrated approach to women's health is highlighted. A service where women could be counselled about all aspects of their health would be most beneficial.

Family planning clinics, whether based in hospitals or community health services, are an obvious possible source of HIV testing, both for women who do not want to get pregnant and women considering pregnancy.

Since 1986, the contraceptive and sexual counselling clinic of the National Association for Sex Education in Sweden has been offering HIV testing as one of its regular activities. Special sessions for HIV testing put people off, so they integrated testing as a full-time service like any other.

Only about 250 people have asked for and

had an HIV test annually at this clinic, and only a few have tested HIV-positive since the service became available. In countries with a higher prevalence of HIV, the effects on clinic time and resources would be much greater. The proportion of men to women tested increased from 17 per cent in 1986 to 50 per cent in 1990. This suggests that HIV testing may be one way to draw men to attend family planning clinics and talk to them about safer sex.[41]

A survey was conducted in Nairobi to find out how women would respond if offered an HIV test in a family planning clinic. Almost all the 783 women who were asked agreed to be tested as part of the study. The five per cent who refused said they were afraid of blood being taken, afraid to know the test result, afraid of their partner's reaction, confident they were seronegative, or had no time.[42] This indicates the overall acceptability of HIV testing in family planning clinics, though in practice, the number of women who actually ask for a test would probably be lower.

The International Planned Parenthood Federation and many national family planning associations encourage local clinics to offer HIV testing and counselling, and have arranged numerous training courses for this. But most have been very slow to take this up. Many want to avoid the issue. Many do not have the resources, which need to be considerable where HIV prevalence is high. Many are afraid that the link with AIDS would put women off family planning, though this has not been shown to be true.

Family planning clinics are often a separate service from other reproductive health services for women. If family planning providers came together with midwives, antenatal, abortion, STD and infertility services to arrange HIV testing and counselling jointly, family planning clinics would not need to offer separate facilities.

Alternatively, they could collaborate with a specialist HIV testing and counselling service with cross-referrals. Leaflets and posters could be exchanged, and joint posters and leaflets could be developed. Each could train the other to include information about their respective services when they talk to clients. Each could offer advice sessions at particular times or on one day per week, using counsellors from each other's services. Similar collaboration with drug treatment programmes could be organized.

For the population of women in general this may make most sense. There would then be a joint base from which information, outreach work, referrals, support and special services for those with HIV/AIDS and those at risk of infection could be provided.

Independent test sites may be preferable because they are the most voluntary way testing and counselling can be offered and women have to decide to walk in the door. In other clinics, unless trained staff or specialist counsellors are available, there is a risk that staff will not have the knowledge and skills needed.[43] Further, if women sense that other health care depends on accepting an HIV test, they may stay away.

Better policy on testing women needs to be developed and implemented. Testing, like public education on HIV infection, should be available to all women, not confined to or forced on pregnant women, women who use drugs or sex workers.

Why women seek testing or counselling

Most people who are tested, even in high prevalence areas, do not have HIV. Testing should be seen as a form of increased knowledge for the individual, no matter what the result, and not just a way for public health services to 'find' people who have HIV.

Many people ask for an HIV test of their own accord. As public consciousness of HIV/AIDS issues grows, more people have sought an HIV test for reassurance that they are not infected, often before taking a major step in their lives.

In a testing centre in Uganda, the main reasons why people wanted to be tested were: wanting to marry, wanting to study, partner has died, mistrust of partner's sexual movements, partner asked them to be tested (mostly men asked women), sent by a doctor, had been tested before and wants a re-test, feeling unwell, to decide whether to have children, being pregnant.

Among 100 couples who came to be tested together, 42 per cent wanted to get married, 43 per cent were living together or married, and 15 per cent wanted to re-unite after a separation.[19]

A hospital-based clinic in a small city in France found that 18 out of 62 couples asked for an HIV test because they wanted to start a sexual relationship or to stop using condoms for intercourse. Almost half of them were under age 23 and most had had higher education. The women were more likely to propose testing than the men.[44]

Women counsellors in seven HIV/AIDS testing centres in Austria found important gender differences in why men and women attended. The women came:

- because they were afraid of infecting someone else. They considered protection against HIV, as with contraception, their responsibility;
- to confirm closeness to a male partner, especially one who has HIV;
- to get 'permission' to enter a new relationship;
- to draw a line underneath their past and stop worrying about AIDS, with a negative test result as proof that they were safe;
- to have something that allowed them to lay down conditions for continuing a relationship with a partner who refused to practise safer sex.

Male clients, on the other hand, often saw a woman counsellor as someone whose shoulder they could cry on and who could excuse them from responsibility for their situations and behaviour.[45]

Counselling

Before someone has an HIV test, pre-test and post-test counselling are universally recommended. This means many things to many people. Pre-test counselling may be limited to practical arrangements for a test to be done, or it can involve several long discussions about the person's situation and whether they want to be tested. Post-test counselling can range from only giving a person their test results and referring them for treatment or help if they test positive. Or it can provide ongoing support for weeks, months or even years.

Many professionals and activists have been trained or have trained themselves to do counselling with HIV testing. These include people with HIV, activists in voluntary organizations working on AIDS issues, all types of health workers, social workers, psychologists, and other health counsellors. Specialist training is now available in many countries, as expertise has been built up over time.

'Counselling as a routine component of health and social services is relatively new even in highly industrialized countries. In other regions, it is unusual for counselling to be included as a part of ongoing services and, in many cases, it is a new concept, especially where counselling is seen as an extra-familial activity.

HIV/AIDS counselling is predicated on a number of principles and values, including confidentiality and privileged communication and interpersonal relationships between counsellor and client, which may not be acceptable in some cultures.

HIV/AIDS counselling also constitutes a potential strain on national health and social services. In less economically well-off countries, this strain is frequently a major obstacle to developing HIV/AIDS counselling programmes.

The processes of counselling need to be carefully assessed in the context of national and local cultures and resources. Without sacrificing counselling principles, alternative approaches need to be developed and tested.' [46]

Telephone hot lines

Counselling and/or information about HIV/AIDS through telephone hot lines has been available for some years. Some people may prefer to make a phone call because it is totally anonymous. People at low risk may find the fastest reassurance. People at higher risk can be encouraged to seek face-to-face counselling and possibly a test. Hot lines differ in how they are organized and funded, what services they provide, how they are staffed and who their target users are. [47] Some hotlines always have women available to speak to women. Others have specific days/times.

Most developed countries have telephone hot lines. In 1990, 20 of 32 countries in Latin America and the Caribbean had a hot line, mainly in urban areas. [48]

An analysis of the hot line in Trinidad & Tobago found that it was accepted by the public, met a need for counselling and information and provided more than 77 per cent of callers with referrals for more counselling and HIV testing. The ratio of men to women calling was about 3 to 2, about the same as the gender prevalence of HIV in the Caribbean at the time. When only about 800 people called in the first half of 1989, a promotion campaign was launched. [49]

Pre-test counselling for women

Information about HIV/AIDS given to those contemplating a test must be accurate and fairly presented, and include a realistic description of the medical care available for HIV/AIDS-related illness.

From a clinical point of view, it is always worth being tested, especially once symptoms have appeared, and as long as treatment and supportive services are available. There are also many non-clinical issues. One is whether a woman can cope with a positive result, whether the information will help her and those she cares about, how she will take the result back into her life and community, who she can tell without losing love and support if she is positive, and therefore whether it is worth knowing.

It is important to help women assess their own relative risk. A counsellor would ask a woman why she thinks she might be infected and raise questions about her history, current situation and practice; how she plans to prevent getting HIV in future if the test result is negative, or protect others if the result is positive; and whether knowing a test result will help her to do this.

For everyone who seeks testing, there is uncertainty, concern about their actual contact with HIV, and possibly fear and guilt over whether they have infected others.

It is not uncommon for women to become very anxious that they are positive because of actual risks they have taken in the past or because they do not know how much they might have been at risk with specific partners or in certain situations. Unfounded perceptions of risk create unnecessary worry.

Good counsellors can usually distinguish between those who are 'worried well' and those who have good reason to consider a test. Other women may be unworried but engaging in risky behaviour without perceiving themselves to be at risk. For the former, clarification of current risk and ways to reduce risk can quickly reduce anxiety. For the latter, confronting denial and possible underlying self-devaluation can be taken up.[50]

Some people have convinced themselves they have HIV, including physical symptoms, when they really have quite different problems to sort out. A test may be inappropriate for them altogether. However, no one should be refused a test when having the information would clearly put their minds at rest.

Safer sex practices and use of condoms should be explained and ways to get partners to use them explored. For pregnant women or those contemplating a pregnancy, pregnancy-related transmission and its consequences should be explained. Other reproductive health decisions, such as use of contraception or having an abortion, should also be brought up, even if abortion is clandestine.

To help to avoid problems in relationships, it is important to offer women the opportunity of bringing their partners with them to be tested. A discussion on how to approach a partner with this suggestion may be welcomed by women, especially if they are afraid of resistance or aggression. A discussion on how to cope with telling a male partner a test result should also be included in case he will not come for testing.

Discussion must allow enough time for questions on both sides. Women may want to think about and discuss with others what they have learned during counselling, before deciding to be tested.[51] Only then should a decision whether to be tested be taken.

It is not ethical to use incentives or disincentives to induce someone to accept a test they would not otherwise agree to have, e.g. by making the test a condition for access to experimental drugs, medical care or other help. Women must be able to decide of their own accord, without pressure one way or another, to have a test or not, in their own time.

If the decision is yes, arrangements should be made for testing and returning for the result and post-test counselling.

Post-test counselling

The period of time between testing and getting the result should be kept as short as possible.

Not everyone returns. If they have given a false name or address or no name at all, they cannot be followed up. It may be that they were talked into the test, and not returning is their only way of refusing it. Or they may have changed their mind about wanting to know the result in the meantime. They may return at a later date to ask for their results. These should be retained and the door always open to them.

Those who return are probably very anxious. The first part of post-test counselling involves dealing with the result, negative or positive. Prevention of getting or transmitting HIV from/to others should be raised again at some point, no matter what the result is.

A negative result can be a pleasant shock to someone who has good reason to fear infection and who has expected to hear the worst. A positive result is obviously immeasurably worse.[52]

'When men get AIDS, they're angry with the world, with everyone. This is part of the grieving process necessary to an eventual acceptance of any fatal disease and one's eventual death from it. But when women get AIDS, they're angry with themselves. They feel guilty. They blame themselves for not having done something they should have to prevent it.'[53]

For women, especially where a pregnancy or a newborn baby may be affected, the added guilt and pain of possibly hurting the child may be the most difficult aspect to cope with.

When partners are tested and counselled

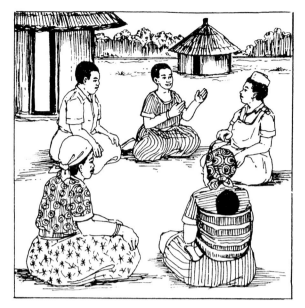

Ministry of Health, Zimbabwe

- ability to give accurate and consistent information;
- trustworthiness;
- credibility;
- ability to ensure privacy and confidentiality, and create a safe environment for talking;
- commitment to patient care;
- objectivity;
- empathy for people;
- professionalism;
- ability to assimilate new information;
- ability to listen;
- ability to talk and hear about sensitive issues such as sexuality, death, violence, divorce, etc.;
- ability to mobilize community resources for counselling;
- familiarity with the client's socio-cultural environment and circumstances;[55]
- awareness of and sensitivity to gender issues in counselling.

together, few feel relieved for themselves and many feel guilty if they test negative but their partner tests positive. Women particularly may feel they should be sharing the pain.[54]

If it achieves nothing else, counselling must help people deal with this knowledge in as supportive a way as possible.

People need to hear that they can survive a long time with HIV infection, because most will still see a positive result as an imminent death sentence. People generally want as much information as possible. A counsellor must find a balance between false reassurance and being alarmist.[51]

Most importantly with a positive result, women will need support in thinking about, finding help, and coping with changes in their lives. Women will have multiple needs and will require referrals for support and care.

Who should be a counsellor

Counsellors need to be informed about HIV/AIDS and have certain personal qualities. These qualities include:

Counsellors have to overcome their own fears of HIV and AIDS, assess their own risks of infection, realize that they are not immune, get over discomfort about sexual behaviours and experiences, combat their own feelings of helplessness and despair, realize that they cannot make everything better, be able to stand back from the grief they feel with their clients, cope with anger, blame and guilt about what is happening to people, know how far to push someone to deal with their own emotional reactions and behaviour patterns, and know when to stop. The opportunity to discuss these concerns with colleagues makes a counsellor better able to deal with these issues and distinguish their own reactions from their clients.[56]

As one woman counsellor explains:

'The life of an antibody test counsellor is full of limitations. I can only see people once, usually for half an hour. I don't know anyone's name, unless told, nor what they will do when they leave my office. At the beginning, this was very disturbing to me, as I wasn't used to such a format. I am also a psychotherapist in private practice, seeing people on an ongoing basis, and that continuity is a significant part of my professional life. What is striking about the structure of counselling at the test site is how it so aptly mirrors the feelings many of us share who work within this epidemic: feelings of not doing enough, wanting to give more, wanting to have more information, wanting to have more time available, as if the 'moreness' could somehow alleviate our feelings of sadness and helplessness.

Over the past year, however, I've begun to re-evaluate my role and its limitations, and I have learned to respect my ability to be a knowledgeable, astute, caring counsellor, as enough. For the most part, I've also come to trust that those in front of me will get the support they need and will do what's in their best interests. I've learned that taking on the pain of others is not useful to them or to me. I am no longer left with the chronic feeling that I haven't done enough. I've begun to see myself and my role as but one stopover on a long journey for my client. This has helped diminish my own need to appear to be the omnipotent counsellor.'[52]

Who should be a counsellor for women

Programmes around the world have found that people with HIV/AIDS, drug users and ex-drug users, sex workers and ex-sex workers make the best counsellors for their peers. Gender race and class issues also affect counselling. Being a peer and the same sex does not automatically confer sensitivity and understanding, but can make it more likely.

At the very least, women should be given the choice of seeing a woman counsellor. Women's increasingly outspoken preference for medical treatment by women carries over into HIV counselling.

An example of how this can be quite astoundingly ignored is contained in a report from Brazil in 1990 on the response of 27 women with HIV/AIDS when women doctors referred them to male psychologists for crisis counselling.

More than half the woman were embarrassed, unwilling, or very angry about seeing a male therapist. Almost a quarter of them refused the therapy because they could not accept it from a man at that time.[57]

There should be no need to re-invent the wheel in HIV/AIDS counselling. The choice to see and be helped by a woman should be the first choice a woman is given when she asks for an HIV test or counselling.

Prototype leaflet for women about HIV testing

Women and HIV/AIDS: Protecting Yourself and Others

If you think you may be infected with HIV, you need to decide whether you want to know for sure. The following are some of the reasons why you may or may not want to have an HIV-antibody test:

Reasons to take the test:

- You think you would feel better if you knew the result than if you remained uncertain.
- You are not feeling well and want to know what is wrong, so that you can get the right medical care.
- You think that knowing will help you to avoid unsafe sex, sharing needles/syringes, or engaging in other unsafe behaviour which puts you or those you are close to at risk of infection.
- You are thinking about starting a sexual relationship or getting married, or whether to continue or resume a relationship with someone if either of you has had sex with others, and the test result could influence what you do next.
- You are thinking of having a baby or you are pregnant, and the test result may make a difference to whether you start or continue pregnancy.

Reasons not to take the test:

- You do not feel able or ready to deal with the feelings that your test result would bring up.
- You are not feeling ill and do not need medical care.
- You think you can avoid unsafe sex, sharing needles/syringes, or engaging in other unsafe behaviour – without having a test.

- You aren't currently putting anyone else at risk.
- You are afraid to lose the support of your partner, family, friends and/or neighbours if the result is positive and they find out.
- Your job, employment prospects, housing, chances of getting a mortgage or life insurance might be at risk if the result is positive and becomes known.

REMEMBER:
Everyone at risk needs to make changes in their behaviour whether or not they are tested.

ASK YOURSELF:
Will having the test help me to make those changes or make it more difficult for me?

TALK IT OVER WITH AN EXPERIENCED COUNSELLOR FIRST

What does the test result mean?

Positive – Antibodies to HIV have been found in your blood. You can infect another person, even if you feel perfectly well.

Negative – Antibodies to HIV were not found in your blood. Either you are not infected *or* you became infected too recently for antibodies to show up on a test.

Usually antibodies are detectable within 3-6 months from when people are infected. It can take longer in a few people. If you were at risk in this period, a re-test may be suggested.

An infant can carry the antibodies of its mother for up to 18 months. Before then, antibodies only indicate that the mother has HIV.

IF YOU DECIDE TO BE TESTED, TALK WITH AN EXPERIENCED COUNSELLOR AFTERWARDS.

The AIDS Information Centre, Kampala, Uganda

by L. M. Barugahare

The AIDS Information Centre (AIC) is a non-government organization. It was established as a pilot project in January 1990 by a consortium of ten organizations, which form the management committee. Among its other objectives, AIC aims to reduce the number of people who go to blood-transfusion services with the intention of finding out their HIV status.

The Centre was initially established to cater for about 5,000 clients during the first year. By the end of 1990, it had attended to 9,417 clients who were tested for HIV infection. This figure had risen to 15,000 clients by the end of May 1991, with an average of 150 clients per day.

The centre provides pre- and post-test counselling and free, anonymous, voluntary HIV testing to all adults aged 16 and over. In addition, HIV testing is carried out on children aged two to six whose mothers are HIV-positive.

Pre-test counselling is offered to individuals, couples and groups. Post-test counselling is offered to individuals and to couples who have agreed to get their test results together. There are particular advantages to each method.

Pre-test group counselling allows various views to be shared by members of the group. The problem of stigma can also be tackled, as the group discover their common problems and anxieties. Although there are personal matters that individuals cannot discuss in the group situation, many other issues will have been covered in group discussions. This saves time in further, individual counselling.

Individual counselling allows the client to talk about personal issues, and express emotions and feelings freely. The implications of the test and its results, options for the future and behaviour change can be covered deeply. Confidentiality and empathy are emphasized to help the client gain control of his or her emotions. The counsellor is able to establish a personal relationship to offer ongoing support.

Counselling of couples allows them to trust and help each other. Being tested together and knowing each other's serostatus partly solves the problem of who they can tell about their test results. A wide range of options can be considered and potential conflict reduced. Transmission chains can be reduced as a couple can more easily be counselled to adopt safer sex practices and deal with the problem of stigma. With shared discussions about HIV/AIDS, the couple can go on talking outside the counselling room. If they are thinking about marrying they can plan accordingly. If they are already together and decide to stay together, they can trust each other more and help to support each other.

Ongoing education, counselling and support are provided through a Post-Test Club. AIC emphasizes that knowing one's HIV status empowers one to practise safer sex and that knowledge is power.

Through grants, AIC intends to open three branches by the end of May 1992. Each branch will be supported by a post-test club and will operate satellite services for the rural areas.

Data on first-year clients

Among the first 9,417 clients of the Centre, 36 per cent were women and 64 per cent were men; 85 per cent of clients had finished primary-level schooling, 17 per cent had finished secondary school and 18 per cent were still students.

Seventy-two per cent were HIV-negative and 28 per cent were HIV-positive. Of those who were HIV-positive, more than one-third were reporting early signs of AIDS. This is evidence of the still growing dimensions of the AIDS epidemic in Uganda, which supports the need for patient care as a major priority along with preventive interventions.

More women (35 per cent) than men (24 per cent) were HIV-positive. Thirty-seven per cent were married and 7 per cent were poly-gamously married.

Of those who tested HIV-negative, 77 per cent intended to get married or stick to one partner, 28 per cent intended to ask their partner to be tested, 16 per cent intended to abstain from sex, and 6 per cent said they would use condoms regularly.

Of those who tested HIV-positive, 76 per cent decided to stick to positive living, 9 per cent to separate from their partner, 2 per cent to go back to their village, and 1 per cent to

commit suicide. However, there has been no case of suicide.

Of 200 clients who were HIV-negative and who returned after six months for a re-test, only one per cent were seropositive. These admitted to risky sexual behaviour during that period. Sixty-seven per cent said they had remained in unions with one sexual partner.

Data on client couples

Couples who had come for HIV testing were either planning to get married, were married or living together, or wanted to re-unite after a separation.

In the couples where both partners were HIV-positive, the majority intended to separate or to stay together without sex. In the couples where both partners were HIV-negative, most intended to marry or stick to one partner. Only a small number in either group planned to use condoms.

Of the couples who had discordant results (one partner negative and one positive), many more of the women were positive than the men. It was not possible to assess why. Among these, a large majority intended to separate. The rest intended to stay together without sex or using safer sex methods.

Women living with HIV/AIDS: personal histories

This chapter contains personal histories of women affected by HIV and AIDS, written by the women themselves or by someone who has known or worked with them.

Personal statement by a woman living with HIV in the South Pacific

I would like to thank my doctor and her beautiful team for all their love, encouragement and most of all their prayers during these hard times. Without their love, support, encouragement and prayers I don't think I would still be alive today.

I got this disease from my husband, who travels to and from overseas.

I developed sores on my body sometime last year I saw a doctor and he put me on antibiotics for five days. The sores dried away but came back after a few days. I suspected something was very wrong with me when the antibiotics didn't work. I decided to see my own doctor. I was tested and found to be positive. My doctor gave me the results of the tests one afternoon. I was so shocked, I didn't know what to do, whether to cry, scream or commit suicide. I was so lucky that these lovely people came to the rescue. Their encouragement, support, love and most of all their prayers helped me along. When I got home

that afternoon, I saw my children. I cried as if I was losing each one of them. They didn't know what was going on. I would have killed all of us that day if it wasn't for my doctor's encouragement and prayers.

My husband was not in the country when the doctor broke the news to me. This gave me enough time to think about the whole thing seriously. I was 100 per cent sure that if he were tested they would find him positive too. My big worries were my children. I took them to be tested and thank God they are not infected.

I know if I take up the decision to leave my husband, it will only make things worse for him and me. He will find another partner, and there will be another one infected. It took me some time to accept the fact that I'm a carrier.

My husband was happy to see us on his return. I picked a good time to tell him: when the children were in bed. He broke down, but what can we do? He was tested and found to be a carrier too. At the moment I have accepted the fact that I'm a carrier and am very careful about it.

I was aware my husband was having casual sex when not with me, but I was too ashamed to ask him to take precautions. I kept telling myself, next time. My advice to young mothers is, 'Don't ever wait for next time.' Now I have big regrets. I'm so lucky that I didn't have any more children after I was infected.

I'm so concerned about young mothers who might be victimized this way. I went to a private doctor one day and asked to be tested for the disease. I just wanted to see how patients are treated. He asked a lot of questions about why I wanted to be tested. I showed few symptoms of the disease. He suggested I didn't take the test. He tried to tell me that there was no cure for this disease. I think doctors should understand that early detection will save another person's life. I was lucky that I took the tests first. I would have had another child if I didn't know I was infected.

With my doctor's counselling and encouragement, I still live happily with my husband and children. I think doctors play a very important role in this case. I know if it wasn't for my doctor and her team I would have taken my life and my poor innocent children's lives, too. Prevention is better than cure. In my case it's rather too late but I will do all possible to help prevent the spread of this disease.

Women at risk: case studies from Zaïre

by Brooke Grundfest Schoepf

Nsanga

Nsanga is 36 and very poor, the mother of a five-year-old girl and a boy in primary school. Until recently, she contributed to the support of a younger brother in secondary school who lives with an elder brother. A younger sister also lives with Nsanga in a single room with a corrugated-iron roof, part of a block surrounding an open courtyard. The yard contains a shared water tap, a roofless bathing-stall and a latrine, but no electricity. In good weather, Nsanga moves her charcoal stove outdoors to cook.

Nsanga wasn't always the head of her household. Village-raised, she married a schoolteacher in 1980, and managed somehow on his skimpy salary, despite galloping inflation of nearly 100 per cent each year. In 1983 the IMF instituted a series of 'structural adjustment' measures designed to reduce government expenditures so that Zaïre, like other Third World nations which had borrowed heavily in the 1970s, could make payments on its international debt. More than 80,000 teachers and health workers were made redundant by this 'cleaning up' in 1984. Bringing health to the budget, this housecleaning has brought malnutrition and ill health to hundreds of thousands, including low-paid government employees, their families and those whom they formerly served. Many no longer have access to even minimal health care or education. Nsanga's husband was one of those who, lacking a powerful patron to intercede for him, joined the ranks of the unemployed. After six fruitless months of waiting in offices, he began to drink, selling off the household appliances to pay for beer and then *lutuku*, the cheap home-distilled alcohol.

Nsanga tried many things to earn money. Like most poor women in Kinshasa, she has had only a few years of primary schooling. Since she has no powerful friends or relatives either, she was unable to find waged employment. She cooked food for neighbourhood men, she sold uncooked rice in small quantities and dried fish when she could obtain supplies cheaply. These efforts brought in only pennies at a time. Her husband left and Nsanga does not know where he is. The children ate into her stocks and she went into debt for the rent. She asked her elder brother for a loan, but he refused, pleading poverty. Although he has a steady job as a labourer on the docks, he has two wives and nine children.

Without her start-up capital, exchanging sex for subsistence seemed the obvious solution. The first year she had a lover who made regular support payments. She also had a few occasional partners to meet occasional cash needs. Then she got pregnant and the regular lover left. His salary couldn't stretch that far, he told her. So Nsanga had to take on more partners. The neighbourhood rate was 50 cents per brief encounter in 1987 and Nsanga says that if she is lucky she can get two or three partners per working day, for a total $30 a month (at most). Many men now avoid sex workers since the mass media have identified 'prostitutes' as a source of infection.

Nsanga's baby was sickly and died before her second birthday, following prolonged fever, diarrhoea and skin eruptions. Nsanga believes it was because semen from so many men spoiled her milk. Nsanga reports that she has had a few bouts of gonorrhoea, for which she took some tetracycline pills on advice from the pharmacy clerk. About a year ago she had abdominal pains for several months, but no money to consult a doctor. She says that the European nuns at the dispensary in her neighbourhood do not treat such diseases. Diagnosis at the nearby University clinic costs the equivalent of 30 encounters, so none of the women she knows can afford quality care.

Asked about condoms, Nsanga said that she has heard of but never actually seen one. She has heard that men use them to prevent disease when they have sex with sex workers. Nsanga rejects this morally stigmatizing label, and if a lover were to propose using a condom, she would be angry. 'It would mean that he doesn't trust me.' In her own eyes, Nsanga is not a sex worker because she is not a 'bad woman'. On the contrary as a mother who has fallen on hard times through no fault of her own, she is trying her best to meet family obligations.

Nsanga has become very thin and believes that people are whispering about her. In fact, her neighbours are sure Nsanga has AIDS, but then, Nsanga reasons: 'People say this about everyone who loses weight, even when it is just from hunger and worry. All these people who are dying nowadays, are they really all dying from AIDS?' Her defensiveness is shared by numerous women in similar circumstances.

Tango

Tango is a college graduate, aged forty. She has worked for fourteen years in a gender-typed formal sector job. Her work demands considerable technical and public-relations skills. Unmarried, with a slim figure and wearing stylish European clothes, she has had a succession of lovers over the past twenty-five years. These have included fellow-students and wealthy older men from both African and expatriate elites. Four years ago she became pregnant and decided to keep the child, rather than going to a doctor in her network for an illegal abortion. Although formerly her ethnic tradition strongly discouraged premarital pregnancy and imposed heavy sanctions on unwed mothers, Tango's parents were delighted with her decision. They reasoned that she is not likely to marry and will not have many more opportunities to bear a child.

The infant was robust, healthy and much loved. When he was one year old, Tango was hospitalized for pneumonia. The sickness dragged on and she lost weight. Tongues began to wag. Tango became frightened. Then she reassured herself: 'My child is not sick; therefore I am not infected.' After six months her health improved and Tango was further reassured. Nevertheless, her long sickness and the deaths of a former lover and numerous acquaintances from AIDS have made her prudent. Since she has read that condoms are not 100 per cent sure protection, Tango now prefers to forego sex: 'I have my child to think of. My parents are too old to raise him.'

Tango remains unmarried by choice. She has refused to place herself in the subordinate status, and what she feels are the uncomfortable situations that marriage imposes on women – in her culture and in the West. Friends say that she could have married an American lover who was ready to divorce his wife for her. In the pre-AIDS era, Tango believed that she had the best possible sort of life for a woman without wealthy parents. She has a moderate-paying job which she enjoys, health insurance, vacation travel, a low-rent apartment in the centre of town, many friends and relations in the city and the moral support of her parents living in a distant city. In addition, Tango enjoyed the fun of having lovers, with dinner dates, dancing and gifts. She suffered none of the heartbreak that comes from emotional involvement with one (she believes, inevitably) unfaithful man; no jealousy of rivals, nor the galling burden of having to support and care for children while their father divides his resources among several women.

Tango's apartment is old, with unreliable plumbing and indestructible cockroaches, but relatively cheap and very convenient. Tango walks to work and to shops, saving on fares and on waiting time for the collective taxis which supplement the overcrowded bus system. She owns numerous furnishings, accumulated from her salary and gifts. To these blessings – and the pitfalls avoided – Tango has added the joy of a child of her own, a boy named after her father.

Because of AIDS, Tango has given up lovers. She misses both sexual satisfaction and luxuries which her wages cannot provide, such as new clothes, dining out, and replacements for her outworn household appliances. Trade might be an option, but her private-sector job is demanding, and unlike many people in government employment, Tango cannot take off time from work to conduct a business on the side. 'Besides, everyone is selling something these days and nobody has money to buy.' Tango voices a common complaint. Whether she will remain celibate is unknown. But because she is single and can manage on her salary, the choice is hers to make. Moreover, if she decides to take a lover she can insist on regular condom use. Tango might follow the example of her friend Zena, who is divorced, self-employed and apparently well-off.

Zena

In 1985 Zena, Tango and their friends dismissed the news of this mysterious new disease as a 'Syndrome Imaginaire pour Decourager les Amoureux' (imaginary syndrome invented for discouraging lovers).

Which lovers were being discouraged? Africans, of course. By whom? Europeans, of course. Why? Because they believe that Africans have too much sex. Really they are jealous.

This denial served as a cultural defence. Then there were too many cases reported by physician-friends working at the three major hospitals in Kinshasa. By 1987 people in their relatively privileged circle acknowledged that AIDS is real, fatal and sexually transmitted. In 1988 some began to use condoms. Fear of AIDS caused Zena to remain celibate for about six months. Then she took a very young lover to meet her 'hygiene needs'. She initiated him into adult sexuality and believes that she can count on his manifest attachment (and her gifts) to keep him faithful.

Tango and Zena are unusual. Because of their economic independence, they can control their sexuality and negotiate condom use. Since learning about AIDS they, like some married couples, have reduced significantly their level of risk. Not all employed single women are so fortunate, because most women who are employed receive very low wages and for many, sexual services are a condition of employment.

Vumba

Vumba is a nurse, age 25, who in 1987 earned $35 per month. She grew up in Kinshasa and is single, without children. She lives with her widowed mother and two younger sisters, still in school. The rent for two rooms in a courtyard very much like the one where Nsanga lives is $11. However, Vumba's courtyard has electricity and she splits the bill with the neighbours. She pays $5 per month to run her two electric lights, a two-coil hotplate, a radio, a fan and an old refrigerator. Vumba's mother sells beer in the courtyard, 'but with everyone selling something there is very little profit'. She is looking around for something to sell that would make more money. Meanwhile, Vumba is the family's mainstay.

She has a lover, a clerical worker who earns less than she does. Although they have been together for nearly five years, he seems in no hurry to get married. Vumba reasons that he probably sees no advantage to marrying, since

she would still have to use her salary to support her mother and sisters. She talked to him once about using condoms but he refused: 'Because they aren't natural.' He says condoms would interfere with his pleasure. He has never tried one, but friends have complained of reduced sensation: 'They say it's like eating a banana with the skin on.' Her lover already has children with another woman and has no objection to Vumba taking the pill. In her experience this is unusual, and is one more indication that he is not serious, since: 'Children are the seal of marriage.'

In 1986 hospital workers were screened for HIV. Nearly nine per cent were infected, up from six per cent in 1984. Vumba was among those found seropositive. She was not told at the time. 'Maybe they thought I would commit suicide?' When she learned of her test results she was devastated, but thus far there have been no signs of disease. Has she told her lover? 'No, of course not. I proposed to use condoms. But since he refused, the consequences are his lookout! Where do you think I got it, anyway?' she asks.

Vumba's defensiveness arises from a situation of relative powerlessness. She believes that if she were to tell her lover of her serostatus, he would disappear. This assessment is shared by many women, and frequently has been borne out in practice. Since HIV-infected persons may be shunned by friends and even by some family members, Vumba's behaviour is self-protective. She believes that the pleasure she experiences with her lover is essential to her health, and that if she were to worry about her HIV status, the disease would come on right away.

Actually Vumba has had a few other partners (she says she doesn't remember how many). She began having sex in nursing school at age 17. Since she did not experience satisfaction in those days, she has put them out of her mind. Vumba likes to dress well. A six-yard length of locally made wax-print fabric tailored for an ensemble cost two months' salary. These days, AIDS is called 'Salaire Insuffisant Depuis des Années' (acquired income deficiency syndrome). Moreover, Vumba says, 'The doctors at the clinic are demanding and can cause endless complications for a nurse who refuses their advances.' She heard that several doctors are infected, too. Quite a few are no longer at the hospital and two are said to have died of AIDS. 'Others just don't want to be around so many infected people.'

In 1984 when hospital staff began talking about AIDS Vumba was frightened too. Although the nurses were told that AIDS is hard to catch, she would have liked to find another job where she would feel less exposed. 'Maybe, after all, one could get infected from a patient?' But now she asks: 'What's the use?' Vumba is afraid of the pain and the wasting, but she tries to put this from her mind. She would like to have a child because without children she will never become an ancestor. She fears that she will die 'an insignificant person' and that her name will be forgotten, because she will have no children to name their children after her.

Vumba has other worries: 'What will become of my younger sisters?' With men now looking for younger and younger partners whom they believe less likely to be infected, the temptations for girls from poor families are very strong. The deepening crisis leaves less money to pay school fees, buy clothes and bribe poorly paid teachers to give them passing grades. Do her sisters know about condoms? Vumba isn't sure. She hasn't told them, because she doesn't want them to think she is encouraging them to have sex. Perhaps they have learned about condom protection from Franco's song? Vumba sighs:

- 'Even if they know about Les Prudences (condoms), what's the use? Men won't use the things and the girls can't make them. Anyway, a young girl would be ashamed to ask her friend to use a condom. He would

think she was a prostitute. It's the same as with birth control pills.'

Avoidance, denial and notions of propriety combine with gender inequality to increase young women's vulnerability. Although at least half the adolescents in Kinshasa are sexually active by age 17, many adults do not consider their desires legitimate and avoid the subject.

Mbeya

Mbeya is a carefully groomed woman in her late forties, with heavy gold jewellery, many ensembles of stylish Dutch wax-print fabric, expensive handbags and matching shoes. She often drove an elderly Mercedes herself, although there was a chauffeur for running errands and driving her youngest child to school. Two elder children are studying in Europe and one in the USA.

Mbeya's husband was for many years an important figure in the ruling party's inner circle. For such men, the company of stylish young women is a perquisite of the job, a routine part of the socializing integral to politics. Mistresses are also part of the intelligence-gathering networks with which no man in high politics can do without. Mbeya says that she was not too jealous because: 'He always respected me as the first wife, mother of his children, and kept his other women away from the house.' There was plenty of money and she never felt done out of her rights as has been the case with many of her friends whose husbands are unfaithful.

Mbeya had a friend who couldn't abide her husband's outside wives and lovers. 'She harangued him about this so much that finally he left. She divorced him, but he got back at her. He forbade their children to visit their mother when they came home from school in Europe.' Her friend died of asthma, and Mbeya is sure that her condition was aggravated by her chagrin. Mbeya muses: 'Everyone is wondering why that man hasn't succumbed to AIDS!' The fact that some notorious philanderers have remained healthy, and that some people get sick while their spouses do not, causes confusion. AIDS' apparent arbitrariness reinforces beliefs that implicate fate, luck, ancestral spirits and sorcery in disease causation and contributes to denial of risk.

A wealthy physician-businessman living on Mbeya's street, and two of his wives, died from AIDS. Neighbours blamed the first wife because she traded on her own account, travelling to Nigeria to purchase household appliances on commission from friends and acquaintances. Mbeya reflects:

'It could just as well have been the husband who gave her AIDS! Who knows what younger wives do when their husband is away? And did he only sleep with his wives? After all, a doctor has many opportunities!
• Men are always quick to blame women, especially when women earn their own money!'

AIDS has entered the complex terrain of gender struggles and competing moral discourses. Mbeya and her friends wonder where AIDS came from. Several traditional healers claim that AIDS is an old disease which has become epidemic because women no • longer observe the old sexual customs. However, in Mbeya's ethnic group, as in many others, high status women controlled their own sexuality. Tradition has been reinvented in aid of controlling women.

In 1988, Mbeya became aware that her husband was sick and not getting any better. She began to suspect that it might be AIDS, and told him that she wanted to use condoms. Her husband refused. So she said that they should stop sexual relations. Her husband's family was outraged and he refused this too. They threatened to throw her out and keep her youngest daughter. Mbeya acquiesced. Following her husband's death, her in-laws accused her of infecting her husband, despite the logic of the situation. Mbeya protests that she married as a young virgin straight out of convent school and that all through the years, she was a faithful wife.

Recently widowed, Mbeya soon will have to leave her husband's luxurious villa and all the furnishings. These now belong to the husband's family, who have already taken possession of the cars and the businesses and rental properties her husband had acquired. The house will be sold and the money shared among her husband's brothers. Turned out of her home, bereaved and fearing she is infected, Mbeya will go to her brother's where she will become his dependant.

Emotionally Mbeya is still reeling from her husband's unpleasant death and in no shape to face the future. Why hasn't she gone to be tested? Intellectually, she knows that AIDS is fatal, and that if infected she will die eventually. However, Mbeya would rather not think about that just yet. 'If I am seropositive, then worrying would bring on the disease.' Many people use this construction to avoid learning their serostatus.

It is the fact of multiple partners, rather than the type of relationship, however socially categorized and labelled, that puts people at risk. Prevention cannot simply be targeted to sex workers and their clients. Although poor women are at greater risk, the experience of married women dependent on wealthy husbands indicates that gender relations as well as poverty act to prevent women from protecting themselves from HIV. Social structure limits the ability of women to become independent actors exercising social agency, and those who perceive themselves to be powerless erect psychological defences against the pain of risk assessment. Thus, effective, culturally informed empowerment strategies require theoretical and method-ological sophistication.

Black women living with HIV and AIDS in South Africa

by Anna Strebel

'Thembi'

'Thembi' is 25 years old, and both she and her partner are HIV-positive. They are un-employed and live in a male hostel with a young child.

'I did feel a bit bad, but what could I do? Then you must just believe in God, because if it just came like that, it just came, and there isn't a way to come right again.

Before this rash broke out, the people in the house said I was getting AIDS. I said it wasn't AIDS at all, it was a rash.

There are some women who don't wash. There are some women who use something for the men and that causes it. The dirty illness. He got it from sleeping around. He flirted with a woman I didn't know about. The woman who stays in the room with me told me that I must open my eyes. Women come from the rural areas.

So then the people at the hospital told me that he infected me with the thing. Then I came to tell him and he said, "It's my own business." He said it isn't him but me who sleeps around. But after all, the thing is in him. But now he argues that it's not him, but me.

He also didn't want to let the people know what was wrong, so when I was drunk one day, I told them. Then he hit me because I accused him about the thing in front of the people. He was very cross and then he hit me.

We still sleep together, but now, because the bed is small, the child and I lie down below and he sleeps above. We use nothing. I'm so scared of those things [condoms]. Perhaps sometimes it will stay behind inside you. I'm not interested in those things. I don't know about not doing it. They say if you have the urge it must just come. If the urge is there and he wants you, then you must just be there. Because sometimes the men hit you because of it. He won't let me say no to sex. He will just think that I won't sleep with him because I'm flirting or I've got another man.'

'Nomsa'

'Nomsa' is a 35-year-old single woman with HIV. Her partner had tuberculosis and died of AIDS. She has some secondary education, used to work as a cleaner in the hospital, and now lives with her child in her brother's house.

'My whole body itched, so I went to the doctor and got a white lotion in a bottle. I rubbed it on and the thing went away. They didn't tell me anything, so I asked the doctor what was wrong. The doctor said it was nothing, there was nothing wrong with me, but I asked them to test my blood. I knew that this sickness was in the people who don't look after themselves properly, that sleep with the men, someone who has something. You don't know, you sleep with the man.

It was very painful. I thought I would die. Last year, when I heard I had the illness, my head couldn't . . . I looked like someone who was going to die. I also didn't want to look at other people, I was scared of the people. If the people know I'm sick, they will be scared of me. I didn't want to go out, I just stayed at home. Then my family took me home, so that I could forget about it for a bit there.

I don't have boyfriends any more. I don't want to make other people ill any more. I know about condoms and I would use them. I'm not interested in sex any more, because I'm scared of the men. I don't know if the man is sick or not, understand? Maybe I'll get sick again. I would use a condom, but the men don't want to use them. You bring the condoms, you give it to him, he doesn't want to use it. They don't even believe in them, they get angry.

I use nothing. I don't want to have a boyfriend. I don't want to have more children. It is too burdensome to raise a child, buying clothes for the child, food and all that, going to school.

I won't tell other people. Our nation, if you're sick they are funny towards you. They are scared of you, they don't want to talk to you or do for you. You don't have friends, your friends run away from you. No, my child doesn't know about it, he's still a child.

I am sorry about the future. I feel that the sickness has gone. If I look after myself it will stay away. I believe so. Now I am happy, really happy. My heart was sore. I wanted to kill myself, because I saw people who were sick and I thought I would look just like them. They can't do anything for themselves, just sleep and stay in bed. I'm still young. I won't stand for just staying in bed. I want to do everything for myself, understand, because the people get tired of people who look sick. It's better if you can do everything for yourself. If I could study, go to night school, so that I could forget my thoughts. Because it stays here in my thoughts. I just think, if I get sick from the sickness, who will look after me, because the people are scared.'

Reaching within, reaching out

by Marie Marthe Saint Cyr-Delpe

When I went back home to Haiti, I stayed busy all the time. I realized that I was afraid, but I didn't dare voice my fear. In the midst of accusations of being disease carriers, uncertain of our own risks, I was afraid to speak the unfamiliar. To speak the unfamiliar in our country is to beckon its curse upon you.

We knew so little about AIDS. Accused by those who profess to know all, one begins to doubt one's own knowledge and awareness. I left my job and my town and came to New York. I had been offered work with the Haitian Coalition on AIDS.

As a woman, I had learned early in life that I must be silent, and that demanding was for men; as women, we learn to negotiate our demands through subtle means. AIDS demanded open, pointed negotiations leading to change, a skill I didn't have. I felt that I could no longer live my sexuality. Yet harbouring the same feelings of false security as many others, I saw myself as one with few worries. After all,

I am a one-man woman. Unfortunately, for long enough, my partner believed in having as many women as he could get his hands on. I seriously began to worry about my own survival. I remember threatening to kill him if he ever gave me this virus. Our conversations on the subject gave me no real guarantees, but they did give me some sense of assurance that he was concerned. I would fool myself into believing he would be faithful. Of course I hope that he is.

The AIDS crisis has brought forth a twisted interpretation of the role of Haitian women in the transmission of the virus. During my last visit to Haiti in December 1987 to January 1988, I was eager to talk to Haitian people from all walks of life about their perception of the unspoken disease. In the cities of Petion Ville and Port-au-Prince, the overwhelming attitude among those I spoke to was that women were responsible for the transmission of this disease – blaming the victim among the victims.

Success in Haitian society is defined by one's ability to speak the elite language. There are very few employment opportunities or other means to prove oneself. Male sexuality has become a substitute for the social and economic rewards that are lacking. The political and economic hardships have diluted traditional values and allowed violations of social codes. If one sees AIDS transmission as a reflection of the market economy, devised to sustain male economic and sexual power as well as social control, it is not surprising that women are used as scapegoats.

The women with whom I have worked are infected because their husbands are or were bisexuals. In the spirit of self-sacrifice, a highly valued attribute in Haitian family life, these women have maintained their silence. Their anger often is veiled behind a shield of undue commitment, and they are embedded in their prescribed roles. They maintain a passive and subdued facade. Very few have opted to leave these threatening relationships behind them.

I am reminded of Alice. Ever since her husband was told that he was HIV-positive, he had taken to sleeping on the floor. This was before she understood the possibility that she may already be infected or learned the basics of safer sex. She looks fine, and sometimes she forgets all about AIDS. She gets very angry out of sheer frustration at the absence of sexual expression in her life. Generally, she does not talk about her sexuality; she is not used to thinking in terms of her own satisfaction, so she silently accepts her husband's decision to abstain. She finds herself lost in the depth of her own silent fears and hopelessness. And because her self-image is determined by her ability to have and raise children, she was confronted by the worst nightmare of life when her baby died of AIDS.

Traditionally, the contributions of Haitian women to the country, and to the economic and social survival of the family unit, plagued by male absenteeism, have not been acknowledged. The AIDS crisis can do only one thing among Haitian women: awaken them from their state of self-neglect and self-sacrifice, and develop strong advocates for the promotion of the well-being of the whole family.

Asserting myself is still a struggle, but I remind myself that I must always communicate my needs, and actively define and shape my life. I am no longer silent.

Personal experiences in the Bahamas

by Rosamae Bain

Sue

Sue, a 19-year-old woman and mother of four children, was admitted to hospital for a caesarean section. Her partner and only sexual contact in life went to donate blood. On screening, he was positive for HIV. Family testing revealed the young mother, her two-year-old toddler and the new baby were all positive for HIV.

The status of the family three years later: The father is still healthy, working and supporting the family and practising safer sex. The patient changed from a young, beautiful girl to an ill-looking elderly lady. She has lost more than 20 per cent of her body weight, has swollen lymph glands, severe anaemia, amenorrhoea for the past year, skin infections, hair loss, premature ageing, and difficulty in walking. She is a totally different individual from the carefree happy person of three years ago. She is unable to work, has periodic hospital admission and the two children have died.

Roxie

Roxie, a heavily built 30-year-old single mother, is employed in the hotel industry. She was named as a sexual contact of a healthy HIV carrier, who is a married man with four other named contacts. Her last three children are from the same married man, and he is the only sexual contact she had in eight years. Following screening in 1988, she was also classified as a healthy carrier. Her four children, ages 5–11, were all tested negative.

Roxie continued to do well until she developed weakness in her lower limbs, weight loss, diarrhoea and severe anaemia two years later. Within eight weeks of her first hospital admission following diagnosis, she died, leaving her four children in the care of a sister. Today, the courageous sister is coping with her own six children plus those of her dead sister.

Kim

Kim, a 12-year-old school girl, occasionally skipped school with friends and drove around in jitneys all day until time for school to come out. Then she would go home. On other occasions, she would take friends home, as her parents were out at work and younger siblings were at school. Her friends would watch TV, play music, dance and occasionally engaged in intimate sexual relations. This lifestyle resulted in her becoming a mother at age 13. When she came for antenatal care, she was found to have HIV and other STDs.

Within a year, Kim changed from a healthy girl to a case of AIDS, presenting with excessive weight loss, diarrhoea, swollen glands, skin rashes, chest infections and oral thrush. She had frequent admissions to hospital and died when she was 15, leaving behind a young grandmother with a toddler to care for.

Lucy

Lucy, a 45-year-old professional, was referred to the AIDS & Infectious Diseases consultant by her private physician, following a positive diagnosis of HIV. Within two years of her diagnosis, she presented with weight loss, chest infection, skin rashes and diarrhoea. The care her immediate family provided was excellent, spending time, providing care and love. Her mother and a sister took time off work to care for her at home as long as possible. Other family members encouraged and assisted.

Ida

Ida, a Bahamian university student in the USA was still a virgin when she came home for Christmas. She fell in love and had her first sexual encounter, two days prior to returning to school. A month later, her mother got a call saying Ida was ill. She had syphilis and another STD. Further testing showed her to be positive for HIV eight weeks later. The results of one sexual encounter, leaving a depressed though healthy student continuing her education.

Vickie

Vickie is a 9-year-old, beautiful, intelligent student from a cocaine-infested area. She was admitted to the children's ward and diagnosed with pneumonia. On admission, she was found to have excessive, foul vaginal discharge. Screening showed her positive for syphilis, hepatitis B and HIV. Investigation by the STD team and medical social workers resulted in the child being placed in alternative housing. She is having ongoing health education appropriate for her age, health care and emotional support. A social worker is involved as well.

Working with people with AIDS or HIV and their families requires an immense sensitivity to people's needs and a deep commitment to helping others. The main aim of the nursing, medical and ancillary staff assigned to their care is helping patients and their families cope as successfully as possible with their disease.

The women of Grupo Pela Vidda, Brazil

This conversation was recorded in São Paulo, Brazil.

Zia: When a woman tells her partner that she has AIDS, he runs away. He goes to another experience. And she stays alone.

Patricia: Did you ever have a man after you found out you were infected?

Zia: Yes. I told him and he left. I couldn't go to bed with a man keeping this kind of secret. He said that he didn't use condoms, that I should look for another partner who could accept them. Because as much as he tried, he couldn't.

Marta: I had three different experiences. To the first man, I didn't say anything. I only insisted that we use condoms and he accepted this without a problem. But after a short while, he found out that my husband had died of AIDS. Even though he had used condoms, he came looking for me. I heard that he was armed; I heard many stories . . .

The second experience was completely different. He knew my husband. I haven't done anything with him, we have only gone out together. I told him I am HIV-positive. And even so, he wants to go out with me. But I can't. I will not stay with a person just to have his company and to have sex, if I don't love him.

The other man is a policeman. I only met him a few days ago. We went for a beer, and we talked. We talked about a friend whose husband is in jail. Then he said, 'If I was the wife of a bum who went to jail, I would leave him, because there is a lot of AIDS in jail. AIDS disgusts me.' Then I thought to myself, I cannot tell him that I am HIV-positive. But later on, when we were more intimate, I said, 'If you are so afraid of AIDS, why don't you use condoms?' He said, 'I am not going to use those things, no way.' I said, 'So, you are not afraid. If you were afraid you would use condoms. Take me as an example. Do you know anything about me? Do I know anything about you?' He answered, 'No, I don't know.' I said, 'It's right to use condoms. If we are going to be together, I insist on using condoms. Furthermore, I think you move too fast. You don't even know who I am.' He answered, 'OK, you are so wonderful that I will buy a box of condoms.'

He was supposed to call me yesterday, but he didn't. Maybe he thought about it and got frightened. This is the way I try to proceed. I don't tell the truth because the truth makes the person run away. But I look for other ways of guaranteeing that the person will not be at risk: using condoms, having safe sex.

Patricia: So your position is to never say that you are infected?

Marta: Yes. This is very difficult. And you are going to lose many men, the ones you want. Both cases that did not work out well for me were people I felt comfortable with. It is not that I want a commitment from anyone. It's not even sex. But I miss some affection. But no man will give affection to you with 36

years on your face without asking for sex.

Zia: I don't feel the need for sex any more. Even before I found out that I was HIV-positive, I already wanted to be alone. I had so many bad sexual experiences that I thought it would be better to be alone. I don't know if this is the right way, but it is better to be involved in many activities and not to let sex bother me day and night.

Veronica: My boyfriend said that he was infected. Now, after some months, I found out that he is not infected.

Xica: Do you believe he wanted to get infected?

Veronica: Yes. I met him through an advertisement in the paper. He said he was HIV-positive in the advertisement. He was looking for an HIV-positive woman. Now he says he wants to have sex without condoms. I'm still with him, but I don't think for much longer. I don't want to have guilty feelings if he gets infected.

Isaura: I felt that a tractor passed over me after I found out I was HIV-positive. I hate my husband, and I love him at the same time. I want to kill him and I want to be close to him. It is very confusing. It seems that I am going crazy. The hate is because I have always been loyal to him. He always had his freedom and his own life. Now, this happens to me. I am sure he infected me. I only had him. When he was sick, we loved each other very much. Then, when I found out what he had, I started to hate him.

Patricia: Is your husband alive?

Isaura: Yes, he is.

Marta: Ah, your feelings will change. My husband loved me very much. And I was very loyal to him. He used to do drugs before being with me. When he was with me, he said that he was not doing drugs any more. I thought I was very mature and experienced, and I believed him. I don't know if he was already infected or if he got infected after being with me. When he got sick, I started to feel a maternal love for him, even in the face of the disease. I loved him and I wanted him. But eventually I couldn't take it any more. I was always crying, always afraid of his crises. I started to wish he would die soon. Then I felt I couldn't live without him. How could I have wished that he would die soon? I couldn't understand what I wanted.

The doctor said that I had to remain calm, but how could I? I had to take care of him as well as my son, my daughter and myself. I wished that someone would take my children away. I didn't know what I wanted.

My husband died and now I miss him very much. When he was sick, he told me that he already knew he was positive for more than two years, that he had denied to himself that he was putting me at risk. He was afraid of losing me because he loved me very much. And I forgave everything. I loved him too much.

Beatriz: Of all the women I have told about my being HIV-positive, no one ran away. They have all showed solidarity with me.

Maria: I feel happy! I have a lot of friends. We go out, we have fun, we go to bars. I just don't stay out all night any more. At two in the morning, I am at home, and they are still out there. I don't miss having a boyfriend. There are even a lot of candidates, but I am not interested. Before, I let the disease run my life. When I went out, I was afraid of the rain. But now I live normally. Just because it rains, am I going to catch cold? No, I don't live like this any more. Now I have fun.

Beatriz: When I am at home doing nothing, I think: 'I don't know how much time I have left. I am going out. I am going to live.' I take better care of myself. I know that what counts is today. I have begun to like myself more and to do things I like. I am closer with my daughter and with my mother. I want to say something to you, Isaura, whose husband is alive. Try to give him all the love

you can, all the attention. It doesn't help to want to die first. I also wanted it, but he died first because he was already sick. Give him all the love you can, because when he passes away, you will feel that you could have done more. I think all the time that I could have done more.

Margarida: I felt disgusted when I found out I was HIV-positive. I felt like throwing myself under a car. I got really depressed. Because I am sure that my fiancé, who died, knew he had AIDS. He didn't tell me anything. When he died the doctor called me in. I did the tuberculosis test and the result was positive. Then came the AIDS test. When the doctor told me the results, I was calm. Then, afterwards, it struck me. I had never been sick before. I have been to the hospital only to deliver my children. And now, I live from hospital visit to hospital visit. I feel better, but at the beginning I didn't even want to take a shower.

Monica: When my husband died, everybody checked me out and asked, 'Aren't you sick?' And I answered, 'No, thank God, I don't have anything.' Almost four months have passed. Whereas I had been too thin, now I have even gained weight. And the people, the neighbours, the shopkeepers, look at me invitingly. They think I don't have anything any more. They think I didn't die within one month, so I don't have AIDS.

Dora: I am not open about being HIV-positive because of my daughter. I am afraid that she will not get a boyfriend because they will be afraid of her, since her mother has HIV.

Rebeca: At school, if the teacher talks about AIDS, I say that I have many books about it at home. The other kids ask me why I have all those books. I answer that on my street a man died of it and that now everybody tries to learn more about it. Then they ask to borrow my books. But usually they are not serious. They say, 'You are too thin. Get out of here. You have AIDS.' They don't know that a fat person can have AIDS. The young people say, 'I think I don't have it, because only gays and prostitutes get it. I will not catch it. We know each other. We know where we live. We know each others' families.' I can't talk too much about it, because I am afraid they will ask me questions and find out about my mother.

Julia: Something happened to me at the hospital. I went there to have an X-ray and I met a seropositive man who was also having an X-ray taken before me. When I was called, and the technician was positioning my head for the X-ray, he said, 'You know, that guy who just left, he has AIDS.' I said, 'Me too.' The technician got embarrassed and said, 'Sorry.' I think he was afraid that I would tell the guy what he said. I asked him, 'If you are afraid of getting AIDS, do you use condoms?' He answered, 'No. Me? Why should I use condoms, if one can get it from kissing, from tears, from sweat.' Then I said, 'So, you better be careful because you are touching my forehead. It is hot and I am sweating.' He was very embarrassed. I felt I had to say something else. But I realized that he was so misinformed that the few minutes we had together would not be enough to make him understand. I would like to bring some educational material for him.

Patricia: He broke confidentiality. He could be prosecuted because of that incident.

Yara: On a TV programme, it showed an HIV-positive baby and doctor who was wearing a mask and gloves. The programme didn't explain that he was wearing a mask and gloves to protect the baby. No, people got the wrong message that the baby might contaminate the doctor.

My husband died of both depression and discrimination. He didn't die of AIDS. He was HIV-positive, had tuberculosis and recovered from it. He came back home and started thinking only of AIDS. He was a very macho man. People think that because he was in prison, when he was there he was a woman. But it is not true. He did drugs. People wondered, 'What happened? Did his wife sleep around?' He had all this on his mind, as well as the lack of money, his own suffering, then my positive test. Imagine him finding himself condemned to die, and seeing the person he loves, who took care of him, also condemned. He got depressed, he wouldn't take medicines, he wouldn't eat. He entered a convulsive crisis, went to the hospital and died ten days later. On his medical report, it says that he died of AIDS because he had a positive HIV test. But he only had biliary tuberculosis that had been treated two months before. He had gained weight and he didn't have any other infection. He died of depression and discrimination.

Marta: My son is 12 years old. Today we were having lunch at my mother's house and she started arguing and accusing me, 'It is not my fault you have this problem. You got this problem by yourself.' I said, 'What is this, mom? We can't be sure about how I got infected. I may have got infected during the surgery I had. I am not guilty of being sick! When Uncle Batista got hepatitis, he quarantined himself, because he loves us and he doesn't want to infect us. Do you think I want to infect you? I don't want to infect anyone.' Later my son asked me, 'Mom, is it true that you have AIDS?' Then my mother said, 'No, she doesn't. It is all because of that surgery she had. It was a bad surgery.' So, behind my mother I made signs to my son to agree with her and I also agreed with her. Later on, I told him that I am HIV-positive because I believe he has the right to know the truth. He is already a young man; he hugs the girls. So he needs to know about these things. I'd rather he learned about them from me.

Yara: I told my son Cristiano about everything. I myself keep the glasses separate, everything. Sometimes when I am eating, Cristiano says, 'Mom, give me a bite.' I used to say no. He would ask why, and then he would come and take some. You understand? He doesn't worry. I am the one who has it.

Proof positive?

Anonymous

When AIDS (as we then exclusively knew it) first came on the scene, I was as distressed and shocked as the next person. 'How awful for them,' I thought. 'They' were, we had been reliably informed, the three 'high-risk groups'. To this list could be added 'in the USA' because none of us saw it as a problem for Britain.

I had a background in social services, thought myself as broad-minded as the next woman and grieved for these unknown souls who were far, far outside my sphere of contacts. Like most other newspaper readers, I ingested, at an intellectual level, more and more information: that there is a difference between HIV and AIDS, that there is high-risk activity rather than high-risk groups.

And this is the level I stayed on until one day, in a pub, which isn't my usual hunting ground, I met a beautiful man. He had just returned from living abroad, and was tanned and golden. As I sat and talked to him, I realized he was the most desirable person I had ever encountered. I admired everything about him. He was lithe and young and kind and chivalrous – and he, it transpired shortly after, admired me. One night, two years ago, we ended up in bed. 'You must use something,' I demanded (not having anything in the contraceptive line with me except the word no, which I had difficulty getting past my lips). 'I'm terrified of getting pregnant.' No thought of safe sex, other than in the sense in which Marie Stopes might have used the phrase, entered my head.

He produced a packet of condoms, and everything, as they say, developed from there. He was, and still is, the best thing that ever happened to me.

You've probably already guessed the rest. Yes, he is HIV-positive. After one of the most confusing and bewildering childhoods I've ever heard of, he turned to drugs in his late teens. He was living with his grandmother, who had brought him up after his mother's death. She was then a very fit and alert old lady of 80, but her sedate and immaculate seaside flat held fewer charms than the chaotic summer squat just down the beach.

He travelled the world – America, India, Afghanistan, Australia, ending up in southeast Asia. On the way, he used everything going, including heroin. He gave up the lot in 1983, but when a couple of his user friends tested positive in 1986, he also decided to take the test. Despite all his precautions, he was infected.

The local doctor offered him what counselling skills were at his disposal. 'You're a dead man,' he pronounced. He tells me that the first few months were appalling, as the reality sank in. Understandably, the thought of returning to drugs crossed his mind – what had he to lose now? But he rejected this idea and decided that keeping in the best of health was the better plan. He then retreated into the pattern of behaviour which he had used to deal with unhappy events in his childhood – he just put the news out of his mind. HIV ceased to exist for him; it hadn't happened.

It was two years after this that we met and then began my coming to terms with it. I wasn't afraid of my own physical wellbeing – we should all know by now what does and doesn't transmit the virus. The question that gave me sleepless nights was whether I could cope with the emotional turmoil of getting involved with someone who might die and leave me bereft.

In the end, there was no choice. I was already involved and leaving him of my own accord would cause me more grief than his leaving me involuntarily. At least if we stayed together I could love him and look after him to the best of my ability. Which is what I do, making sure he eats properly and sees his consultant a couple of times a year. It is I who scans the papers for HIV/AIDS news, who nags him to collect his food supplement drinks.

He is in excellent health and has put on a little weight since we met. No one except me and a couple of long-standing ex-user friends knows about his status and that's how he likes it. I sometimes wonder how others, envying us our extraordinarily close relationship, would react if they knew that all isn't roses in our particular garden.

We now read that everyone who tests positive may not go on to develop AIDS, which gives some hope. In the meantime, we lead very normal lives and perhaps appreciate our time together much more than most couples do. All in all, I'm a very lucky person.

Witness

by Misha

This text came to us one misty evening when we were discussing AIDS, drug addiction and sex work. Charged with emotion, this account turns the spotlight on a very particular yet very real situation, giving us a dreadful glimpse of the unacceptable and the sordid. While sex workers are among the most involved in prevention of HIV infection, and among the best organized, especially in client-related projects, there are particular *situations that we must admit to, to open our eyes to the reality of drug addiction combined with sex work. It would be wrong to generalize. It would also be wrong not to talk about it. – Aspasie*

It is nearly two years ago now and like so many other times, I was once again without an apartment to work from. So I had to entertain my clients in a hotel used by sex workers in

Geneva in the Paquis district. There were about 20 of us in that hotel. Twenty women from all over the world, of different races, young, old, beautiful, not so beautiful and also drug addicts.

We would look for business right in front of the hotel. There were about 15 of us that evening, working the pavement along a 150-metre stretch. The customers would pass up and down, look at us, size us up, discuss prices and what they could get.

For quite a while I had been watching a good-looking man, very well dressed. He stopped at nearly every girl, said little, then quickly moved on to the next. I said to myself that he had to be very complicated, taking so much time to make up his mind.

Nearby was Marie. Half sitting, half lying, her legs stretched out in front of her to keep from falling off the car she was leaning against. Her arms hung at her sides like dead weights. Her head was down, her mouth half open, and a little saliva dribbled on to her breast. Her eyes were shut. I knew Marie well enough to guess that she had just had a fix of heroin and was really high.

The client I was talking about came up to me, but just as he opened his mouth to speak to me, his eyes fell upon Marie. Without wasting any more time on me, he made straight for her. To talk to her he had to bend down low, since Marie had neither the strength nor the will to lift her head. The man turned his back on me and I couldn't hear what he was asking her. But I could see her clearly and I heard her mention the sum of 150 francs. Apparently they agreed on this because Marie, with help from the client, hauled herself up on to her wobbly legs. They both headed for the hotel entrance. As they passed me, I could hear the client de-manding: 'You will keep your word? For this 150 francs, I can have and do what I want?' Already the hotel door was closing behind them.

That such a smart and intelligent-looking man should single out Marie interested me a great deal, as did his insistence on really having all he desired for 150 francs.

I decided to wait for this client to come out. Forty-five minutes later I see him leaving the hotel in a great hurry. Someone who, a short while ago, didn't give a damn about what people would say, taking all his time to choose, now looking as if he has only one wish – to leave, to get out of the street as quickly as possible. I rush up to him and stop him by grabbing on to his sleeve. Irritated, he looks at me. I ask if I can put one question to him. He looks at his watch, glances left and right to make sure no one is watching us, tries in vain to free his sleeve which I'm still gripping tightly, then glares at me, but consents to hear me out: 'If it's really necessary, but hurry.'

I ask him then why he chose Marie when he could have had any of ten or more better-looking girls and all of them in a normal state. He stares at me hard and his eyes light up cynically. 'Would you or one of your girlfriends have let yourself be fucked up the backside without a condom? Would you have let me beat you while I pushed my cock into your mouth until I came and then forced you to swallow it? And all for 150 francs?'

I can't answer him. I feel like I'm going to be sick on the spot, from rage and disgust. He sees the effect of his words on me and adds, eyes full of hatred and contempt: 'What do you think? If I come for a prostitute, I want the services of a real one, one who will give me something for my money.'

I can't stand much more of this, but ask him if we are still women in his eyes. On this he replies: 'Do you think that that' – (and he points to Marie's window – 'is still a human being?' I let go of his sleeve and through my tears, watch him disappear into another street.

I turn round, hurry over to the hotel and go up to Marie's room. The door is open. Marie is lying in bed completely naked. She is asleep, gently snoring, half turned on her stomach. Across her back I can see red marks, obviously made with a belt. From her mouth flows a thin thread of saliva. Her make-up has run. I can see she's been crying in spite of the state she is in. I cover her and close the door behind me and slip away.

Today, two years on, Marie has no further need to let herself be abused in this way. She's been dead for six months. Of AIDS.

23 March 1988. Fribourg.

Translation from French by Philip Bickle and Graham Fletcher

In her own words

by Jacqueline Revock

In 1987 I was diagnosed HIV-positive. I was an injection drug user and the doctor just confirmed what I already knew in my heart. I thought I was prepared to accept what he had to say. Fat chance! What he said was that since I was 'just' HIV-positive, there was nothing that could be done for me. His only advice was that I should have myself sterilized immediately, so that I could not bring any sick children into the world. I left his office and cried all the way home, and then I gave up. I spent the next month trying to kill myself via a monster heroin habit. Lucky for me, I ended up in jail instead of a grave.

In September 1990, I was incarcerated on Rikers Island. In jail I found hope, not much, but enough to start trying to live. I realized that not only did I not have to die, but that I did not want to die. I found out that my T4 count was exceptionally high. After three years of street living, I was asymptomatic. I spent 8 months on the Island and began to acquaint myself with the virus that decided to take up residence in my blood. I learned that I was not just a walking death sentence.

In May 1991, I was transferred to the Union County Jail in New Jersey. Unfortunately, UCJ

is not quite as enlightened or medically advanced as Riker's Island. During my first medical examination, I informed the doctor of my status and began to explain to her a number of physical complaints I had. She cut me short and asked me if I took AZT. When I said no, I do not require AZT, she became quite robotic and perfunctory. I had again fallen under the 'nothing can be done' category.

I requested that my T4 count be done again and she mumbled something about not worrying because I 'looked so healthy'. I wrote the medical director about my request. During my interview with her I was told the test was very expensive and I 'looked so healthy'. I said I would like to remain looking this healthy, and T4 monitoring was an important part of my care. Finally, in July, they drew my blood to do a T4 count. Two weeks later I asked for the results and was told they were confidential. I would have to sign a medical release form through my lawyer to get the results. When I was informed that my count was 857, I was chastised for being worried.

Everything is a battle for me and every other inmate who is HIV-positive or has an AIDS diagnosis. There is no doctor in attendance after 4pm or on the weekends. I have witnessed two extremely chilling incidents of apathy on the part of the jail personnel. One HIV-positive woman walked around with active hepatitis for five days here before being hospitalized. She became jaundiced and complained of abdominal pain. They told her to rest and put her on a liquid diet. Her requests to see the doctor were ignored. The officers would not go near her, and most of the nurses were only concerned with her ability to swallow her aspirin. Finally, after countless calls to the jail from her family, she was placed in the hospital. Upon her return to the jail specific medical orders from the doctor were lost, and medications ordered were either substituted or not given at the prescribed time.

The second inmate I need to tell you about is a friend of mine who has an AIDS diagnosis. She had been having trouble breathing. For weeks she wheezed and coughed and became paler. They moved her into a single room so her breathing wouldn't disturb her roommate. She became too fatigued to eat. Again, numerous requests for medical attention and numerous family phone calls. She almost died of PCP before they took her to the hospital. When she came back, she was housed with an inmate who had an upper respiratory-tract infection. My friend contracted PCP again and had to be rehospitalized. She was put on aerosolized pentamidine therapy. Her monthly trips to the hospital clinic involved her being handcuffed and shackled and escorted by the sheriff's department. Privacy during treatments is out of the question. She had to receive these treatments and any other in all her 'jailhouse jewellery' and with a female officer present. This is the routine even when the inmate is hospitalized. No matter how sick or debilitated, at least one ankle is shackled to the bed. You are not even allowed to go to the bathroom alone. There are no allowances for privacy or dignity.

As far as any type of counselling or education is concerned the administration feels our hearts and our minds are nonexistent. Unless an inmate writes to outside agencies, there is no way to obtain information about HIV/AIDS. Those of us who are willing to tell others about our diagnosis counsel and support each other. There is no medical or prison employee we can turn to. There is no one to speak to about our fears and questions. There is no way to make any kind of informed medical decision for yourself. If your T4 cells are low enough, you can get AZT. That's it.

Infected inmates all over the country are facing my problems and much more severe ones every day. I have to start small, here at the county jail. I'd like to see some kind of understanding and compassion here. We are entering the second AIDS decade. I hope and pray it won't take another ten years before people begin to care. Sometimes I could kick myself when I realize that it took jail to make me care. Other times I thank God I'm here and not still out on the streets. In the past 13 months, I've become more educated, more informed. I refuse to just wait to die, or try to hasten the moment any longer.

While I have been here, I've tried to help anyone who asks. I pass out pamphlets and information. I write officials and politicians. There are times when I feel like the tree that falls in the middle of the forest and I wonder if anyone hears me. Others times I feel like I could do anything. The only thing I am certain of is my will to live, to live healthy and productively for as long as possible.

Women-centred projects, action and services: some examples

A wide range of groups and individuals are engaged in HIV/AIDS prevention and care for women. Some projects are mainly or only for women; others are not but show an awareness of gender issues. They are variously involved in self-help and caring for others, advocacy, research and education. They provide a rich source of ideas and models for action, and show just how much women can and are achieving internationally in HIV/AIDS work.

The Women & AIDS Support Network, Zimbabwe

by Sunanda Ray

WASN was set up following the first SWAA meeting in Harare in May 1989. Our objectives are:

- to disseminate information on how HIV infection specifically affects women as infected persons, as carers, as mothers of infected children and children who may become orphans;
- to encourage women in organized groups and clubs to support women with HIV infection and to support each other in protecting themselves against infection.

In 1989 WASN held a major conference with the theme 'AIDS: an issue for every woman'. Over 100 delegates from both urban and rural areas of Zimbabwe attended, including representatives from women's organizations, government, AIDS service organizations and individuals. One of the aims of this conference was to break the barriers created by the first wave of anti-AIDS messages, which separated women into the 'good' and the 'bad'. The conference report and recommendations were circulated to all governmental and non-governmental AIDS organizations and programmes, to promote gender sensitivity and empowerment of women.

WASN has focused discussion about AIDS on sexual relationships. We talk to men about supporting other men, for instance in the workplace, to be monogamous, and not to be violent if their wives ask them to use condoms. We try to work through the problems couples have if one or both is HIV-positive. We talk with women in church groups and sewing cooperatives about supporting their friends if they find out they are HIV-positive, rather than laughing at them or chasing them away. We talk with rural women about not feeling threatened by urban women and not to blame them if their husbands are infected. We hold educational sessions with schoolgirls about feeling proud about their bodies. We participate in radio and TV programmes, and write magazine and newspaper articles, with emphasis on positive images of women as strong and sensitive rather than passive, helpless victims.

For World AIDS Day on women in 1990, we worked together with the AIDS Counselling Trust and the National AIDS Control Programme to produce a booklet *Why should women be concerned about AIDS*, which was published in the three main languages and distributed all over Zimbabwe. Its main purpose was to encourage women to talk to each other about their fears, their anxieties and their anger about what AIDS meant to them, as a way of softening some of the taboos relating to sex and death. On World AIDS Day in 1991, we launched a collaborative publication between Noerine Kaleeba of TASO (The AIDS Support Organization) in Uganda and WASN about her personal story of living with AIDS in her family. It is called *We miss you all; Noerine Kaleeba: AIDS in the family* and was written to give courage and hope to those living with HIV and understanding to those who are not.

A WASN workshop in 1991 was on 'Images of women and AIDS in the media', where we looked at stereotyped images of men and women. Contemporary messages asking young girls to say no to sugar-daddies were discussed, with a challenge to health educators also to ask sugar-daddies to leave our young girls alone. We talked about why many women who see themselves as 'good' distance themselves from other women who they consider 'bad', in case they are somehow tainted by them. We recognized that having more women doctors, lawyers, magistrates and so on, does not seem to have reduced these stereotypes or reduced incriminations against women.

WASN has worked hard at challenging and changing the images used in drama for mobilizing people and educating about AIDS. Several existing plays used for health education centre around male characters who get HIV by visiting sex workers or by having casual affairs and who then take infection home to their wives. Men are seen as agonizing over which woman gave them HIV rather than recognizing and feeling sad about how many women they might have infected during their many relationships. We rarely find out what happens to the women in these stories, except perhaps the wife, who tragically watches as her baby dies of AIDS and wonders when it is her turn. Audiences watching these plays are typically composed of men who laugh at every stereotyped line ('I have five girlfriends and they are all faithful to me') and women who sit quietly, looking aghast, wondering what they have done to deserve such humiliation. The 'bad' women in the dramas are the sources of infection and the 'good' women, the wives, are passive, helpless recipients. We have argued for more progressive attitudes towards community theatre, in which drama is used to promote positive behaviour and images, rather than reflecting negative attitudes prevalent in society. We want to see women shown mobilizing together, not just weeping at funerals. To encourage more women-centred images, we support initiatives by women's theatre groups to write and perform poetry, songs and plays about women's experience of living with HIV/AIDS. We are making a video about images of women and AIDS which will be used all over the region, in urban and rural settings, to promote debate about empowerment and support.

We try to help women caring for others with HIV, either formally as health workers or in their homes caring for relatives. We give practical information about prevention of infection and personal protection, through booklets in three languages and/or demonstrations. With health workers we have been involved in discussions on facing and dealing with fear of infection.

WASN also acts as an advocacy group for basic human rights for women, such as the right to work. We became involved in discrimination against women with HIV in the workplace, when several women with HIV lost their jobs after their HIV status became known. Women are often employed as domestic workers, looking after young children in creches and pre-schools. The Minister of Health has issued a directive that HIV infection is not a valid reason for dismissal. But there is still a lot of anxiety about this, even on the part of health workers. When children are involved, the issue becomes particularly emotive. WASN has organized meetings with legal groups and trade unions to clarify the rights of workers.

WASN has a small core of active women involved on a daily basis, and a wider membership of women and men interested in our work. We have discovered that the stigma attached to AIDS carries through into our work. Some of us are HIV-positive, some are negative, and some don't know. We know of women who have wanted to join us but were afraid to be thought of as HIV-positive. We know of schoolgirls who wanted to join us but were afraid their parents would worry that they were at risk. We know of other women whose husbands would not allow them to come to meetings, and still others whose long working hours prohibited another journey in the evening. One of our main achievements has been to influence others so that our messages are incorporated into their daily working activity, whatever work they do. Our meetings are also a source of support for many members involved in HIV-related work, whether as health workers, teachers, in laboratories, the army or social work.

WAMATA: People striving to control the spread of AIDS, Tanzania

Theresa Kaijage talks to Sunanda Ray

We spent a long time working on what the name WAMATA should stand for. The name was all right, but we kept changing the wording. I had written in the draft that it should reflect the caring, the loving of a member who had HIV or AIDS. One man said, 'As you have put it, it sounds really feminine.' Some said this loving, this tenderness and caring do not reflect the African male and that AIDS needs to be conquered by more than love, care and tenderness. It is a struggle. So in the name of WAMATA we show how the family is struggling against AIDS in Tanzania, *Walio Katika Mapambano Na AIDS.*

We started in June 1989 with five families, as a voluntary non-sectarian, non-governmental grassroots organization, based on the spirit of solidarity, love and hope, to provide medical and home nursing care, counselling, and to some extent material assistance to people living with HIV/AIDS.

All the gender issues we had never tackled came up at once. Initially we ignored them or thought they were irrelevant. We thought it was Eurocentric to tackle them in Africa, because we thought our African culture was different and dealt with things in a different way. All the agendas that we had ignored – legal, educational and health problems, inequitable gender relations – suddenly we are dealing with these multiple issues, which people have not learned to analyse in a way that promotes equal sharing of both resources and power at all levels. In order to deal with AIDS, we have had to confront these.

In WAMATA it has been an uphill battle, in terms of full participation of men and women, both in the organization and at family level. There are women we are trying to support materially because there is nobody else to support them. AIDS has left them with fewer alternatives. Because their husbands have died of AIDS, it has not been easy for them to seek re-marriage and support from a new husband as an option. Therefore, the organization has to step in. During the period when a woman and the organization are working towards helping both their families to accept that her husband died of AIDS, the woman herself may be dying of AIDS. Their children need support and both families need to work together to negotiate joint custody of the orphans.

Then there is the question of property rights and inheritance for the widow. In some communities, she is taken over by the husband's brother because that is the way property is kept within his family. The children need the right to their father's property, but they are too young. If the woman is not staying in the father's family, who is going to look after the father's property and therefore the children?

WAMATA is engaged in constant negotiations with the families on both sides, acting as mediator, helping widows work on their wills. We have members who are lawyers to advise us on legal issues, particularly regarding the rights of inheritance.

There was a woman who had disputed refugee status. She came to WAMATA because she had to be admitted to hospital and had nowhere to leave her children. We helped to place the children in an orphanage. When she got well she wanted her children back, so we managed to find her a place to stay. It was meant to be temporary residential accommodation, but she has been there for a year and a half now. She is a woman in a desperate situation, with no relatives in Tanzania and children from men who were not willing to take responsibility and have since walked out of her life. She has no support of any kind except from WAMATA. We are all volunteers, so we cannot be with her as back-up support all the time. We do what we can.

Another of our members was diagnosed HIV-positive in 1989. She has a husband and six children. She is employed by the University as a supplies officer. Her husband was diagnosed HIV-positive in 1988. She was the first to be told by his doctor. He was not told. She was not counselled, but she had the responsibility of disclosing the diagnosis to his family. She was warned by his family not to tell him. Their reaction was that she had caused it.

When the tension between her and her husband got worse, she realized that staying together was not good for either of them, and she moved out. They still live close to each other and she tries to keep in touch with him and the children, giving as much support as she is allowed to give. Just before they separated, she went for voluntary testing and learned that she too was HIV-positive. She told her sister, who has been very supportive ever since. It was during this period that a friend introduced her to WAMATA. She joined in 1990 and said:

'I could not believe it when I found people discussing their HIV status freely and sharing information on treatment alternatives and support. My husband and I are still separated, but as I accept my status better, I also accept his situation more. He

has not accepted his diagnosis, but now he allows me to support him more.'

This woman has a good job so she mainly needed emotional support from us. She had to come to terms with her anger at her husband's family for rejecting her at a time when she felt they needed each other most. She has learned better ways of persuading him to do things other than blaming him, and he is no longer reacting in an angry, defensive way. The children are at secondary school and know what the diagnosis is for both their parents. The oldest child sometimes goes to get their medicines for them. This woman is trying to sort things out legally, but sometimes a case might be won in court but not at home! Things will not always go smoothly, but she is now strong enough to deal with it and her children will always be there for her.

For women who have been widowed by AIDS, whose husbands were their sole support, we have tried to set up a revolving, income-generating loan fund. It has not worked very well. Many members were not engaged in self-sustaining activities, so they could not pay back the loans when the initial money was finished. It was so little. When you give people such little money and ask them to return it, it is ridiculous. All we give them is seed money, to get projects off the ground. No one usually manages to pay it back.

One woman had five children and was guardian to a sixth. Her husband died of AIDS. He was her second husband, and only two of the children, both daughters under age 5, were his. That was problematic in terms of inheritance. She felt that traditionally, she did not have the right to impose herself on his family. So she moved in with her own family and stayed with her mother, who was also a widow and had moved to stay with her own parents. So in fact this woman had moved to stay with her maternal grandparents with the six children.

She had been dismissed by her employers for being sick. She joined WAMATA, who tried to help her get her job back, unsuccessfully. We gave her some money to start an income-generating project in the village. We also gave the children some food supplements and paid the school fees for one of the sons. She started in her grandparents' house, selling a few supplies that she felt were needed in the community. Soon it led to her being able to purchase a piece of land and one thing led to another. She was no longer afraid to say that her husband died of AIDS and could approach other people for help. She managed to buy corrugated-iron sheets and build her own house on her piece of land, and now she and her children are living there. She feels that if she dies of AIDS, at least her children will have their own home and land and this feels good. She has also helped to start a local branch of WAMATA there and is on the committee.

Another woman was selling peanuts when she came to WAMATA, because her husband's family had kicked her out of the house. All she owned were the clothes she and her one-year-old child were wearing. We gave her some money for a project. The first thing she bought was a black dress, because she said she never had a black dress to mourn her husband properly. It served two purposes. She had an extra dress, and she fulfilled cultural expectations on her behaviour, and that was important to her.

Very few people are in a position to pay the money back. The people who usually qualify for this aid are those with absolutely nothing. People who have a job or relatives to support them do not qualify. Some donor agencies feel disappointed by this failure to 'revolve' the funds, but it is unrealistic. It is not because the participants have not tried. It is very hard to generate a surplus, enough to pay back the original money. In many ways, we are happy if they are able to support themselves on the proceeds and to look after their families. That is a bonus.

The contribution of churches and other NGOs in Tanzania to AIDS work

by Kari Hartwig

A number of national church bodies in Tanzania, in particular the Catholic, Episcopal and Lutheran churches, have begun AIDS programmes since about 1989. The churches have been among the first organizations within Tanzania to begin doing AIDS education work and support for people with AIDS and their families. One of the reasons for the strong role of churches in AIDS prevention is their history in providing medical assistance. Their stance has rarely been moralistic or condemning, thus offering a safe environment for information and support. The example of one programme is illustrative of the kinds of activities in which the churches are involved.

The Evangelical Lutheran Church in

Tanzania has established a five-year AIDS prevention and action plan. Medical activities consume most of the budget. Lutheran hospitals, health centres and dispensaries are being supplied with HIV-test kits to screen blood donors and patients with clinical symptoms of AIDS. Other equipment includes adequate sterilization facilities and protective gear such as gloves, aprons, and boots for staff. Continuing education seminars on AIDS for health workers are given at least once a year.

Though the greatest portion of funds is directed towards medical equipment and support, the main stress of the programme is on education. The primary target groups are pastors and evangelists, women's groups, church youth groups and choirs, health workers, community health workers, and primary-school children. Pastors and evangelists are trained so that they may in turn teach their congregations. A special training for evangelists in how to teach primary-age students about AIDS will be included at their annual meeting.

Another primary objective is to counsel AIDS patients, their families, those who are HIV-positive, and those seeking premarital counselling. Again, the main people targeted for training are pastors and evangelists. A number of counselling and training programmes have already begun.

This and other non-governmental programmes are young and still learning which policies and programmes are most effective. These programmes all have government permission to operate, and most agency representatives spoke positively about the support of government for their programmes. Each of these agencies share in common the fact that they are largely supported financially by outside donors. The longevity and size of their programmes will largely be based on continued donor support.

With the exception of the churches, gender appears to be an incidental consideration in most of these programmes. In the case of WAMATA, their support groups have tended to attract more women, even though women are not a specific target group. The African Medical and Research Foundation programmes are focused primarily on men by the nature of their target groups, truck drivers and STD clinic attenders, who are primarily men. Although neither organization has a stated objective specifically to give services to men or women, that has been the outcome.

The churches have targeted women's groups to receive information about AIDS. As women fulfil the role of primary caregivers, it would not be surprising in future to see or hear of church women's groups being trained in counselling and support skills for people with AIDS. Some women's groups are already taking this initiative upon themselves.

For example, a Catholic women's group in Mwanza requested a guest speaker to talk about women and AIDS. In particular, they wanted information on:

- the numbers of women in the area who were HIV-positive;
- what efforts were under way to prevent AIDS in women;
- what type of support there was for women suffering from AIDS;
- how the women at the seminar could help others work through their grief about AIDS deaths if they or family members had AIDS;
- how they could help reach youth and teenagers.

Church-based AIDS education for women is important. Women's access to mass media is more limited than men's. Women therefore rely on informal sources of information. Religious groups can provide a safe and acceptable environment for women to receive information if the messages are not blaming or moralizing.

Approaches to AIDS education for the grassroots in Nigeria

by Adepeju A. Olukoya

In Nigeria, health-education efforts for controlling AIDS have mainly relied on the use of the mass media, both print and electronic, and primarily in urban areas. Nigeria is 85 per cent rural, with a 54 per cent illiteracy rate among males and 77 per cent among females. It therefore is very important to make attempts to reach the grassroots with the message of AIDS prevention in a language they can understand.

What to call AIDS

The initial problem was selecting a vernacular name for AIDS. Although it has been referred to as 'slim disease' in some parts of Africa, no colloquial name existed in Nigeria, as far as I was aware. After much reflection, it was decided to use a descriptive phrase. The Yoruba people in Southern Nigeria have a name for sexually transmitted diseases, and this was used as the basis for reference to AIDS. It roughly translates: the STD that does not respond to any treatment.

Fathers' Clubs

The Family Health Clinic of the Institute of Child Health and Primary Care of the College of Medicine in Lagos provides comprehensive family health services to a target population of 30,000 people in a predominantly slum area of Lagos. One of the ways of gaining acceptability for the clinic's programmes – and getting the men involved – was to start a Fathers' Club. The club meets monthly. Health topics are treated at some of the meetings. One of the health topics treated at one of the meetings was AIDS. In addition, key points about AIDS, its symptoms, and prevention of transmission were translated into the local language and made into posters displayed at the clinic. It was felt that if the mothers attending the clinic knew about the disease, they might talk about it at home. Some of the fathers also use the services of the clinic, and so they were reached by these posters as well.

The Fathers' Club meeting on AIDS generated a high degree of interest, and the discussion continued long into the evening. Condoms were made available to the Club Secretary, who served as an agent for distribution. Each father was asked to tell at least ten other people at home or at the workplace about AIDS. A tally sheet was given to each club member present, to note the number of people spoken to about AIDS. Initial feedback has indicated that some of the men not only reached, but exceeded their targets.

This same approach was used with the Fathers' Club of a non-governmental organization, Regina Mundi, as part of their primary health care project situated in Mushin, one of the most densely populated areas of Lagos. Feedback from that attempt showed even better results. In both cases, many of the club members admitted to never having heard of AIDS before. The few that had heard about AIDS were happy to have a forum where they could ask questions, and to learn about the disease in their native language.

Marketplaces

The initial success in the Fathers' Club led to the idea of carrying the AIDS message to other public arenas, such as the marketplace. The first opportunity came during the 'Health Day' activities of one of the medical students' clubs. The students made plans to set up a booth in one of the big markets in Lagos on a Saturday. Services at the booth included: family planning (condoms, foam tablets, an initial packet of birth-control pills for eligible women), blood pressure screening, counselling and treatment for any health ailments, continuous talks on various health topics including hypertension, anaemia, etc. Loudspeakers were used so that market vendors who could not leave their stands could nevertheless benefit from the information provided. The highlight of the programme was a talk on AIDS. It was estimated that over 1,000 people listened to the talk (which was given an impromptu translation, at popular request, into other traditional languages by students and bystanders).

The response was so enthusiastic and there were so many questions from the audience, that the author and some of the students were kept standing on the roof of the van for almost three hours talking about AIDS. The presentation included a demonstration on the proper way to use a condom (the neck of a beer bottle donated by one member of the audience was used as a model). Simultaneously, students handed out condoms to any of the listeners who wanted them. This initial experience led to the inclusion of such activities in the required fieldwork for final year medical students of the College of Medicine, Lagos, as part of the maternal health/family planning unit of their primary health care training.

Club talks

STOPAIDS, a voluntary non-governmental organization, began a programme of lectures on AIDS for recreational clubs around Lagos. Pamphlets and other information on AIDS were taken along to informal discussions on the subject, held at convenient pre-arranged times with selected clubs. The discussions have demonstrated a good deal of success, in providing an opportunity for those who had read about AIDS in the press to ask questions. It has been interesting to note that some of these men were concerned about the right way to wear a condom, and had many questions about the disease.

AIDS and sex work: an Indian perspective

by I. S. Gilada

At the Indian Health Organization (IHO), we seriously question social interventions which attempt to reform or rehabilitate sex workers. Nor can we see any lasting value in the types of social protection which have been initiated. While we strive to eliminate forced and child prostitution, we do not take a position against sex work per se. Thus, we appear to be confused, and from within that confusion we locate the women in sex work. From within our own frail perceptions and hopelessness, we locate ourselves. We have chosen to provide help and support to these women, who are probably the most underprivileged in contemporary society. This paper attempts to represent the reasons for our confusion and a hope for a beginning towards change.

Living conditions

Women who sell sex in Bombay and most other urban centres live in a territory and world beyond the pale of description. Words can only minimize and discount the squalor and neglect in which they live. An average of 10–12 girls stay in one small room. Most eat in filthy cafeterias or buy food from street vendors. Commodities are sold at double the cost in their locales. Most of the young girls abuse drugs or alcohol and smoke.

Sex work and sexually transmitted diseases

At the STD clinic in a large teaching hospital about half a kilometer away from Bombay's largest area of sex work, I was surprised to learn that within the space of a year, not more than 300 women sex workers would seek treatment, whereas the number of male STD patients at the same clinic was about 100 per day. Yet our surveys estimate that Bombay has about 100,000 women sex workers in a population of 10 million.

I visited the locality and encountered weird treatment methods for STDs used by quacks who were practising in the area, including some who inject coloured water into the vagina and uterus as treatment. I decided to try to organize appropriate health care for the women and their children. To this end, the first

health camp was organized by the IHO in 1982 at Kamathipura, Bombay's largest locale for sex work. We continue to run camps to this day at regular intervals, and also have two mobile clinics in the red-light areas. Through the camps, we offer specialist care and diagnostic facilities to the women, but for us the situation was an eye-opener. Our analysis of data on more than 800 women showed that:

- About 15 per cent of them were below the age of 18.
- About 15 per cent had entered sex work through 'Devadasi', a system of dedicating girls in the name of a goddess and later pushing them into selling sex.
- Each woman sees an average of four clients per day and their average income is about Rs 400 (US$15) per month.
- Most of them know nothing about contraception and STDs.
- Most seek medical care in their locality from unqualified quacks, who constitute 90 per cent of all medical practitioners in the red-light areas, and who often give injurious treatment.

Clinically, we found that 80 per cent of the women who attended our camps suffered from STDs and laboratory investigations showed that 90 per cent of the women had demonstrable STDs. Over 50 per cent had two or more STDs at a time. The most common STDs seen are syphilis, chancroid, gonorrhoea, donovanosis, and venereal warts. The incidence of genital herpes is also increasing.

During the camps, medical social workers interviewed the women. From these, we concluded that the problems of women in sex work required medico-social solutions and not purely medical ones. Since then, the IHO has been actively involved in providing social relief as well as medical care, including to child prostitutes, eunuchs, Devadasis, senior sex workers, and their children.

HIV infection and sex work

It is but natural that sex workers are vulnerable to HIV infection. In fact, nearly 15 to 25 per cent are already infected with HIV. Nearly 29 per cent of registered HIV-infection cases in India are women sex workers. Yet at the end of 1986 among 600 sex workers screened by IHO for HIV, only three were HIV-positive. The continuous rising trend in HIV prevalence among sex workers since then suggests the beginning of a major AIDS crisis in India. At the beginning of 1992, HIV prevalence in Bombay sex workers was 32 per cent.

The denial of this trend, and complacency and inaction by government authorities is likely to make India top of the world for AIDS cases by the year 2000. This is partly because of our large population and partly because India already leads the world for STDs with 50 million of the estimated annual 200 million cases of STDs internationally.

The first case of AIDS among sex workers in India was reported from Bombay, a 32-year-old former Devadasi. She died of multiple infections with tuberculosis and candida in 1988. Till her death, the sex workers of Bombay were not convinced that AIDS was so close at hand, as previously only asymptomatic cases were detected. Her death was used to educate sex workers and pressure government authorities to do something. The attitude of sex workers changed to a great extent, but then they began asking why they should bother about the society that had never bothered about them. They complained that when they insisted on the use of condoms, their clients went next door.

Are we equipped to tackle an AIDS epidemic in India? No. At present, AIDS cases are underdiagnosed, underreported and ill-treated. There is no system of follow-up once someone is found to be HIV-positive. Counselling, outpatient care and inpatient services are far from developed. Ninety-five per cent of the national budget until 1991 on AIDS was spent on testing services. After the tests, nothing is done for those with HIV. As a consequence, sex workers testing positive continue in the profession, and professional donors continue selling their blood and organs.

A new trend is that sex workers are not even told about their test results, let alone counselled or educated on safer sex. Nor can they be expected to stop their only source of livelihood on becoming HIV-positive unless they are rehabilitated.

Over 60 per cent of the Hijras (transvestites, transsexuals and eunuchs) are engaged in sex work. In Bombay alone there are 2,000 Hijras in the red-light district. The prevalence of HIV among them was 10 per cent in 1987, according to an IHO survey. Further studies could not be done because of lack of facilities. The Hijras entertain up to five clients a day, that is, 10,000 persons visit them daily, of whom many may be bisexual. The Hijras also attract a lot of foreign clientele.

Despite this, AIDS is seen as a disease of the poor and illiterate, the sex workers and deviates. It can rightly be said that AIDS in India is being spread through sex, blood and ignorance.

Explorations into needs and action

For the past ten years, we at the IHO have tried to use various strategies in an effort to evaluate vectors of possible change. Needless to say, these have scarcely made a dent into the lives of sex workers, nor do we feel that we can resist conventionality alone. We have no doubt that an integrated movement by the government, society and sex workers themselves is the only way toward total social change. IHO has given top priority to the prevention of forced and child prostitution, safer sex campaigns among sex workers and their clients, distribution of free condoms, counselling services, the treatment of STDs and minor ailments through our mobile clinic and media support.

In addition to the regular medical camps and the mobile clinic, we cherish the dream of a network of clinics exclusively for women sex workers, since health care remains our point of entry and helps to establish a personal rapport with the women and allows for an exchange of views.

We have campaigned against the Devadasi system and publicized and filed cases against abductions of women and children, using contact tracing to try to trace kidnappers.

We have run a day-care centre for the girl children of sex workers in central Bombay for the past two years, including school drop-out intervention, counselling of mothers and a health-care programme. We are planning a residential school for the children of women sex workers on the outskirts of Bombay.

We run an education and awareness campaign about incest and rape, which explores myths and misconceptions around these, with the aim of reducing their incidence.

We organize social programmes to foster brother-sister relationships and get-togethers and the response is encouraging. Besides the warmth and joy that religious festivities provide, relationships of befriending and showing that help and support are available are developed.

We often approach the press on issues related to sex work and AIDS with the hope of creating public awareness and highlighting the social aspects of sex work and the dangers of HIV/AIDS. The press has played a great role in the past nine years in educating the masses and creating public support.

We invite active political representatives, including concerned ministers, with the hope that some political will may be created and utilized to resolve the problems. Recent responses have been encouraging. We also recently published a document entitled *AIDS: A Nation at Risk*, specially targeted at policymakers and planners.

At the instigation of IHO, a union for women sex workers has been formed in Bombay with the name 'Asahaya Tiruskrit Nari Sangha'. Similar such unions have also been started in Nagpur, Pune, Kolhapur, Surat, Jabalpur and Latur. The Bombay union has organized public demonstrations against police harassment of sex workers and government apathy. In a short span of time, the efforts of the Bombay and Pune unions have resulted in minimization of police harassment, with members of the unions no longer having to pay protection money to the police. They have raised awareness of and some reduction in forced and child prostitution and some reduction in the Devadasi system among members. Self-protection and self-direction are probably the most valuable first steps taken. Efforts are ongoing to educate them about the seriousness of diseases like AIDS and the usefulness of safer sex practices.

Last year we launched 'Project Saheli', a new project on AIDS control, run and managed by the sex workers themselves with the technical guidance of the IHO staff. A three-tiered cadre of caregivers – a Saheli (friend) for each 25 sex workers, a Tai (sister) for each 10 Sahelis, and a Bai (motherly lady) for each 8 Tais – are managing the project with the support of social workers and health educators from IHO.

Outreach to bar workers in Bangkok

by Werasit Sittitrai

Most bar workers come from rural areas of Thailand and from poor families, and have a low educational level (primary or secondary school). They therefore have low bargaining power with the authorities, the bar owners and their clients. They have little contact with sources of information such as the media because of their low educational background and the time limitations of their work.

Working conditions

Most bar workers are women, but there are some men (in gay bars), while transvestites or female impersonators may also work alongside the women. Workers in gay bars serve primarily male clients and some female clients. In other bars, female bar workers serve male clients and female clients are rare exceptions. In massage parlours, female clients, though few, are not unusual. There are also a few bars with male workers serving only female clients and some which have both male and female workers.

Women in bars earn money in several ways: as monthly salary, as part of the money clients pay for the women's drinks, as a share of the money that clients pay to the bar in order to take the women out, and as direct payment for sexual services. The amount of money and type of earnings may differ depending on the type of bar and area.

Bar workers have a relatively high rate of turnover. Workers in gay bars stay in their occupations for a few months to a year or so. Bar girls stay longer. Some work for a while and then leave the job to do other things or to go home and get married. Others work for a period of time in one place and then change to another, depending on the income that can be earned in each place, their need for money, health conditions, and how they feel about continuing to exchange sex for money. Female workers may move from one bar to the next and then to a massage parlour or bars abroad. Some male or female workers are sponsored by Thai men or foreign men as regular partners for a period of time.

Private lifestyles

Outside the bars, bar workers lead private lives like the general population. Some of them may have other daytime jobs as factory workers, waiters and waitresses, or store clerks, even though working at night makes it difficult for them to keep these jobs. Some workers are students either in the regular school system, in college, or in vocational education to prepare them for new occupations, like hairdressing and dressmaking.

Many bar workers are married and have children, or are living with lovers. Others live with parents, relatives, or friends with similar occupations, or live alone. They may have sex with casual pickups from discotheques or shopping malls or a regular sexual partner, whom they support financially. Many of the women are divorced and have to support their parents as well as their children. It is not unusual for a worker in gay bars to live with a wife or lover who works in a female bar or massage parlour. Of 141 male workers in gay bars questioned on their sexual behaviour in a two-week period, sexual intercourse was most frequent with male clients and non-client females, followed by female clients and non-client males.

Since bar workers' lives consist of two dimensions, work and private life, an outreach programme must be a full package that covers both aspects.

In the bars

The programme should not only engage the bar workers but should include others in the bars as well (such as owners or managers, captains or mamas, cashiers, waiters and waitresses, doormen, janitors and clients). If all these groups are informed about the programme this will encourage cooperation and facilitate the work of AIDS education. Each of these groups must be exposed to the same set of information, education and services, so that they say, share and repeat similar messages. Experience in the field shows that different groups can often be exposed to contradictory information from different sources, which creates a situation that disrupts the whole educational campaign.

Attempts to reach clients must be made through the above core groups together with using appropriate media and other strategies. The aim of this comprehensive approach is to set up a network of education, encouragement and reinforcement in a bar. For example, when a bar girl is changing her clothes in the dressing-room, her peer group encourages her to use a condom. When she goes out, the cashier gives her two condoms to use with the client. At the door as she walks out with the client, the doorman says 'Come back safely' or 'Do it safely'. Finally, if the girl refuses to have sex with a client who does not want to use condoms, the manager supports her decision and does not take sides with the client when he complains. Additionally, some clients may decide to use condoms after seeing sexy posters promoting condom use in the bars. The girls they go out with will also have been taught by outreach workers many ways to convince clients to use condoms and be able to enjoy sex at the same time.

Outside the bars

Outreach workers must approach the bar workers at home as well as approaching the other people in their world, especially spouses and lovers, hairdressers and health clinic personnel. By doing this, the outreach programme can create a consensus of favourable opinions and understanding about risk behaviours and the prevention of HIV. In addition, these people can help by encouraging and reinforcing appropriate attitudes and behaviours for the bar workers through face-to-face interactions.

Outreach workers and materials may reach bar workers in two different ways. One is for the outreach workers to grow close to the bar workers and so ask to visit their homes or hairdressers or their neighbourhood. In this approach, the status of the bar worker is clearly acknowledged. Another approach is for outreach workers to select areas or apartments where many bar workers live and to visit the area to conduct an outreach programme. The outreach workers then interact with the bar workers as if they are part of the general population. Risk behaviour and AIDS prevention are explained with an emphasis on sexual contacts. Unless the bar workers reveal their occupation the outreach workers will not expose them or hint that they know or suspect their profession.

Preparing for an outreach programme

The following is a list of crucial preparatory work for setting up an outreach programme:

- Visit the bars and get acquainted with everyone. Always show respect and courtesy.
- Learn about the work situations in the bars: bar rules, how to get clients, private dealings with clients, bar workers' private lives, background, love, family, mobility, future plans, trouble at home, sex life, health conditions, etc.
- Figure out what would be the things or persons or relationships that touch their feelings and hearts most.
- Learn about their knowledge, attitudes, beliefs and practices concerning HIV transmission and safer sex.
- Choose the best time and place for each outreach activity. This is difficult, therefore good plans and strategies are needed to solve likely problems: before work (they have to get ready); during work (too busy, too noisy); after work (too sleepy, many workers have gone with clients); at home (shy to expose their private life and embarrassed about their living conditions).
- Work with the management, do not be hostile to them.
- Ask the cooperation of government authorities but do not rely on them for outreach work.
- Seek internal networks to assist with the outreach work, e.g. a group of girls all coming from the same geographical area.
- Show the target audience clearly how outreach activities are beneficial and yet not disruptive to their work or their life.
- Do not copy any outreach strategy or method without studying its adaptability and applicability. Not every activity can be applicable to every bar, for example, bar workers may not be able to function as outreach volunteers in a bar where most bar workers are hostile to each other as they compete for clients.
- Finally, but most importantly, the outreach workers must show that they do this work because they care. Only wholeheartedness leads to long-lasting change.

Positively Women, England

by Kate Thomson

I have been asked to talk about Positively Women, so I will give you some idea of how we started. It was almost four years ago and I had recently been diagnosed HIV-positive and was feeling completely isolated. After eight years or so of heavy drug use, I'd been 'clean' for about three and felt like I'd really got my act together. All the court cases, probation orders, etc., were out of the way. I'd made new friends, found a job, and was doing evening classes, planning to go on to university. A whole new life, a new start, and I felt really proud of myself. I'd come a long way, so I told myself.

At that time there was more and more talk of AIDS on the TV and in the papers. Although I thought I was probably OK, I realized that I might well have been at risk in the past through my using, and I suppose, though I didn't think about it then, through unprotected sex which I was still having. Anyway, when I came down with shingles, I was sure that it could be a sign of HIV infection. As I was feeling pretty run down anyway, I decided to be tested. I never really believed that I would be positive. I think I just wanted confirmation that I was in the clear. So when it did come back positive, I was stunned and completely unprepared. That is not to say that you can ever be totally prepared for a positive result, but you can definitely be more prepared and informed than I was at that time. I was not counselled either before or after my test.

I felt utterly alone, not knowing anyone else who had been diagnosed, and I wanted to talk about how I was feeling. But I didn't really think my friends would be able to understand, not having been through the same experiences themselves. My relationships and friendships really suffered because of this. I was sick of hearing social workers, health advisers and doctors saying they understood. I didn't really see how they could, if they had not had a positive diagnosis themselves.

I met some gay men who were positive and that was great – a real relief to be able to talk about my fears around dying, and other things like that. Yet it wasn't really enough. There were still so many issues untouched upon and concerns which we did not have in common. What I really wanted was to meet other HIV-positive women who I could talk to about my fears about having children, or rather, not having children, about sex, relationships, and so on.

This, however, was not so simple as it might at first sound. Trying to locate another positive woman in the London area at that time was about as easy as finding a needle in a haystack. Eventually I found an advertisement placed by another positive woman, saying she was trying to set up a support group. I made contact.

Walking into the room the first time we met,

I experienced an incredible feeling of relief – of being able to let go for the first time since I walked out of the hospital where I had been given my result. By the time we left it was as if I had been able to shed most of the tremendous isolation I had been feeling and throw off the layers of sadness and fear I had been carrying since my diagnosis. For the first time, talking to other women, I regained hope for the future and I realized that I wasn't necessarily going to die an early death. I realized that HIV doesn't necessarily equal AIDS, and AIDS doesn't necessarily equal death. That was our first meeting.

From then on, for the next two years, we met regularly each fortnight and gradually, as they heard about us, more and more women joined us. It became a real social network rather than just group meetings. We did loads of things outside the group times and exchanged phone numbers, went to visit each other at home, in hospital.

We had no funding so we had to rely on the goodwill of other individuals and organizations for office space, stamps, envelopes, photocopying, and help with our phone bills, which were always very high and impossible to pay on Income Support, which most of us were on. Little by little the demands made on the time of those of us who were actively involved grew, and we were often asked to participate in training days and conferences.

One of our main problems at the time was getting the trust and acceptance of other AIDS organizations and AIDS professionals. It certainly didn't help that most of us, at the beginning, were drug users or ex-users, that none of us came from professional backgrounds, and that we had no experience of dealing with funders.

The fact that we were women also didn't help. Although from the start there have always been friends who have supported us, many others just seemed to be waiting for us to fail. They seemed to be under the impression that they were already doing everything that needed to be done. Significant numbers of women who eventually contacted us told us they had been warned not to approach us at all – that we were a bunch of chaotic, drug-using women. Apart from anything else, this tells us a lot about attitudes towards drug-users in the AIDS field at that time – and I am not really sure how much that has changed today. I suppose those kinds of attitudes just made us all the more determined to prove them wrong.

For most of us, throughout our personal involvement with AIDS and with Positively Women, it has been anger – anger at people's attitudes, anger at the lack of appropriate or accessible services, anger at needs not being recognized or met – that has provoked our responses. If you suggested to any of us a few years ago that we would be speaking in front of conferences we would never have believed you. It was only the anger at having sat through two days of experts talking about things which didn't seem at all relevant to our lives as HIV-positive women that I, for the first time, got up and spoke in front of a conference. Eventually, you just have to say something about the reality of people's lives, about getting food and adequate housing, about childcare or the lack of it, and about the need to provide us with those things, before spending thousands and thousands of pounds on dodgy research and flying people halfway around the world in club class to present the results of their work.

For a lot of us, becoming involved has been a way of reclaiming a degree of control over our situations, situations where all too often it seems that the power to make informed decisions over our lives has been taken away from us or disallowed. Becoming involved has been a way of coping with our diagnosis, of creating a path through the chaos and uncertainty that a positive diagnosis can bring.

Membership of Positively Women is increasingly diverse and the women come from many different backgrounds, lifestyles and cultures: grandmothers, heterosexual women, lesbians, bisexual women, 14-year-olds, famous people, not so famous people and so on. Many of us were already very lacking in self-esteem and self-confidence, sometimes because of drug use or involvement in the sex industry, and having been told for so long that we were worthless. Others because of having been subjected to physical, sexual or mental violence within or outside the home, often from an early age. Often a positive diagnosis alone is enough to shatter how someone feels about themselves. Far too frequently, contact with services can make things worse because of the discriminatory attitudes of some health professionals. Often these professionals define our behaviour as anti-social, deviant, or downright irresponsible. In actuality, it is merely the result of a rational response within the confines of our own individual personal situations.

Sadly, many women are made to feel that they have brought HIV upon themselves. A situation obviously not helped by society's negative, discriminatory and inaccurate images of women with the virus. We always seem to be seen as junkies, sluts, or deviants, irrespective of what we do, which again also highlights negative attitudes towards women who choose to use illegal drugs, or who are sexually active. Blaming them for being positive also neglects the realities of many women's lives – the fact that for many of them, it is just about impossible to insist that their partners wear condoms, and impossible therefore to take the responsibility for their own protection.

At Positively Women we try to emphasize the positive value of the different experiences we all bring to the groups, hopefully allowing people to talk freely, without fear of being judged or put down for their beliefs or their actions, past or present. We try to help them realize that in the same way that there are no innocent victims of HIV, no one is guilty for having been infected. As people have been around for a while, they often find themselves counselling others in similar situations and helping them to come to terms with things in the same way, often doing it better than professional counsellors with no personal experience of the issues. We found that this was what women wanted – to be able to talk to others with the virus in a situation where they could be frank and honest about the reality of their lives whatever choices they were making, however others might view those choices.

By the beginning of 1989, we were overwhelmed with the numbers of individuals getting in touch. I was still studying at the time and Sheila, who had until then been the main point of contact, had just had a baby. We couldn't cope. We realized that unless we were able to secure minimal funding, we would have to give up. There was no one person who could put in adequate time on a voluntary basis. Luckily, Caroline was able to make a full-time commitment and we were able to get a grant and free office space. That was our first real home, and from then on it has all moved almost too quickly. Sometimes it is frightening, and we look around and ask ourselves, 'What have we created?'

We now run two weekly support groups. There will be three or four from January 1991 onwards, including a bi-monthly African women's group. We do home and hospital visits whenever possible, one-to-one peer support in person and by telephone. We have a children's fund so that we can give small grants to women with HIV who have children. We hope to have groups starting up outside London in the near future. We produce our own range of leaflets and are in touch with women from all round the world.

However, we don't think that support groups are necessarily enough. We will be organizing far more social activities in the future, because this is what people want. We also see Positively Women as a stepping stone to other services. We get a lot of referrals from other organizations and we work closely with them, referring people back to them, or on to them, for expert advice when we actually can't deal with the issues, or if we don't have the expert knowledge. Basically, we are there to provide whatever women want. It's their organization.

Obviously, all this expansion has not come without major problems. For example, funding never comes without strings attached and obligations – the need for evaluation and monitoring of our services far more closely than we ever bothered to do before. We have to learn to grow from a support group into a structure where we have paid workers and volunteers and women using the services. It's really changed the whole nature of what we are doing and how we are doing it. We are very conscious that we are in danger of setting up an 'us' and 'them' situation, which we certainly do not want.

It's very easy for us as women to fall into a caring role and take on too much, do too much for other people. Those of us who are full-time workers have to be aware of the dangers of burn-out. There are very few of us who are able to put in time, partly because many women are frightened of doing things actively for us. They are afraid of being identified and becoming public. They may have kids or jobs or family to protect. So we find ourselves doing very long hours and getting burnt out, overtired and sick, and then having to take time off work.

Therefore, we have to build into the work really good systems of support and we have to ensure that we are not overdoing it. It's often very frustrating. The services we are offering are never enough. The services that other people are offering are never enough. What we and other people have managed to achieve is just the tip of the iceberg. Services are still nowhere near matching the need. There are still only a few places which actually consult women and ask them what they want and fewer still which use that information to make changes. There is such a long way to go.

I think of our fight as a support and self-help group as concurrent with the general fight to get women's issues on the AIDS agenda. But getting recognition on the agenda is not enough. Having our voices heard is not enough. Words are great and important and can save lives, but actions can save a hell of a lot more lives. What we need is appropriate services that women living with HIV will use. We need accurate information that is culturally sensitive. We need legal protection against discrimination. We need more information through research on the effects of HIV on women's bodies, which will enable informed choices in respect to treatment options. We need to safeguard the rights of women with HIV to have children without being morally judged or discriminated against. We need to strive towards creating an environment where those of us with HIV or AIDS can be as open about our diagnosis as those with other medical conditions are able to be, without fear of rejection, blame or stigma, without the fear that our children's playmates will no longer be allowed to play with them, or of people putting graffiti on the sides of our houses. We need more options in how to continue drug use or in how to come off. We need housing, food, enough money to live on.

Just because HIV has been made into a moral issue, doesn't mean it should remain so. If we can't change the world, at least we can get angry about it. And we can use that anger in constructive ways to make changes as individuals where we can. It all adds up in the end.

Women with HIV need good, informed, sympathetic doctors, social workers, drugs workers, researchers, lawyers, and so on. But these professionals also need us and they need to listen to us and to value what people with HIV have to say, if they want to do their jobs effectively. We need to build up relationships of trust and partnership and cooperation. Some of this two-way process is beginning to happen in small ways. But it's still not happening fast enough and a lot of us are getting impatient. Having HIV does tend to make you impatient, not surprisingly. I suppose you never really know if you'll be hanging around waiting till it's too late.

Sometimes I want to forget all about HIV. I get sick of it. I would just like to disappear where it's not mentioned. But then some small thing makes me angry again and I realize it's not going to go away by just ignoring it. If we know anything for certain about AIDS, it is that. We have ignored it for long enough already and it's still here.

Women as carers, Scotland

by Jane Wilson

Doing good and feeling bad just isn't good enough. – Jean Baker Miller

Historically, women have always been carers both within their family systems and in society as a whole. I have little doubt that it will be women who increasingly carry the weight of caring for those affected by HIV and AIDS. As we in Lothian enter our fifth year of responding to the human needs of an inhuman virus, many women who are caring both professionally and personally have begun to voice concerns about how they function in this role. Who are these women? They are:

- Women living with HIV and AIDS who, via self-help or informal support networks, will share their strength, experience and vision with others affected by the virus. These women will continue to come forward regardless of whether they are unsupported or under-supported in this task.
- Women in their family and social settings who, as mothers, wives, sisters, grand-mothers, daughters and friends, will carry the emotional and practical responsibility for tending to themselves and their loved ones with the virus. These women will carry this burden whether sufficient back-up or respite care is available or not.
- Women in the community or statutory settings who provide their caring either as low-waged support and ancillary workers or unpaid volunteers. The value society places on women's work is often reflected in their pay packets. Along with this, the increasing trend towards using volunteers to offset the the escalating cost of caring for those with

the virus will mean increasing demands on women, who constitute the majority of volunteers in the community. The exception to this is the commendable work done by the gay male community. They have been the vanguard in mobilizing an effective response to HIV.
- Women working in health, social services and the voluntary sector who have brought their caring skills to the fore in an effort to support those affected by HIV and to halt its spread. These women occupy the field work and base level positions rather than the managerial or policy-making ones, in disproportionate numbers.

Unequivocally, the caring provided by all these women should be acknowledged, validated and supported. However, in all the literature available on HIV and AIDS, the role of carers – and more pointedly, their needs – receives only cursory mention. In addition, suggested guidelines rarely seem to be translated into an active reality.

Women as carers receive limited support, recognition or validation. But do women collude in this from the start? Unlike men, women may place themselves in a 'no-win' situation as carers, which should concern us as well. Paradoxically, women involved in caring work talk constantly about the need for support, while at the same time feeling unable to assert these needs in a way that allows them to be met. They often comment on how they 'cheat themselves' in this regard. If we assign our caring attributes to our 'nature' or our 'natural ability' as women, then it would be questioning our own natures if we admit that we need a great deal of support in this role.

The issue of status is also involved. Few would argue that a division of labour exists between men and women, with caring overwhelmingly ascribed to women. Although caring is a necessary activity for the healthy functioning of society, it is often separated off from the 'mainstream' activities of men. It is often seen as a supportive element to the male task of acting upon and changing the world. If we see caring as a 'secondary' activity, this will have an impact on how we view both our work and ourselves. If we listen to women describe this work, there is no doubt that they often perform their caring with an uneasy sense that it is not as useful as what men do.

To evaluate caring on the basis of quality and quantity, women may often feel that their giving is insufficient and inadequate, and again self-image and self-worth will suffer. The social assumption that women's caring is ever plentiful can leave many women feeling that others are asking too much of them. This dilemma may give rise to feelings of resentment and internal conflicts. Guilt may result, as women often believe they should be able to fulfil this role without difficulty. In order to avoid guilt feelings, they may deny that they actually resent these excess pressures. Consequently, it becomes difficult to take even small steps to limit demand on what they can cope with. Women will find themselves trapped in the scenario: 'I can't give any more, but I don't feel allowed to stop.'

There are clear implications for HIV/AIDS work. It could be said that women may be much more vulnerable to burn-out and stress-related illnesses than men. Support may be either non-existent, haphazard, inferior, or as one manager described it 'a luxury which could not be afforded'. Women will not only devalue their own contributions, but perhaps also those of other women.

Thus, we must not only continue to demonstrate our capacity to care, which we should be proud of, but also allow our own needs to be met and to legitimize our right to have such needs.

In several workshops held by the Scottish Women and HIV/AIDS Network and in preliminary research being carried out on this subject, the following demands seemed to surface over and over again regarding this work:

- Formal and public acknowledgement of the role that women play.
- Clear guidelines as to what our responsibilities and tasks are in the work we undertake.
- Comprehensive supervision which covers developmental educational and supportive functions, as well as monitoring and supervision of organizational, professional and personal roles. Protected time and consistent arrangements which would allow this to happen.
- Access to both formal and informal consultation in work, time to advance the work and have access to expertise on the difficulties that arise within the content of the work.
- Provision of a range of support structures which would allow carers to defuse and discharge the emotions that arise.
- Sufficient back-up coverage to allow a rest from caring, so that carers can renew their energy and process feelings of grief and bereavement.
- Provision for one-off and ongoing training at all levels, to be able to develop knowledge, skills and competency.
- Substantial increases in funding for this work, to reflect a commitment to caring by funding bodies.
- Opportunities for women to bring our experience and expertise into the decision-making arena, allowing us to participate fully in shaping the direction and development of services.

Salud Integral para la Mujer, Mexico

by Ana María Hernández Cárdenas

SIPAM means 'Integrated Health Care for Women'. SIPAM is a non-profit, non-governmental organization, founded in 1987 in Mexico City. SIPAM takes up the issues of reproductive health, sexuality, AIDS and public health policies. SIPAM's members have a range of social and academic experience.

Our aims are to:

- struggle to develop and strengthen women's dignity, especially regarding their health, in order to contribute to the development of a more democratic and just society, without any kind of discrimination;
- contribute our knowledge and work to strengthen the women's and feminist movement from a gender/class perspective;
- participate in the development of a whole-body concept of women's health;
- advocate the active participation of women in government health policy development and implementation, and the incorporation of feminist proposals on health into public policy;
- undertake joint activities with health workers in unions and institutions to improve the relationship between health workers and patients and improve the quality of health care for women;
- influence public opinion in favour of the causes and demands of women, particularly regarding health issues.

At present, there are 30 women from various professions involved in coordination, administration, and four programmes for health promotion. These programmes are:

Women's sexuality and AIDS programme

This programme focuses on education through prevention workshops and instructor training.

In September 1991, we opened a centre that offers HIV/STD-detection services, which include counselling before and after testing. This centre has the support of the Ministry of Health and is the first of its kind, run by and for women, in Mexico. In its first ten months, 142 women have been tested. Thirty-three per cent have had sexually transmitted diseases but none has tested HIV-positive. These women were invited to join our AIDS and Safe Sex Workshops.

These workshops have been run since 1991 for health workers, male and female students, teachers, secretaries, housewives, lesbians, men, and women from poor communities. We have participated in conferences, presented our work experience in several radio and TV programmes and in the press. We provide continuing training for our members in the latest developments in AIDS research and methodology of educational work with women.

Integrated health care programme

This programme offers inexpensive, alternative physical and mental health care for women in which women play an active role in their own healing process. We offer gynaecological consultations three times a week and provide information about contraception, pregnancy and childbirth, infertility and other health topics. For two years, we have offered childbirth preparation classes, especially directed to women from poor economic backgrounds. We also provide individual and group psychological therapy.

This year, for the second time, we are offering a seminar for health workers on health politics and gender, and are planning two workshops on issues concerning women health workers and another on the relationships between health workers and patients.

We have plans to develop a clinic where students from medical schools and health workers will be trained in and exposed to specific health needs of women and quality of patient care. We also have a plan to train a group of women health trade unionists to raise gender issues in their unions and workplaces.

Self-run, primary health care programme in Ajusco

Over a two-year period we have organized a group of 15 housewives in this poor neighbourhood in the south of the city who we will train as medical assistants in childbirth preparation, AIDS, mental health, publicity, women's health rights, and administration. The goal is for them to open a self-run community centre in 1993.

Publicity and communication programme

We publicize our activities through interviews in the press, and on radio and TV. We have a weekly radio programme since September 1991 called 'Let's stop being patients' on Radio Educación, a government station. This programme has helped publicize the proposals of the different women's groups in Mexico. So far we have dealt with topics such as AIDS, maternity, abortion, infertility, and reproductive rights. We announce women's activities and analyse issues in depth. And we have published several issues of our health bulletin *La Trenza* and given papers for national and international conferences.

Association for Women's AIDS Research and Education, USA

by Judith B. Cohen

I would like to share some history and present some findings from the first US community-based study of women and AIDS, an ongoing programme of research and prevention that began in San Francisco in 1984. Project AWARE has demonstrated that:

- women at high risk for HIV can be found;
- they will join research and intervention programmes;
- they will share sensitive information about the risk circumstances in their lives;
- they will continue in follow-up;

they can make significant changes in risk behaviour, as demonstrated by only one HIV seroconversion among more than 600 women who made at least one follow-up visit out of 1,800 women we have seen to date.

If our experience has made us sure of anything, it is that the process of how programmes operate is the key to their fate as research or prevention efforts.

Project AWARE began as a descriptive epidemiological study of women and AIDS, but from the beginning, it differed from the usual epidemiological studies in that the design and operation of the programme was based on participatory research and evaluation. Conventionally, research and intervention programmes operate from the top down. Investigators make the decisions, and staff and subjects are expected to perform as specified by the investigators. Participatory research, on the other hand, has subjects/participants making the decisions about design and operation. AWARE is between these, with staff and those being studied as cooperating participants in the process.

The philosophy and the process grew from the realization that the standard 'objective, rational' model of scientific inquiry was not relevant in a situation where the participants and the issues were already stigmatized, scapegoated, and necessarily hidden from conventional research strategies.

There was nothing objective or rational about a research situation where a woman discovered that her partner had been diagnosed with AIDS, infected as a result of behaviour that she may not have known about. Then someone wanted to ask her a lot of questions about things that were at least personal, if not downright threatening, such as her sex life, her drug use, and her own possible HIV-related symptoms.

It was clear before we began that for such women, the situation was already full of threat, fear, and possibly shame and guilt. The challenge for us was how to work with women in a context of caring and respect, supporting their own values and their challenged self-esteem. It was also clear that the questions asked and the issues discussed had to be realistic, grounded in the realities of their own lives, and not in the expectations of others.

So, from the beginning, participatory research happened from necessity. In 1984, little was known about whether women in the community would respond favourably to a programme asking questions about their sexual life and sex partners, and also about other sensitive and illegal behaviour, such as drug use and sex work. We thought that if we wanted to know what would make it possible for women to participate, the best way to find out was to ask them.

Before the programme began, we sent letters of invitation to everyone we knew who might be interested in women's AIDS risk in our area. They were invited to discussions held in the community, and were encouraged to invite others who they thought might be interested.

Participatory research also occurred because of community initiative. The community meetings were attended by hundreds of women, and some men who wanted to talk about AIDS from many perspectives, including social work, women's health, gay and lesbian rights, drug abuse, maternal, adolescent and perinatal health. The meetings reinforced existing networks, and established new alliances. It helped that we were meeting in a city with a history of active community participation in health and social programmes.

There was a commitment to listening to what was expressed, and to acting on that information. At the meetings and privately, women at high risk and those concerned about them, made their concerns and conditions on the research known:
- Women wanted to talk with people who spoke their own language, who would not

put them off with medical or technical terms.

- They wanted interviewers who were familiar with the realities of their own lives, who could listen, understand, and not expect impossible things from them.
- They were not interested in being 'guinea pigs', used only to give information.
- They wanted help in meeting their own needs, and not just those related to AIDS.
- They were very concerned about their own privacy and confidentiality since they were being asked to confide so much intimate information.

Most importantly, staff were recruited who were women who had themselves been in the same risk situations. They were women of all ethnic groups, who had been sex workers or drug users, or who had been in relationships with a bisexual or drug-using partner, or who had worked on behalf of such women. These staff still represent these concerns, and have been able to develop and provide appropriate referrals for drug and spouse abuse, medical and counselling needs, and other social and community services to participants in AWARE.

Staff also participate in community activities that help to build and maintain resources for women. Their presence, in the programme and in the community, is an ongoing force for commitment to doing the right thing and they are also the ideal models to demonstrate to women in the programme that behaviour change is possible.

Despite the prediction that women would be reluctant to come forward, once word of the programme became widespread, women called to request appointments faster than they could be scheduled. Many preferred to come for an initial session to a location other than our base at the AIDS programme at San Francisco General Hospital. They were afraid to be seen at the AIDS clinic. In fact, the preferred location for many was at some more

general health clinic that was not near their homes, for fear of recognition by those who knew them.

The earliest participants were often women who tended to be well-informed and active politically. They were at very high risk for HIV infection from sexual relationships, usually with bisexual men, but they were also very knowledgeable about sexual practices and their potential for STDs. Some of them had much more knowledge about sexual behaviour and how to discuss it than we did, and they were extremely helpful in increasing our knowledge about the many varieties of sexual behaviour and language. In addition to wanting the HIV-antibody test, they had very specific goals for behaviour change. They did not want to stop their diverse sexual activities, but they did want the most current information and advice on how to practise these activities safely.

A second, larger group were women who entered the programme because they had already had large numbers of sexual partners, and had heard of AWARE from the local news, care providers, or the local AIDS hotline. Unlike the first group, they did not know each other, and they were isolated in their concerns about AIDS because of personal and social circumstances. For them the programme was their only opportunity to talk to someone about their personal fears. In fact, their fears rarely were realized. They were the most likely to be seronegative upon testing, and their primary behaviour change has been to reduce the number of sexual partners that they have.

The other large sub-group includes women who knew or feared that they were at risk because of a specific relationship with a man who was a bisexual or an injection drug user, or who was already known to be infected. Some of them were isolated because their current partner did not know of their past relationship. Others were struggling with discrimination as part of 'AIDS families' in which a spouse or child was already ill. Either way, their psychological and social shock and trauma were severe, and often prolonged. Their ability to achieve behaviour change has often been limited by the need to deal first with more basic and immediate survival issues.

Another group of women, in addition to the risk circumstances already mentioned, exchange sexual services for money or drugs. They are a very diverse group, from those who provide very specialized sexual services to a limited clientele, to those who survive on the streets, including runaways and addicts.

In 1985, soon after AWARE began, the Centers for Disease Control issued a request for proposals to do a collaborative study in several cities of HIV infection among female sex workers. We have been awarded some funds, but these funds are only for laboratory testing and examinations, and other funds had to be found to cover the social aspects of the programme.

The key to our participation in this study was our collaboration with COYOTE, the sex workers' rights organization, active in San Francisco since the 1970s. Members of COYOTE met frequently with us, and we worked together to design the study, including how to recruit, development of research interviews, and counselling services. Women who had worked as sex workers were hired as AWARE staff, and became an essential part of the community effort, responsible for outreach and preventive education. Now, they have also learned to interview women for the study and are certified to do HIV-antibody tests and counselling.

I would add that one of the most challenging efforts at behaviour change in AWARE was getting our University administration to agree that women whose employment applications did not include even one steady job in the past were still well suited to become successful university employees.

For the women hired, this has become a

sustained behaviour change. All of the women originally hired have been with us for at least four years now. The only one who has left has done so to direct her own sex worker prevention education programme, with its own funding.

Now let us look at what we have found out. Among both seropositive and seronegative women, there were high levels of behaviour that could expose them to HIV at entry into the study. Virtually all women reported vaginal intercourse, and nearly half reported some anal sex as well. Using condoms with partners was quite rare, except among sex workers, who were fairly likely to use them with customers, but not with their steady partners. Sex workers were also more likely to report that they only had oral sex with some customers.

At follow-up, three kinds of change were possible. A woman could report that the high-risk relationship had ended. Or she could report that specific risky sexual practices were no longer being used. Or she could report that safer sex was achieved by consistent condom use by the partner or partners.

In general, most women reported significant behaviour change. That change was more likely to be the end of a relationship or stopping a form of behaviour, such as vaginal sex, than increased use of condoms.

For example, although nearly half of the cohort reported at least some anal sex prior to entering the programme, 70 per cent of seronegative and 80 per cent of seropositive women had stopped this behaviour at follow-up. Among the few who still reported this behaviour, condom use increased dramatically, from 8 per cent to 86 per cent among seropositive women, and from 9 per cent to 78 per cent among seronegative women.

The most difficult change was to get partners to use condoms more, and this was especially difficult in relationships that had been in existence for a long time. Even women who found out that they were infected with HIV, and who shared this information with their sexual partner, were not always able to convince their partner that condom use was necessary. Nearly a third of them lost the relationship, and almost as many stopped vaginal sex. Among the rest, 25 per cent still reported condom use rarely or never. While this last group included some women whose partners were also infected, it also included and still includes women whose partners refuse to believe that they can become infected by having sex with an infected woman.

Some of those concerned with AIDS prevention have recently warned of relapsed behaviour, where initial gains in preventive behaviour have not lasted over time. In this cohort, women have the opportunity, if they wish, to be reassessed every six months, so we now have data on behaviour for as long as three years of follow-up. Once behaviour changes, it is unlikely to relapse in this group. Some were not able to change initially, or left a more risky relationship and later established a new, safer one. But once change has occurred, it appears to be lasting well. Of course, the test is the rate of HIV infection over time. The best news is that among the more than 600 women in follow-up, we have seen only one seroconversion to HIV infection in the time the study has been in operation.

There is also some limited information on what happens to drug use over time. Change in drug use has been more gradual, and only about half have stopped using injection drugs entirely. However, with the availability of education, cleaning materials, and in some areas clean-needle exchanges, the few who still share needles tend to do so only with their steady sexual partner. Almost everyone reports cleaning injection equipment with bleach and water.

Before I let you think that things in San Francisco are going so well, it is necessary to share with you two severe problems that are still facing us, which I think we are not alone

with. The first has to do with what happens to women in the natural history of their HIV infection. We noticed some time ago that once women were diagnosed with AIDS, they seemed to die much sooner after diagnosis than men with the same diagnoses. This was not because they did not know they were infected. When we analysed the data, it did not appear to be due to drug use or not, or pregnancy or not. We have now looked at survival experience among all San Francisco women diagnosed with AIDS, and I am sorry to report that more than one-third of them die within one month of diagnosis. Among women diagnosed before 1989, only one is still alive. This pattern was there before treatments like AZT, but it is still there. Clearly, we need aggressive research into why this large difference in survival persists.

The other problem is among younger women. There have been alarming increases in sexually transmitted diseases, especially syphilis, and now HIV rates may increase as well. Those at highest risk are young women who use crack cocaine, the least expensive of the addictive drugs, although their alcohol use is also high. They tend to be women who live in the poorest areas, and they do not know anyone with AIDS, nor think they are at risk. Their experiences with public health agencies and the law are such that they do not seek health care or treatment, except in emergencies, and neither pregnancy nor STDs are seen as emergencies, especially when local care is limited or non-existent. We are working in some of these areas now, and acute syphilis infection rates are in the range of 25–30 per cent among the young people we are seeing for the first time.

So let us not be complacent that progress made is sufficient, or that new and even more challenging community efforts are not called for. Let us also remember that the education and prevention that needs to be achieved often happens in an environment that sometimes seems to be as unfavourable as possible to the success of these efforts.

Recently, in a national news magazine, a picture appeared of a woman we know well. No effort was made to protect her identity. Her name and work location were given, despite the fact that the text under her picture quotes her as saying that revealing her HIV status would be suicide. The picture appeared on a Friday. On the Monday she was arrested by the local police, who asked the courts to order HIV testing against her refusal to be tested. They said they would ask for her to be charged with attempted murder if she was found to be HIV-positive. In our state, this is possible because a state ballot proposition was passed last year that allows mandatory testing of those arrested for sex crimes. If there is evidence that the person knew of their positive HIV status, they can be charged with committing a major felony instead of the usual misdemeanor charges. So far, this has only been used against those arrested for sex work.

We are outraged because we know her very well. Never mind that she has been unable to get into drug treatment, or that she obtains condoms regularly from our outreach staff, or that her work is now nearly all oral sex. The magazine staff offered her money to pose for them, and did not advise her of the risk involved. Would they have done this with one of their own employees, or even with a gay man?

This is happening with a sex worker now. Tomorrow it may be an HIV-infected drug user, or a poor woman with HIV infection who becomes pregnant. In our efforts to try to understand and change infection risk, let us never forget that the world of those we try to understand is full of many more risks and realities than just AIDS. These determine what is heard, and what can be changed, and how effective our efforts will be.

South Carolina AIDS Education Network, USA

by Ellen Spiro

Doing grassroots AIDS education in the Bible Belt of the USA is very personal. In Columbia, South Carolina, cosmetologist DiAna DiAna realized that her clients at DiAna's Hair Ego were practising unsafe sex – lots of it – from conversations at the beauty parlour.

'I'm like a priest,' she explains. 'They confess everything to me. I know what they're doing and who's sleeping with whose husband, wife, or girlfriend.' Out of an immediate concern for the wellbeing of her largely black clientele, DiAna created the South Carolina AIDS Education Network.

In 1986, after reading an article on AIDS prevention recommending condom use, DiAna tried to get the local newspapers to carry condom advertisements. One publisher told her that the people of South Carolina didn't need to know about AIDS because they weren't susceptible to it. Thus began her condom crusade. She started giving out free, gift-wrapped condoms (because 'the ladies were just too embarrassed to take a naked condom'), along with her homemade AIDS pamphlets, from baskets in her beauty shop.

DiAna met Dr Bambi Sumpter, a public health educator, at an AIDS workshop, and the two began to collaborate on ways to get information out to school kids, adults and college students. They launched a full-scale campaign, which included lectures, at-home safer sex parties with sex-toy prizes, six-hour AIDS prevention training courses, plays written by DiAna, talent shows, and educational pop songs written by local, young musicians attracted to the cause by its eccentric, upbeat leaders. The campaign was funded by beauty shop tips.

In 1988, DiAna and Sumpter applied for grant money from the state for their educational programmes. South Carolina, where people with AIDS can be quarantined by law, denied them funds. The state health agency accused them of 'trying to sexually arouse young boys'.

DiAna and Sumpter videotape their work, including question-and-answer sessions with schoolchildren, to say to an adult parent, 'Look at the questions these kids are asking. Then make a new evaluation as to whether or not you feel they need to have this information,' says Sumpter. DiAna wanted people to know 'how we're doing grassroots programmes in the black community' which accounts for about 60 per cent of the local AIDS cases. 'When we made our first videotape,' recalls DiAna laughing, 'Bambi was sitting in the grass, giving the whole basic AIDS presentation, and I was running the camera. We were literally out there in the grass with the fire ants. Now that's grassroots!'

Today at DiAna's Hair Ego, clients can watch AIDS-related videos as they sit under dryers or get combed out. DiAna says 'They don't have to have a hair appointment to watch an AIDS video. I tell them to come in any time and to bring their kids too, because we have all kinds of videos – for adults, kids, and the ones in between.'

DiAna and Sumpter have just begun to take their safer sex parties on the road, adapting the living room event into a hilarious game-show-style extravaganza, complete with applause meter. With uninhibited volunteers participating in a series of games, both audience and participants are effectively educated about the pleasures of safer sex. Fundraising efforts have recently expanded to include a few entre-preneurial pursuits: the Safer Sex Get Acquainted Kit, condom fashion jewellery, and a new safer sex board game.

'People are dying,' says Sumpter. 'Our people are dying. We can't just wish this away.' DiAna, rinsing the shampoo from a customer's hair, agrees. 'If someone's always got to take some gossip out of the beauty shop, maybe now they can take something useful – information about AIDS.'

AIDS Counselling and Education Organization, USA

ACE is an organization in New York for women at the Bedford Hills Correctional Facility, a maximum-security prison holding about 750 women. Many are at high risk of HIV infection and in 1989, up to 20 per cent of incoming prisoners were estimated to have HIV.

ACE was started in 1985, as the result of staff and prisoners' fear of casual contact with women with HIV. Guards were using masks and gloves and prisoners were demanding that women with AIDS and those rumoured to have AIDS be put in isolation. As a result, a group of twelve women sent a letter to outside groups and the prison administration asking for education about AIDS and information about prison policy. The administration responded by bringing in medical professionals to provide information and training for the women. These women then began to offer a series of educational seminars for other prisoners, which are now mandatory for all incoming prisoners. The group was formally established at the end of 1987. The prison librarian acts as a liaison and the women are sometimes given leave to attend meetings about AIDS outside the prison.

By 1989, 30 women were involved in ACE's work, about half of whom were HIV positive or had AIDS. One woman had tested positive and thought she had HIV for nine months. She was tested again and found negative upon entering the prison and asked for a re-test before she believed she was not positive. She joined the group because she understood the pain and stigma others were experiencing. Some of the women watched close friends die in virtual isolation in the prison infirmary. Others admitted to an initial lack of sympathy which changed as they came to know women who were infected. They learned that prisoners with AIDS were dying much more quickly than other people, from lack of appropriate care and treatment.

The aims of ACE are to save lives, create more humane conditions for women with HIV/AIDS, provide counselling and education, and build bridges to outside community groups so that support will be available to women as they leave prison. They campaign to get clemency and early parole for women with AIDS-related illnesses. The prison infirmary used to be a place no one wanted to go to. Thanks to ACE, that has changed and medical care has improved. A specialist now visits once a week. Some ACE members help women with HIV who are ill with laundry and cooking, and offer companionship and recreation.

The group began lobbying for the prison to be used as a base for studies of HIV disease progression in women. A Spanish-speaking group was started by one member. The materials the group have developed have been published and videos about their seminars have been made. There is also a peer support programme for women who have been victims of domestic and family violence. Women who maintain contact with this programme have been found to do better after release.

The workshops for incoming prisoners include roleplaying about negotiating safer sex between women and with men, cleaning needles, helping a friend to decide whether or not to have an HIV test, and supporting another prisoner who is being stigmatized for having AIDS. Their work has helped to create a sense of community inside the prison.

Housing: a critical need for people with AIDS

by Helen Schietinger

Housing has been a critical problem for a disproportionate number of people with HIV infection throughout the world. Two factors have contributed to homelessness among people with HIV and AIDS:

- The public's fear of contagion.
  Because people are afraid of 'catching' AIDS, many people who are known (or suspected) to have HIV infection are evicted from their homes or harassed to the point of having to move.
- Financial difficulties of the person themselves.
  An HIV infected person may not be able to afford to pay for housing. A healthy person who is known to have HIV infection may be fired from his or her job. A person with HIV infection who is chronically ill may be unable to work and thus no longer have an income to pay for housing.

In the USA, the deterioration of the extended family, especially in white and middle-class communities, means it is rare for a household to contain three generations – grandparents, parents and children. Most adults work outside the home. Therefore, a very ill person often cannot be cared for in the home by family and requires other placement.

Another issue is the crisis of homeless people in urban areas. There is a growing number of urban homeless who sleep in shelters or doorways at night and are served by soup kitchens or eat from garbage cans. A large proportion of these people are mentally ill or addicted to drugs or alcohol. There are also long waiting-lists to get into government-funded housing programmes for the poor.

Housing programmes for people with HIV usually cannot handle the behaviours of addicted people. Therefore, applicants are screened and those with active drug and alcohol addiction are referred to treatment programmes if these are available.

While there are problems, there are also resources which have contributed to the development of special housing programmes for people with HIV and AIDS. There are well organized homosexual (gay and lesbian) communities in most US cities which have responded to the needs of people with AIDS. Also, philanthropic and church organizations have responded with resources.

Many people with HIV infection would not have lost their housing if adequate home care services were available to them where they were living. A variety of volunteer, home care and hospice services, as well as social services, must be available in order to maintain debilitated people with AIDS in the community.

Models

Various models of housing have been developed in the USA. This is both because of differences in available resources and because of the differing characteristics of people with HIV infection who are homeless.

In developing a housing programme, a needs assessment will help determine what model is appropriate. It is important to learn from people with HIV/AIDS who are homeless:

- their particular characteristics – Are most of them single or in couple relationships? Do they have children? Are they gay or heterosexual? Do they have special problems such as addiction or mental illness?
- their needs in relation to HIV infection – Are they physically independent or chronically ill? Do they have family, lovers or friends who will provide nursing care? If not, are home care services available?

Independent group living

The most common model is sharing a house or apartment in groups, with each person having their own bedroom for their personal items and visitors. They can cook meals and establish social contact with other residents as desired. There may or may not be a 'house manager' living on the premises and staff may be paid or volunteer. Residents may or may not have the option of having a partner live with them in their rooms.

The Shanti Project was the first programme of this kind. Damien Ministries in Washington, DC, manages a house for HIV-infected women which accepts women who are enrolled in a methadone-treatment programme, providing them with additional support to remain in recovery.

This model requires that people be able to live cooperatively with other people in a group living situation. Managing such housing for people with HIV infection is a serious responsibility. Ensuring the safety of the physical facilities requires constant vigilance. People who are ill may not be aware of hazards and may not be able to remove garbage or clean the premises adequately. Providing housing requires monitoring the physical and emotional status of residents. Staff must be able to obtain personal care or nursing services, or

arrange placement in nursing-care facilities or a hospital, for residents who are unable to care for themselves.

Staff must be able to mediate in disagreements among housemates, distinguishing between normal domestic disputes and inappropriate behaviour by a resident. They must have the authority and training to deal with behaviour which endangers or humiliates another resident. They must be able to identify and deal with dementia caused by HIV infection, as well as problems caused by alcoholism or drug addiction.

A programme of group housing requires a trained and very dedicated staff, and well-supervised volunteers. The staff does not usually live on the premises. They work out of an office located elsewhere, but are available for emergencies after working hours.

This model has proved itself successful in providing excellent housing for certain groups of people with HIV and AIDS. It has enabled people to establish a quality of life and level of security which they had lost following diagnosis.

Residence hotel

If people with HIV infection have social problems that lead to chaotic and disorganized lives, e.g. those with addictions or mental illness, independent group living is not appropriate. They require a more structured housing situation in which the premises are continually supervised. A model which serves this group well is a hotel in which people have individual rooms, are served meals, and share bathrooms. The presence of a manager on the premises 24 hours a day assures that someone is responsible for the facility and can intervene in the event of a crisis.

These individuals often have complex health problems besides HIV infection, and they often have difficulty using the health care system. They may be estranged from families, have no networks of social support, and not be a part of communities that generate volunteer services. Therefore, it is even more important that this type of housing be part of an integrated system of social services, including drug treatment programmes, and medical and nursing care.

Family housing

A family's need for housing differs from that of a single individual. A family may be a person with HIV or AIDS who has a lover or spouse and/or children, or a child with HIV infection or AIDS who is being cared for by parents, foster parents, or other relatives.

Most US cities have housing projects which provide low-rent apartments for poor families. This is often not a solution. For example, one woman who lived in a housing project with her two children was forced to leave by her neighbours when they discovered that she had AIDS. There are also long waiting lists for this housing – a person who becomes homeless after a diagnosis of AIDS has needs made more urgent by illness.

A good model for families in this situation is a building with individual flats, with separate living quarters for each family group. The staff needed to manage this type of programme is similar to that of the independent group-living model, except that a strong childcare component is advisable to provide support for parents. The AIDS Action Committee in Boston has such a building, that includes both family and individual apartments.

Foster care

Special mention must be made of children with HIV or AIDS whose parents have died of AIDs, or who have been abandoned by their parents and families. Many of these children do not need to be in hospitals, but remain in hospital from birth because they have no place else to go.

Foster-care programmes in some cities such as New York have prepared themselves to accept identified HIV-positive children. They address issues such as confidentiality of HIV test results, and they educate staff and specially chosen foster parents about HIV transmission issues and care. Foster parents who accept ill HIV-infected children receive additional compensation for the added work involved in caring for their health needs. However, there are not enough foster parents identified to care for the children needing placement.

An alternative to the existing system of foster care is that of group homes specially for children with HIV infection. This type of programme provides continuous staff. This either includes nurses to care for children who are ill, or close liaison with a community nurses' agency. The staff and other children provide a home-like atmosphere in which normal opportunities for growth and development can occur more readily than in a hospital. The cost of this type of programme is much less than keeping a child in a hospital, and may provide more comprehensive care for ill children than foster care. In New Jersey, the Department of Health contracts with the AIDS Resource Foundation for Children to provide group homes for babies with HIV infection.

Emergency housing

The homeless person with HIV or AIDS often has an immediate, emergency need for housing. Some programmes provide temporary emergency housing while permanent accommodation is found. The San Francisco AIDS Foundation, for example, has leased an apartment where people with AIDS are allowed to stay for one to three months while social workers assist them to find permanent housing.

Other solutions

Other solutions include providing funds to pay for part of a person's rent so that they do not lose their accommodation for financial reasons. Others keep lists of possible flat-shares, to keep costs down.

Community-based organizations have responded to the needs of people with HIV and AIDS in creative ways. Many organizations are simple and small. People have become concerned and then joined together to do whatever they can to help the people in their community with HIV and AIDS. Housing is only one of the problems they have tried to solve, but if a person does not have a place to live, it is impossible to provide for his or her other needs.

Some activities in the Pacific Islands

by Karen Heckert

Pacific island populations are so small that the influence of key personalities can be pervasive, so it is important to mention the work of individual women.

In Western Samoa the recently named Minister of Education, Youth, Sports and Culture, one of the few women '*metai*' or chiefs, is a strong supporter of AIDS education and hopes to ensure that it becomes part of the family-life curriculum in schools, despite opposition from a number of churches and parliamentarians.

In Tonga, the nursing and health education staff, primarily women, have provided the majority of AIDS prevention and education activity in the villages, researching knowledge, attitudes and behaviour, producing educational materials and assessing infection-control practices among health workers.

In French Polynesia, the community social worker at the STD clinic has established a support network for men and women who have casual sexual relationships and sex workers who seek HIV counselling and testing at the clinic. The director of the nursing school has offered specialized courses in STD/AIDS prevention and adopted WHO regional materials into nurse training.

Nursing staff in the Cook Islands, especially the Director of Nursing, play an active role in AIDS prevention programmes. The woman head of the Health Education Unit has worked effectively with local NGOs and churches. The woman director of curriculum in the Ministry of Education has worked hard to integrate a Maori language AIDS curriculum in the schools.

In the Marshall Islands, the woman director of Family Planning coordinates an innovative youth theatre project that includes AIDS prevention messages in drama and musical presentations in the villages.

Women's Committees exist in many of the islands at local level and within national structures. In Kiribati, AIDS issues have been integrated into local gatherings and trainings.

In Western Samoa, the women's committees are highly respected. They are responsible for identifying and resolving health and education issues at village level. Representatives from Western Samoa's women's committees have attended workshops on AIDS awareness.

In Fiji, some of the nursing staff in Nadi and an STD physician in Suva work and meet regularly with small groups of gay-identified and bisexual men, as well as women involved in casual sexual relationships, on AIDS prevention issues.

A number of women's groups in Fiji have started local AIDS prevention projects. The Suva YWCA plans to develop outreach efforts with local women involved in multiple sexual relationships, and a national Indian women's group began providing community education for Indian women.

The Women's Crisis Centre (WCC) in Fiji has incorporated STD/AIDS awareness and HIV counselling training into their national and local training programmes. At these, WCC discuss ways to support women who may become infected with HIV as a result of abuse or rape, and strategize on how to educate medical professionals and law enforcement personnel. The Fiji Women's Rights Movement has integrated STD/AIDS education into their national and local workshops on rape and violence.

A number of women in Suva became very involved as caregivers for a woman with HIV-related illness in 1990, through the encouragement of the woman physician who treated her. This doctor mobilized the STD clinic staff, the woman's family, their local church members and the community in supporting and caring for her until her death. She also presented written recommendations to the National Advisory Committee on AIDS for national case-management policies and practices based on her experience.

This woman's case generated a great deal of public controversy, as well as compassionate response, when her husband died of AIDS in hospital and her own HIV status was publicized in the media. A church official forbade church members to be involved in caring for her, but the local minister, the church members and particularly the minister's wife, who organized her care, stood united in supporting her. Her husband had been admitted as an emergency at night. His primary-care physician informed hospital staff of his HIV status the next morning when she learned he had been admitted. Although there were members of the National Advisory Committee on AIDS in prominent positions in the hospital, and most of the nursing staff had received introductory training about HIV, there were vehement emotional reactions about not being informed when he was admitted. Media publicity of these reactions prompted the woman to remain at home until her death three months after her husband's.

The STD physician herself has been discriminated against by some of her colleagues because of her involvement in AIDS work. She is standing steadfast, both in her private practice and as an occasional consultant for the South Pacific Commission and others, to promote AIDS awareness and activities regionally. She frequently gives talks to employers and employees' groups, members of the military, prison officers and inmates, women's organizations, schools, churches and synagogues, local health centres and at conferences. She is the only trained venereologist in Fiji.

The private family planning clinics funded by the International Planned Parenthood Federation have done a good job of taking up AIDS and STD prevention activity. The IPPF's training and resource materials have been widely distributed throughout the Pacific. While condoms are available in government family planning clinics in most Pacific island countries, their use is not universally promoted, at least with women. Usually, clients must ask the nurse for condoms, and only a few are given to an individual client at any one time. Men do not routinely attend FP clinics though they can get condoms from STD clinics or hospital outpatient services. Again, having to ask for condoms is a significant barrier to their use. In spite of donor support and government efforts, government supplies of condoms have run out in several countries, e.g. in Fiji for several months not long ago. In Kiribati, there were plenty of condoms but the expiration date was long past before a new supply was requested and available. A range of problems must be overcome to improve this situation.

The Global Programme on AIDS Health Education Specialist in Suva, Fiji, and local counterparts developed and pilot-tested a community health worker (CHW) training approach. The educational materials were compiled into a workbook called *The Community Health Worker: Our Key to AIDS and STD Prevention in the Pacific – A Training Workbook*. Women nurses and health educators in leadership roles in Kiribati, Tuvalu, Western Samoa, Tonga and Fiji helped to create and field-test these materials in their local languages, to teach small group communications skills for STD/AIDS prevention. The materials and participatory learning approach are being integrated into CHW training in primary health care.

The Fiji Red Cross Society have an active CHW volunteer network throughout Fiji, the majority of whom are women. In late 1991, 225 of these workers were given training in HIV prevention using the CHW training workbook. The Red Cross also developed a flip-chart and script as educational tools for CHWs to use in villages. A nursing sister at the Youth Employment Office in Suva provides frequent educational programmes for youth workers and youth throughout Fiji.

A useful set of materials for training nurses about all aspects of AIDS, called the *HIV/AIDS Reference Library of Nurses*, was also developed in the WHO Western Pacific Regional Office. These materials were widely distributed, and nursing tutors and practitioners from each country attended one of several regional training workshops to learn how to use them. A number of nursing schools in the Pacific have incorporated these materials into their basic training courses. They have also been used in the continuing education of practising nurses.

Personnel from Ministries of Health, national NGOs such as the Red Cross and the Girls' Brigade, schools and church counselling programmes have participated in training workshops on pre- and post-test HIV counselling in Fiji, Tonga, Western Samoa, the Cook Islands and Kiribati. Specific skills for counselling women who attend antenatal or family planning clinics have been addressed, along with counselling of women who are partners of men at risk.

The WHO/UNESCO School AIDS Education Project in the Pacific was funded for three years, from 1989 to 1991. Prototype training manuals were developed for teacher training and for student curricula. Several regional workshops were held to develop materials, adapt them to individual country needs, secure the commitment of government health and education ministries to work together, train teachers and carry out project evaluations.

All Pacific island countries participated actively in this project and most now provide AIDS education at upper primary and secondary school levels. For example, Vanuatu adapted the prototype materials, added new creative lesson plans and translated the manuals into French. In Papua New Guinea and Fiji, evaluation data from students, parents and teachers were collected and analysed. In a few of the countries, where there is no family life or health education curriculum in schools, it has been more difficult to incorporate the AIDS curriculum.

The Pacific YWCA Regional Office in Suva, Fiji, includes AIDS information in their quarterly newsletter. In 1990, national officers of the YWCA Information Network from at least eight countries went on a training course that included STD/AIDS prevention information.

The Commonwealth Youth Programme (CYP) South Pacific Regional Centre integrated STD/AIDS education into the didactic and fieldwork components of its youth-worker training at the University of the South Pacific in Fiji. In late 1990, two students developed a questionnaire to assess condom attitudes and use among STD patients at the Suva STD Clinic. When these youth workers returned home to Tuvalu and Vanuatu, they conducted the same survey. Several other youth workers from the same programme carried out similar surveys in their home countries.

CYP publishes a bi-monthly newsletter that regularly features AIDS activity updates from island countries. They have just initiated a worldwide small-grants project called 'Young People in Action on Health Issues' to stimulate AIDS and drug prevention activities by local young people. Three women from Tuvalu, Nauru and Tonga, youth workers with CYP, made presentations on issues affecting young people in their countries, including how HIV affects young women, at the 5th Regional Meeting of Pacific Women, in Guam in December 1991.

This regional meeting focused on health and was sponsored by the South Pacific Commission (SPC). SPC have a regional information and communication project for the prevention of STDs/AIDS in the Pacific. They publish a bulletin and newsletter, *Pacific AIDS Alert*, which include features on women. Prior to the Guam meeting, they convened an STD/AIDS problem-identification meeting for women in New Caledonia, to formulate a Pacific regional strategy. Work for the future is likely to develop from this meeting.

All these efforts are increasing AIDS awareness and stimulating changes for Pacific women and their ability to protect themselves from AIDS.

With thanks to Mridula Sainath, who provided information about Fiji.

Women Talking about AIDS Project, Australia

by Di Surgey

This is a project of Women in Industry and Community Health, a migrant women's organization in Melbourne, Australia. The project has taken three main directions:

• training ten bilingual/bicultural women community workers to take HIV/AIDS edu-cation to industrial workplaces employing women from their own communities

• working with Vietnamese, Spanish-speaking and Arabic-speaking women to provide a language-specific women's telephone in-formation service

- working with women from Arabic and Islamic communities to develop information resources that put HIV/AIDS education into the context of women's lives.

These resources include a 60-page booklet in Arabic and English called *Women Talk . . . about AIDS, sex and sexual health*, and an audio-cassette of information in Arabic for non-reading women. They are intended for communities of women who have previously had few opportunities to get information.

I have worked with groups of women, mainly from Lebanese, Syrian and Islamic communities, to produce these resources. HIV-infection risks for these women are highest from non-disclosing male partners who have sex with men or who use injection drugs.

During the process of preparing these resources, I found it essential to acknowledge and mark out prejudices and misinformation before these prejudices could be challenged and before the challenge could inspire the women (and the reader) to locate information and work towards better choices. It was also important to make sure that information about AIDS and STDs did not override or overwhelm a basic appreciation of safety in relationships for us as women. Our beginning has to be about finding ways of talking with each other. Writing and illustrating this booklet in direct response to women's expressed needs meant that learning was well shared among us.

Apart from the benefits of assuring cultural accessibility, this process has made a number of women enthusiastic and capable of carrying out peer education at an informal level. The audio-cassette will cater for the needs of 'leaders' of established women's groups for use as a discussion starter.

The best part of the process has been watching barriers between community members and community representatives slowly dissipate, until it is grassroots women themselves saying clearly 'We want this information'. Previously, there was a prevalent view that 'the community is not ready for this information'. This posed a difficulty for me as a worker who is not from these communities and did not have a pre-established credibility base. Support has grown considerably among community leaders as well as grassroots women during the project.

Women Talk . . . about AIDS, sex and sexual health

The following text is from the booklet Women Talk . . . about AIDS, sex and sexual health. *In the booklet, it is divided into five parts, interspersed with information about HIV transmission and prevention, sexuality, safer sex and relationships, reproductive health, contraception and STDs:*

I.
Amira told me that children are born with AIDS from their mother and that you can get AIDS from sharing needles if you inject drugs. She also said that you can get it from having sexual intercourse with a person who has the virus that causes AIDS.

Rana said that if a woman has AIDS it means she has had sex with a person who is not her husband. She said that only 'promiscuous' women get AIDS.

Alia told me that a woman can get AIDS from having internal examinations. Another time she said that wearing secondhand underwear will give you AIDS and that some people get it because they are dirty with their plates, their food, and the toilet. But mostly, she said, AIDS is the anger of God against 'corruptive' people. She said that these people were men who had sex with other men, women who had sex with other women, people who have anal sex, women who have sex during their menstrual period and all people who have no religion.

It seemed to me that some of the women I knew were saying that AIDS is caused by sin and that the people who were living with AIDS were immoral. But then other women were saying that you could get AIDS from toilets, from having a manicure done, from having internal examinations or Pap smears, from wearing secondhand underwear, from plates or from not keeping your house clean. Some women were even saying both things – and that's when I realized that all these conflicting ideas came about because whatever facts we had, we weren't sharing them. What we had was a lot of fear.

I knew that Alia was wrong, but I needed to be respectful to her. All the same, what she was saying made me feel more clear that I needed to get some facts together to share with my community. I wasn't sure about what Rana was saying, so I knew I needed the facts for myself too. This is what I found out . . .

II.
I thought about these facts and how they fitted in with what Amira, Rana and Alia said. It seemed to me that what Amira said was right – that you can get AIDS from sharing needles and syringes if you inject drugs, if you have sexual intercourse with a person who has the virus and that some babies can get AIDS if their mother is HIV-positive.

I found out that Alia believed what she did because she didn't have the facts and she had a lot of fear. She had heard that there are many millions of people with AIDS around the world and she had no other way of explaining why this should be so.

Alia knew that there are some sicknesses that can be spread through poor hygiene and she had no understanding of the difference between HIV and the germs that carry other illnesses.

When she also heard that women can get AIDS she thought it must be because they had been sinful. Now I know that AIDS does not happen because of sin – it happens because of a virus. And I know that anyone can get AIDS – it depends on whether the virus has got into their blood, not on who the person is or whether they have been sinful.

I still wondered a bit about what Rana said – that only 'promiscuous' women get AIDS, but then I heard the story of May. May is the older sister of one of Amira's friends from school. When May was 22 she married a man who came from overseas. When he first arrived in Australia he had an HIV antibody test, just like all migrants. The test was negative, meaning there was no sign that he had been infected with HIV. They had a wedding a few months later. After that, May became pregnant with her first child. She was very healthy and so was her baby, but after a while May became very tired. She would take a long time to get better when she caught some simple illness. The doctors couldn't tell what was wrong with her, but eventually one doctor suggested she have an HIV antibody test. May was convinced that she could not have the virus – she had only had sex with her husband and she knew that her husband's test result, before they got married, was all clear. But May's test result was positive – she had been infected with HIV.

May was amazed and upset – but three years later she is very well and she puts a lot of energy into making sure that she keeps healthy. Her daughter Rose does not have the virus and there is no reason why Rose should ever get HIV or AIDS.

It turned out that May's husband had had sex with another partner not very long before he came to Australia, and his partner had the virus. But May's husband did not have time to develop the HIV antibodies before he had the test and he did not know he was HIV-positive when they got married. She believes he does not have sex outside the marriage but she cannot know for sure. Nobody can know for sure.

May's story also reminded me that a woman does not need to have sex outside of marriage to get AIDS – and I found out that in Africa, where so many women have AIDS, some of the women never had sex outside their marriage.

I also found out something interesting – there are many women who have sex with a lot of different partners but they do not have HIV. These are the women whose job means they sell sex for wages. There are several thousand women sex workers in the state where I live and they see about 45,000 clients each week. According to Bella, a prostitute, her clients are men who come from every culture and religion and speak every language, including Arabic. Bella says they also come from all walks of life, that some are very successful businessmen, some are ordinary labourers, others work in hospitals or universities. Bella does not have the AIDS virus because she protects herself by having what is called 'safe sex'. Bella works in a brothel where all the other prostitutes also have 'safe sex'. Bella says a person can find out which brothels are good at making sure that sex is safe by telephoning the Prostitutes' Organization in each state.

A community worker I talked with also explained that there are tens of thousands of people who sometimes use drugs that are injected – some inject every day but most only inject drugs from time to time. People who inject drugs may not talk about it but they do come from all walks of life. The drugs do not cause AIDS, but sharing a needle or syringe with someone else can spread the AIDS virus. The infected blood of the first person can get directly into the blood of the second person through the needle. People need to know, she said, that if they ever inject drugs they should use a clean needle and syringe of their own which they can get through 'needle exchange' services or from some chemist shops. If they can't get clean equipment, they must clean the needle and syringe they are using with water, bleach, and water again before they inject. They should also know that if they have ever been exposed to the AIDS virus in any way, they should only have 'safe sex' so that their partner is protected. This is because a person can get HIV by sharing needles or syringes and pass on the infection during sex.

Finally, I talked to Shaadi from an organization called the Gay and Married Men's Group. Shaadi has a wife and three children, but sometimes he has sex with other men. Shaadi says he knows a lot of men who sometimes have sex with men but who are also married to women. Shaadi's wife does not know that he has sex with other men, but he protects her and his other sex partners from the HIV/AIDS virus by always having 'safe sex'.

Bella and May both told me that the most important thing is to protect yourself whenever you have sex with anyone unless you know they have not been exposed to HIV in any way.

I was intrigued by this idea of safe sex and decided to find out more . . .

III.
'So,' said Amira, 'it is all really very simple – if there's a chance that your partner has been exposed to HIV in any way, you either don't have sexual intercourse with him – or you always have to use a condom.'

Rana, who is already married, got angry with Amira. 'No, my husband would never have sex with anyone else – he knows that if he came to me with a sexually transmitted disease that would be it – for ever, I would throw him out, I would never let him touch me again!' Rana has been with her husband for one and a half years and she said that 'anyway, my husband would do anything for me. If a man really loves and understands a woman he will accept anything she wants – even condoms – but that's not the point. The point is that if a woman gives a man what he needs at home, he won't have to go elsewhere for sex. Why would he go out?'

'Well, who gets to decide what he thinks he needs? And what if your needs are opposite to his? You always have to start by looking after your own health!' Amira made it sound so simple.

'Amira, what would you know – you're not even married yet, and you think you know so much about sex!'

Just then Alia heard Amira and Rana. She just looked to the sky, then she turned to me and said, 'This is not necessarily true for all men. Some men do go out no matter what – they are just men, and anyway asking for a condom might lead to divorce or he might just say "bad luck for you, I can go anywhere I want for sex". These younger ones like Rana – they think life is so simple that you can just ask for what you want. They think that being in love protects you forever. Our mother would say she is just "showing off her gold"! And Amira, she gets all this information from school – she thinks she knows it all!'

The three women argued amongst themselves for a while, and I had to wonder why they each had such different attitudes and why the issue made Rana sound angry and Alia sound tired. I realized that, with my sisters, we had never really openly discussed AIDS or other sexually transmitted diseases before – not even sex really. I mean, we knew the facts about sexual intercourse, but we had never really talked with each other about our feelings about sex or about how it is for us, as women . . .

IV.
The more I talked to different women, the more it seemed to me that for sex to be really 'safe' for all women, we would need a change in the attitudes of a lot of people. As just one woman, I was not sure what I could do about other people's attitudes. But it occurred to me that getting more information about my body and talking with other women is a good thing I can do for myself. Maybe then I could fit this idea of 'safe sex' into the whole idea of looking after my health . . .

V.
It was easy to understand the idea that sexual health is about having respect for yourself and looking after yourself. And I came to learn that safe sex is just one aspect of sexual health. But I wondered how easy it would be for some women to discuss these issues with their partner.

Most of the women I knew said they would never have the courage to raise the subject of safe sex. Amira, of course, thought that she might be embarrassed but that it was worth it. 'If I say yes to something I don't really want, then I will only end up hating him, and probably myself. Anyway, we are going to be married and I wouldn't want to be living with someone for a long time if I ended up not liking him or myself.'

But a friend of ours said that if a woman thinks she needs to protect herself she should just tell her husband that she needs to use condoms because of pregnancy. Another woman said, 'No, go to your doctor and ask him to talk to your husband about condoms the next time he comes in to visit. The doctor doesn't have to say you went there.' Another woman said, 'I don't say anything to my husband. But I asked my brother to tell my husband to use condoms if ever he has sex when he's not with me.'

Maybe Amira was wrong to make safe sex for everyone sound so simple, but one thing is true. Safe sex is a health issue, it's not a moral judgement.

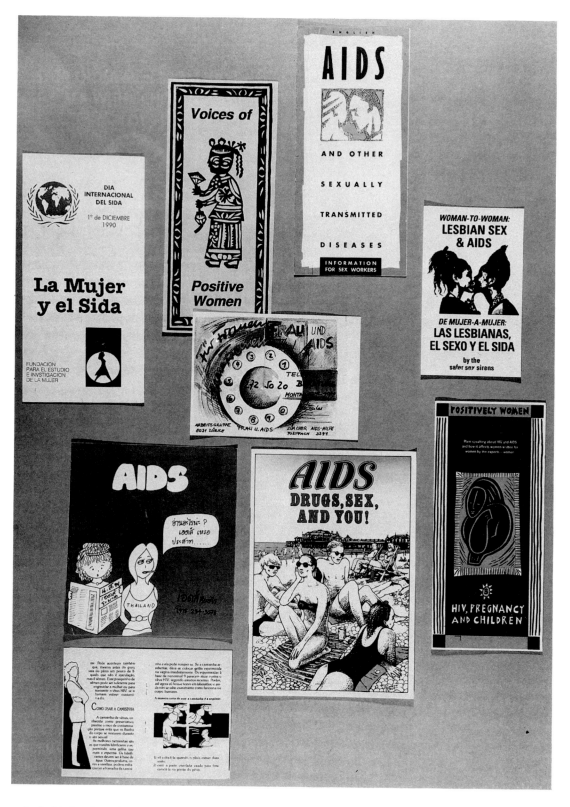

Credits (clockwise): Fundacion para el Estudio e Investigacion de la Mujer, Argentina; Voices of Positive Women; Canada, Commonwealth of Australia; Safer Sirens, Out! DC/,USA; Postively Women, England; Brighton Health Promotion Unit/Health Authority, Sussex AIDS Centre/Helpline, Drug Dependency Unit and Drug Advice and Information Service; Instituto de Estudos da Religiao, Brazil; Empower, Thailand; Zurcher, AIDS-Hilfe, Switzerland

Groups, organizations and resources

This section was compiled and edited with Barbara James

The following is a selection from among the many groups and organizations and their resources that exist internationally. Limited space did not permit us to include everyone we had heard from or knew of. We aimed to include: a broad range of projects, services, activities and resources by and for women, and those who could provide further contacts in their country/region or internationally. We concentrated on those which focus primarily or exclusively on women and women's issues, but included others which we thought were relevant to women, particularly for children. We left out many, many excellent groups, projects and resources. However, information about everyone we heard from during the course of the project and all the resources they sent will be kept in AHRTAG's resource centre in London, and hopefully will become part of a forthcoming global directory that

will be more comprehensive than this could be.

The activities and services described are primarily, but usually not exclusively, for women, unless specifically noted. Some, but not all, of the resources produced by and available from each group or organization are listed with them. The section on publications at the end are mainly those of publishers or special, one-off publications.

Descriptions of resources are included where we had these. Where it says only 'leaflets' or 'pamphlets', these are usually general about HIV/AIDS and aimed at the people/issues the group/organization addresses. The language is only noted if the material is available in more than one language or is in a language other than that of the group. Many of these resources, especially books and videos, cost money. Orders usually need to be pre-paid. We suggest you write for details first.

International HIV/AIDS-Related Networks

The International Community of Women Living with HIV/AIDS

Kate Thomson, Coordinator
c/o Positively Women
5 Sebastian Street
London EC1V 0ME, England
Tel: (44-71) 490-5515

Newly formed international network of women living with HIV and AIDS, set up in July 1992. Aim to gather and disseminate women-specific information on the effects of HIV on women's health and lives. Several coordinators in each region will set up regional networking. Plans for developing a global list of contacts so that women with HIV will never have to be alone when travelling.

Network of Sex-Work Related HIV/AIDS Projects

c/o AHRTAG
1 London Bridge Street
London SE1 9SG, England
Tel: (44-71) 378-1403
Fax: (44-71) 403-6003

A new global network of those providing HIV/AIDS services to sex workers and clients. Proposed activities: a newsletter, training activities, technical consultations, programme policy development, and information dissemination.

International Women's Health Networks and Organizations

Latin American & Caribbean Women's Health Network

Isis International
Casilla 2067
Correo Central
Santiago, Chile
Tel: (56-2) 633-4582
Fax: (56-2) 638-3142

Participate in Chilean activities on women and AIDS. Worked with the Pan American Health Organization to organize the 1st Latin American & Caribbean Symposium on Women and AIDS in 1990. Organized a regional women's health conference in Chile in October 1991 – women and AIDS was one of four main priority issues for the region. Large documentation centre on women's issues, including women and AIDS. Materials mainly in Spanish and English. *Revista* and *Women's Health Journal* include women and HIV/AIDS issues and violence against women, along with all women's health issues.

Women's Global Network for Reproductive Rights

NWZ Voorburgwal 32
1012 RZ Amsterdam, Netherlands
Tel: (31-20) 620-9672
Fax: (31-20) 622-2450

International network campaigning for reproductive rights. Coordinate solidarity action and annual International Day of Action for Women's Health on 28 May. Newsletter includes women and HIV/AIDS issues, along with all reproductive rights issues. (English/Spanish/French)

Inter-African Committee

147 rue de Lausanne
1202 Geneva, Switzerland
Tel: (41-22) 731-2420 / 732-0821
Fax: (41-22) 738-1823

International network of medical professionals, researchers, and organizations on traditional practices which affect women and children. Have held an international meeting on and encourage research projects on the potential inter-relationship between traditional practices and risks of HIV transmission.

Boston Women's Health Book Collective

Box 192, 240-A Elm Street
W. Somerville, Massachusetts 02144, USA
Tel: (1-617) 625-0271
Fax: (1-617) 625-0294

International women's health documentation exchange project. Information and documentation on all women's health issues. Public education, workshops, advocacy, women's health publications. *The New Our Bodies, Ourselves,* 1992. The classic women's health information and resource book. Includes information about women and HIV/AIDS. In several language editions.
International packet on women and AIDS. Articles and abstracts on medical, social and public health

issues; risk factors for transmission; HIV testing; prevention/vaccines; treatment; international perspectives. Unbound.

Annotated list of some of the groups active in women and HIV/AIDS work and resources in the USA, by region and subject, 1992.

International Women's Health Coalition

24 East 21st Street
5th Floor
New York, NY 10010, USA
Tel: (1-212) 979-8500
Fax: (1-212) 979-9009

Promote women's reproductive health and rights in alliance with women's health advocates, health professionals and government officials in Southern countries and Northern institutions.

Reproductive Tract Infections: Global Impact and Priorities for Women's Reproductive Health, edited by Adrienne Germain *et al.* New York: Plenum Press, 1992. Fourteen papers from an international conference in 1991.

The Culture of Silence: Reproductive Tract Infections Among Women in the Third World, by Ruth Dixon-Mueller and Judith N. Wasserheit, New York: IWHC, 1991. Reviews the data on RTIs and makes recommendations for action by policy-makers and service providers.

Special Challenges in Third World Women's Health: Reproductive Tract Infections, Cervical Cancer, and Contraception Safety, New York: IWHC, 1990. Papers from a conference in October 1989.

Reproductive Tract Infections Among Women in the Third World: Challenges for Practitioners and Policymakers, New York: IWHC, in press 1992. Research findings and insights into women's lives by four women professionals from developing countries, and strategies to prevent, manage and control RTIs.

Africa

Regional Networks

Society for Women and AIDS in Africa
Dr Eka Esu-Williams, President
University of Calabar
PMB 2470
Calabar, Nigeria
Tel: (234-87) 22-42-28   Fax: (234-87) 22-11-37

The network aims to undertake sex education, safer sex workshops, health education, counselling, workshops, public education, home care, childcare, support services, training, research and other HIV/AIDS activities designed for the socio-cultural background of African women, to explore ways of reducing the severe effects of HIV infection and its related diseases, to increase AIDS aware-ness and action by women throughout Africa and to collaborate internationally with govern-ments, NGOs and other agencies in the fight against AIDS. Recognizing the need for women to act for their own protection, SWAA aims to mobilize women, address practices that put women at risk, confront superstitions than create stigma, and change traditional norms that make women and girls submissive, in order to make sex and sex work safe.

Education for teenagers and high school students is undertaken in Senegal, Zambia, Zaïre and Nigeria. Safer sex workshops are organized for sex industry workers in Nigeria, Zaïre, Senegal, Cameroon, Ivory Coast, and Guinea. HIV/AIDS counselling takes place in Senegal, Zaïre, Nigeria and Zambia. Workshops and meetings are held annually. Focus on sexual practice, STDs and pregnancy-related transmission. Also target men and children. (Regional coordinators, officers and national SWAA branches are listed under their respective countries.)

Workshop reports: *Mobilisation of women to control AIDS,* 1989. *Coping with the impact of AIDS on women,* 1990. *Barriers to prevention and control of AIDS,* 1991. *HIV/AIDS and the African family,* 1992.

Pan-African Action-Research Network

c/o Brooke Schoepf
13 Spencer Baird Road
Woods Hole, MA 02543
USA
Tel: (1-508) 548-2953

Angola

Society for Women and AIDS in Africa
Teresa Cohen, Assistant Treasurer
Rua Eduardo
Mondlane 130
Luanda

Cameroon

Society for Women and AIDS in Africa
Stella Anyangwe, Vice President
Department of Public Health
C.U.S.S.
Yaoundé
Fax: (237) 31-51-78

Society for Women and AIDS in Africa
Henriete Meilo, Treasurer
c/o Dispensaire Anti-Vénérien Douala
BP 5413
Douala

Guinea

Society for Women and Aids in Africa
Bintou Bamba, Western Africa Coordinator
c/o Hôpital Donka Conakry
P.O. Box 713
Conakry III
Tel: (224) 46-21-18

Kenya

Positively Women of Kenya
P.O. Box 76618
Nairobi
Tel: (254-2) 78-60-51 / 78-57-92
Fax: (254-2) 23-23-92

Department of Community Health
Dr Elizabeth Ngugi
College of Health Sciences
University of Nairobi
Kenyatta National Hospital
P.O. Box 19676
Nairobi
Tel: (254-2) 72-63-00 x 2376

Educational project with youth out of schools, sex workers, and condom use. Focuses on STDs, injection drug use, traditional practices, pregnancy-related transmission and blood transfusion. Pamphlet on STDs/HIV and use of condoms for women sex workers.

AMREF
Wilson Airport
P.O. Box 30125
Nairobi
Tel: (254-2) 50-13-01
Fax: (254-2) 50-61-12

Outreach education programme for lorry drivers and women sex workers along major trucking routes in Kenya, Tanzania and neighbouring countries.

Nigeria

Women's Health Research Network in Nigeria
c/o Centre for Social and Economic Research
Ahmadu Bello University
Zaria
Tel: (234-69) 51248

Research and mobilization on STDs and other reproductive health issues; workshops, focus group discussions and awareness activities among grassroots rural and urban women. Focus on sexual practice, STDs and infertility. Target sex workers, young and adult women, market women, and women in purdah.

Rwanda

Projet San Francisco/Kigali
c/o Center for AIDS Prevention Studies
University of San Francisco
74 New Montgomery
Suite 600
San Francisco, CA 94105, USA
Tel: (1-415) 597-9100
Fax: (1-415) 597-9213

Education, counselling, practical support, referrals and research on HIV risks among pregnant women. Joint project with the Rwandan Ministry of Health. Videos:
AIDS Education Video for Urban Rwandan Women, and AIDS Educational Video for Urban Rwandan Men, by Susan Muska. The videos portray women and men teaching each other what they know about HIV/AIDS and taking this information back into their families.

Senegal

Environment & Development in the Third World
Women & Development Synergy Network
B.P. 3370
Dakar
Tel: (221) 22-42-29 / 21-60-27
Fax: (221) 22-26-95

Information for women, public conferences, sex education, reproductive health information, condom promotion and distribution, outreach, phone help line, training, research and articles on sexual and social behaviour, workshops, meetings, public education and media campaigns, weekly radio broadcasts, self-help groups, advocacy. Focus primarily on sexual practice, STDs and pregnancy-related transmission. Target women who sell sex, both legal and occasional, mothers, and young women students.
Report: *Femmes et SIDA en Afrique de l'Ouest*. Other resources (French/English).

Sierra Leone

Society for Women and Aids in Africa
30 Wallace Johnson Street
Freetown

Information, condom distribution, outreach, individual counselling, public education, workshops, training workshops for skills development and information-sharing for women at all levels. Focus on sexual practices and traditional practices. Services available for men although women are primary target. Leaflet. Plan to do video and newsletter.

South Africa

Women's Health Project
Centre for Health Policy
Department of Community Health
University of the Witwatersrand Medical
    School
7 York Road
Parktown 2193
Tel: (27-11) 647-2635/2184
Fax: (27-11) 643-4318

Project to promote and collect research on women's health, including abortion, contraception, cervical cancer, pregnancy and childbirth, mental health, teen pregnancy and HIV/AIDS. Networking nationally. Research into appropriate HIV/AIDS education for rural black women for purposes of policy intervention and activism. Provide information and sex education for women, including workshops on knowing your body and HIV/AIDS. Focus on sexual practice and STDs. Target mostly poor and working class black women.

Progressive Primary Health Care Network
9th floor, Cavendish Chambers
183 Jeppe Street
Johannesburg 2001
Tel: (27-11) 337-8539   Fax: (27-11) 337-9206

A national programme by local AIDS working groups to start AIDS education programmes in the communities; help communities care for people with AIDS; train, employ and support regional community AIDS workers (CAWs), who will train others and promote local AIDS programmes; and encourage cooperation with different projects. CAWs will come from the communities they serve. They will do needs assessments; identify and mobilize community resources to meet those needs, in consultation with community organizations; and pressure government and businesses to support these efforts. Target groups for prevention programmes include squatters, rural areas, women, hostel dwellers, and youth. Condoms will be promoted and distributed at local meetings. There will be a coordinated national media campaign using a national logo, posters, pamphlets, audio cassettes and videos, taking into account literacy levels in the communities and using key political and entertainment figures. This campaign will contextualize AIDS in South Africa by addressing issues such as single sex hostels and poor recreational facilities in townships.

Society for AIDS Families and Orphans
228 Smit Street
Johannesburg 2195

A registered charity to help to meet the needs of AIDS families and orphans in Soweto. Publicize the impact of HIV/AIDS on women, families and children, e.g. through the media. Raise money for the necessities for life and dignity for families in which at least one parent is ill or has died as a result of HIV infection, and for children who have lost one or both parents to AIDS. These include food, clothing, housing, basic funeral costs, education, and support for surrogate parents of all ages.

Tanzania

Waliokatika Mapambano Na AIDS Tanzania (WAMATA)
P.O. Box 35133
University of Dar es Salaam
Dar es Salaam

Information, outreach as a grassroots-based organization, HIV testing, counselling, training, research, workshops, self-help groups, home care, childcare and services within the family setting, legal advice especially for widows and orphans, hospital visits, financial help depending on available funds, housing and HIV/AIDS clinical services. Open to both women and men.

Tanzania Media Women's Association
P.O. Box 6143
Dar es Salaam
Tel: (255-51) 32181/29089/29904
Fax: (255-51) 29347/41905/29904

Provide information for women, sex education, research, public education and media campaigns, emotional support, anti-discrimination and human rights campaigns, workshops and meetings. Work on teenage pregnancy, maternal mortality, violence against women, sexual abuse, women's health and HIV/AIDS. Newsletter: *Sauti ya Siti*.

Society for Women and AIDS in Africa
Hores Isaack-Msaky, Eastern Africa
  Coordinator
Muhimbili Medical Centre
Paediatrics and Child Health Dept
Box 65001
Dar es Salaam
Tel: (255-51) 34364   Fax: (255-51) 46163

Information, sex education, HIV/AIDS counselling, workshops, public education, home care, childcare, human rights campaigns. Focus on sexual practice, STDs, pregnancy-related transmission, blood transfusion, circumcision, tattooing, vulvectomy. Target school-age youth, elderly women who teach girls about sex at menarche, traditional birth attendants, village women, women political leaders. Men, particularly those who perform circumcisions, are educated in villages. Newsletter and training guidelines for trainers of secondary school children.

Uganda

The AIDS Service Organization (TASO)
P.O. Box 10443
Kampala
Tel: (256-41) 231138   Fax: (256-41) 244642

Counselling and support for positive living; outreach, visits, and practical support for people with HIV/AIDS and their families and children; peer training and education; clinical services and referrals; day centre with activities and meals for people with HIV/AIDS.

Society for Women and AIDS in Africa
c/o Ministry of Health, MCH/FP Division
P.O. Box 8
Entebbe
Tel: (256-42) 20537

Plan to provide sex education; condom distribution; HIV testing/counselling; support for women at risk; home care and clinical services; training for community-based women and youth counsellors, traditional birth attendants and healers; establish family planning and AIDS-related activities; examine traditions and socio-cultural practices and whether these might put women at risk or make it difficult to cope with HIV/AIDS; and establish appropriate communications approaches, e.g. songs and drama. Focus on sexual practice and STDs. Training manuals of maternal/child health and AIDS for family planning providers, community health workers and mid-level managers.

Experiment in International Living
AIDS Education & Control Project
P.O. Box 9007
Kampala
Tel: (256-41) 24-24-29/23-49-00/23-32-37
Fax: (256-41) 23-17-43

Support, referrals and education for women. Emphasize sexual practice, STDs and pregnancy-related transmission. Target adolescents and rural women. Training guides for AIDS workers.

AIDS Information Centre
Baumann House
7 Parliament Avenue
P.O. Box 10446
Kampala
Tel: (256-41) 23-15-28

HIV testing; counselling for individuals, couples and groups; post-test clubs; education; research projects in coordination with university researchers; and referral services. Plan to open satellite clinics in several rural areas.

Zaïre

Society for Women and AIDS in Africa
Manoka Abib Thiam, Central Africa
  Coordinator
B.P. 1793
Kinshasa 1
Telex: (243-12) 21405 USEMB ZR
Fax: (243-12) 21856

Zambia

Society for Women and AIDS in Africa
Dr Nkandu P. Luo, SWAA Secretary
University Teaching Hospital
P.O. Box 50110
Lusaka
Tel: (260-1) 25-29-04   Fax: (260-1) 26-39-61

Information, sex education, safer sex workshops, condom distribution, outreach, HIV/AIDS counselling, training, research, workshops, public education, self-help groups, home care, childcare, practical help, financial help. Focus on sexual practice and STDs. Target women and children in distress.

Society for Woman and AIDS in Africa
Patricia Ndele, Southern Africa Coordinator
School of Medicine
Dept of Post Basic Nursing
Box 50110
Lusaka
Tel: (260-1) 25-05-54

Copperbelt Health Education Project
P.O. Box 23567
Kitwe
Tel: (260-2) 22-27-23

Information, sex and health education, condom promotion campaign and distribution, training regional resource workers and for people in the mining industry and businesses, research, public education, media campaigns. Courses for young women street sellers, covering health and social issues. Setting up a network of families who will adopt or help orphaned children. Focus on sexual practice and STDs. Increasingly target school-age children and young women. Posters, booklets, leaflets and video on HIV, STDs, TB, etc.

Salvation Army Chikankata Hospital
Private Bag S-2
Mazabuka

The first home care programme in Africa for people with AIDS in conjunction with hospital support and community volunteers.

Zimbabwe

Women & AIDS Support Network
P.O. Box 1554
Harare
Tel: (263-4) 70-03-43

Organized the first meeting on women and AIDS in Zimbabwe and have been active since then in AIDS education, workshops and information for women. Challenging images in the media of 'good' women as victims and 'bad' women as transmitters of HIV. Pamphlet for women (English/Shona/Ndebele).
Conference Report: *AIDS: An Issue for Every Woman,* November 1989, edited by Brigid Willmore and Sunanda Ray, WASN, 1990.
Book: *We Miss You All: Noerine Kaleeba: AIDS in the Family,* by Noerine Kaleeba, Sunanda Ray and Brigid Willmore, WASN, 1991. A personal history of Noerine Kaleeba's involvement in AIDS work following her husband's illness and death from AIDS, how The AIDS Service Organization in Uganda was set up by her, their work, and her reflections on the personal and social issues raised by AIDS.

AIDS Counselling Trust
Box 7225
Harare
Tel: (263-4) 79-23-40

Training courses in counselling for social workers, church groups, health workers; counselling services, home visiting; self-help group; information leaflets, newsletter and resource centre, public meetings, talks, discussion groups and workshops.
Poster: 'Girls can say no to sex'.
Publications: *AIDS: Action Now,* by Helen Jackson; *Let's Talk AIDS; AIDS: It's a Family Affair.*

Women's Action Group
Health Information Programme
Box 135
Harare
Tel: (263-4) 70-29-86   Fax: c/o (263-4) 73-19-01

Information, sex education, condom distribution, outreach, public education, policy development, human rights campaigns. Focus on sexual practice and STDs.

Magazine: *Speak Out*.

Book: *AIDS – Let's Fight It Together*, Women's Action Group, Harare, 1988. (Shona/English or Ndebele/English). A story with drawings and dialogue of a whole community as they find out about HIV/AIDS from staff at their local clinic. Various community members express their worries and questions, which are then answered. The book is based on comments and questions from both rural and urban men and women of all ages in Zimbabwe.

Asia

India

South India AIDS Action Programme
O.P. Block
V.H.S. – Taramani
Madras
Tel: (91-14) 41-68-86

Gram Bharati Samiti
S-3, Govind Nagar (West)
Jaipur 302 002
Tel: (91-141) 62560   Fax: (91-141) 56-33-57

Project for women sex workers and their families throughout Rajasthan. Work around other health issues, e.g. disability, leprosy, environment, and with the aged.

Population Services International
FWT & RC
332 S V P Road
Khetwadi
Bombay 400 004   Tel: (91-22) 388-1724

Information for sex workers including group discussions on HIV/AIDS and other health issues, condom distribution (markets own brand of condom – Masti – at traditional and non-traditional outlets), outreach through trained inter-personal communicators, workshops with brothel owners, media campaigns (such as an advertisement on condoms and AIDS screened in video parlours and cinemas). Focus on sexual practice and STDs. Target sex workers, brothel-owners. A professional dance group performs in red-light districts, using song, dance and humour to teach about HIV. A restaurant/bar has been adopted which has video entertainment and education in Hindi. Resources: booklets, leaflets and posters (Hindi).

Indian Health Organisation
Municipal School Building
J.J. Hospital Compound
Bombay 400 008
Tel: (91-22) 371-0819
Fax: (91-22) 371-9020

Mobile clinic that goes into red-light districts of Bombay to offer STD treatment and clinical services, education about health and HIV/AIDS among sex workers, support for self-help groups and rights of sex workers, anti-discrimination and human rights campaigns, media and public education work, lobbying, condom promotion.

AIDS Research Foundation of India
20/2 Bhagirathy Ammal Street
T. Nagar
Madras 600 017

Condom campaign among clients of sex workers on roadsides in Madras. Men use condoms to fix leaks in trucks; women use condoms to carry water. Condom messages based on this, i.e. condoms are for preventing leaks.

Philippines

Health Action Information Network
P.O. Box 10340, Broadway
9 Cabanatuan Road, Philam Homes
Quezon City
Tel: (63-2) 97-88-05
Fax: (63-2) 721-8290

Research, safer sex workshops, training, information and education work on AIDS. Work jointly with other NGOs on policy statements, advocacy for the rights of women and gay people. Focus on sexual practice and psycho-social issues, particularly in relation to gender. University students are particularly targeted.

Newsletter: *Health Alert*.

GABRIELA Commission on Women's Health and Reproductive Rights
3-G St William corner Lantana Street
Cubao
Quezon City
Tel: (63-2) 721-7954

Information, education, condom distribution, curriculum development (reproductive rights, sexuality, AIDS), research on AIDS from a feminist perspective, general medical consultation and management, including obstetric, gynaecological and paediatric care. Focus on sexual practice, STDs, and blood transfusion. Work with organized grassroots women under the GABRIELA umbrella nationwide. Plans to publish a range of materials.

Buklod Center
1 Davis Street
New Banican
Olongapo City 2200

Outreach to bar workers in Olongapo at their workplaces and during carnivals, with HIV/AIDS information and support. Provide night care for children, which interests many of the women as many are single or abandoned mothers; seminars, health education and skills training for supplemental or alternative livelihood. Have a self-help group/union for women sex workers. Pamphlet: *Hospitality – What Price? The US Navy at Subic Bay*.

Womanhealth, Philippines
3 Legaspi Road
Philam Life Homes
Quezon City

Promote women's right to health and reproductive freedom. Information, seminars on sexuality, women's health. Co-ordinates a community-based health care programme.
Video: *Birthpains: Women and AIDS*.

Thailand

Empower
P.O. Box 1065
Silom Post Office
Bangkok 10504
Tel: (66-2) 234-3078/0398
Fax: (66-2) 234-3078

Information, sex education, safer sex workshops, condom distribution, HIV/AIDS counselling, phone help line, workshops, meetings, public education, policy development, media campaigns, legal advice, emotional support, practical help, human rights campaigns. Drama group performs in bars and on the streets with safer sex and AIDS information. Target women who work in bar areas which cater to foreign tourists. Leaflet, pamphlet and other resources.

Mullaneetee Sune-Hotline (Hotline Center Foundation)
90/269 Soi 20 Viphawadeerungsit Road
Chatujak
Bangkok 10900
Tel: (66-2) 277-8811/7699 and 276-2950/2951
Fax: (66-2) 275-8354

Education, understanding, telephone and individual/joint counselling (including family, marital and psychotherapy). Sex and HIV/AIDS education integrated into general health training. Home visits, legal advice, seminars, workshops, training courses for professionals, volunteers and people with HIV, and self-help group. Part-time physician and nurse who do physical check-ups. Target all people with HIV/AIDS, especially women with children and families, teenagers and students. Leaflet on counselling, poster, book, training manual on their counselling techniques, and video about their services.

Association for the Promotion of the Status of Women
501/1 Mu 3, Sikan
Donmuang
Bangkok 10210
Tel: (66-2) 566-2288/1774
Fax: (66-2) 566-3481

Information, meetings in the north of Thailand, outreach at railway station and bus terminal, HIV/AIDS counselling by social worker and outside resource worker. Emergency home care and shelters, one with facilities for looking after children, practical help, vocational training, human rights campaigns, referrals to hospital for care with follow-up. Plan to build a new shelter. Focus on sexual practice and injection drug use. AIDS information pamphlet.

Duang Prateep Foundation
Lock 6 Klong Toey Slum
Bangkok 10110
Tel: (66-2) 249-4880
Fax: (66-2) 249-5254

AIDS prevention and control, targeting high-risk residents, family members of people with HIV/AIDS and of injection drug users, interest in AIDS education for men as clients of sex workers and because of risk of infection of wives.

Caribbean

Regional Network

Caribbean Epidemiology Centre
P.O. Box 164
Port-of-Spain, Trinidad
Tel: (1-809) 622-3404

Regional epidemiology, research and information centre.

Puerto Rico

Taller Salud
Lafayette 803 Altos, Parada 20
Santurce 00909
Tel: (1-809) 726-5381   Fax: (1-809) 767-6757

Conferences, workshops and advocacy on women's health, reproductive health, self-help, and newsletters and leaflets on women's health issues. Workshops on women and HIV/AIDS. Newsletter: *Boletin sobre mujeres y SIDA.* Leaflets on safer sex.

Casa Pensamiento de Mujer del Centro
Calle Ramon Flores #57
Aibonito 00705
Tel: (1-809) 735-3200

Information, sex education, safer sex workshops, condom distribution, outreach, HIV/AIDS counselling, workshops, public education, policy development, self-help groups, childcare, legal advice, emotional support, practical help, human rights campaigns, reproductive health services. Counselling on domestic violence, rape, sexual assault and legal issues. Documentation centre. Training courses on women and AIDS. Focus on sexual practice, injection drug use, pregnancy-

related transmission and blood transfusion. Research paper on domestic violence and HIV/AIDS by Aida Iris Cruz.
Newsletter: *Pensamiento de la Mujer.*

Trinidad & Tobago

Community Action Resource
P.O. Box 472
Woodbrook
Port-of-Spain
Tel: (1-809) 628-1338   Fax: (1-809) 622-3217

Europe

Regional Networks

AIDS and Youth
European Information Centre
c/o Department of School Health
A. van Ostadelaan 140
3583 AM Utrecht, Netherlands
Tel: (31-30) 54-38-88

New centre, being developed in stages, to promote exchange and collaboration on AIDS prevention and education among young people, inside and outside the school, within Europe. Plans for database of informational materials, activities and contacts, and networking.

European Association of Nurses in AIDS Care
Woodseats House
764a Chesterfield Road
Sheffield S8 0SE, England
Tel: (44-742) 55-10-64   Fax: (44-742) 55-52-01

New organization to bring together nurses in AIDS care, hold annual conferences, promote excellence in HIV/AIDS nursing and the importance of nursing in HIV/AIDS care. Newsletter.

Austria

AIDS-Hilfe Wien
Wickenburggasse 14
A-1080 Vienna
Tel: (43-1) 408-6186/6187   Fax: (43-1) 403-6411

Information, sex education, condom distribution, outreach, HIV testing, HIV/AIDS counselling, phone helpline, training, research, workshops, public education, self-help groups, emotional support, financial help, anti-discrimination and human rights campaigns, HIV/AIDS clinical services, reproductive health services, training and supervision for women working in health and health-related fields. Women counsellors have studied and identified gender differences in counselling men and women. Particularly target young and immigrant women. Part of national network of similar services.

Denmark

Kvinder og AIDS (Women against AIDS)
Tordenskjoldsvej 20
3000 Helsinger

Information, education, advocacy and meetings on women and HIV/AIDS issues. Forum for women to exchange ideas and discuss sexuality, sex, children and HIV/AIDS; make women visible in the fight against AIDS; support women trying to take control of their lives; lobby government and officials; and stimulate more research on women and HIV. Working groups on women, sex work and drug use; after-work meetings with women employees in their workplaces; and women, HIV and children. Participation in local events and media discussions. Plans for a public hearing with women sex workers and politicians, policewomen and other experts. Hope to train sex workers as peer educators. Seeking to establish contact with other women's organizations, e.g. the Danish Housewives Society, to set up meetings for women around the country who are not typically reached in HIV/AIDS campaigns. Leaflet and booklet for women.

England

Positively Women
5 Sebastian Street
London EC1V 0HE
Tel: (44-71) 490-5515

Self-help support groups, counselling, social events, advice, referrals, speakers, small fund for care of children, organized by and for HIV positive women. Leaflets: *HIV/AIDS Prevention; Women, Drugs and HIV; Positive Result – Look After Yourself; HIV, Pregnancy and Children; African Women's Health Issues.*

Terrence Higgins Trust
Women's Development Programme
52 Grays Inn Road
London WC1X 8JU
Tel: (44-71) 831-0330
Fax: (44-71) 242-0121

Information, advice, help for people with HIV/AIDS. Phone and face-to-face counselling, welfare advice, library and information service, health education, women volunteer group, interfaith group, drug users' group, family support network and work with lesbians and HIV health education. Coordinate Women & HIV/AIDS Network which meets every three months in London to discuss political, policy and medical issues. Leaflets: For women; about mothers and children with HIV/AIDS; symptoms and treatments for HIV-positive women; information for lesbians.

Praed Street Project
c/o Jefferiss Wing
St Mary's Hospital
Praed Street
London W2
Tel: (44-71) 725-1549

Information, sex education, condom distribution, outreach, HIV testing and counselling, phone helpline, workshops, emotional support, practical help, drop-in, HIV/AIDS and other clinical services, reproductive health services. Focus on sexual practice and STDs. For women sex workers only.

Institute for the Study of Drug Dependence
1 Hatton Place
London EC1N 8ND
Tel: (44-71) 430-1991
Fax: (44-71) 404-4415

Research, numerous publications and resources on HIV and drugs, including on women. Books: *Women, HIV and Drugs: Practical Issues,* 1990. *AIDS: Women, Drugs and Social Care,* 1992. *Women, HIV, Drugs and Criminal Justice Issues,* 1992.

Barnados Positive Options
354 Goswell Road
London EC1V 7LQ
Tel: (44-71) 278-5039
Fax: (44-71) 833-4858

Support for HIV-positive parents and people with HIV-positive children, to help them work out the children's future. Advice on fostering and adoption if required. Training, open meetings, childcare, legal advice in conjunction with Terrence Higgins Trust, direct work with children. Memory Box, a project which helps HIV-positive parents collect mementos for children whom they may not see through to independence. Particularly target mothers of dependent children, HIV-positive women contemplating pregnancy, families with haemophilia and HIV. Several projects throughout England.

Leaflets about this work. Booklet *AIDS in the Family: Information for Parents and Carers of Children and others for children aged 11+ about the social effects of HIV.* From: Barnados Public Affairs Office, Tanner's Lane, Barkingside, Ilford, Essex IG6 1QG, England.

Midwives Information and Resource Service

Institute of Child Health
Royal Hospital for Sick Children
St Michaels Hill
Bristol BS2 8BJ
Tel: (44-272) 251791
Fax: (44-272) 251792

Comprehensive resource centre and library with information about pregnancy, childbirth, midwifery and related health issues, including HIV. Database and enquiry service. Focus on pregnancy-related transmission and infant feeding. Target midwives, ante-natal teachers and childbirth activists.

Journal: *MIDIRS Midwifery Digest.* Reprints and abstracts of research and articles, with commentary on new research, including HIV/AIDS and maternity care issues.

AVERT (AIDS Education and Research Trust)

11 Denne Parade
Horsham, W Sussex RH12 1JD, England
Tel: (44-403) 21-02-02
Fax: (44-403) 21-10-01

Booklets: *Women Talking about AIDS,* 1990. *Taking Control of Your Diet If You Are HIV-positive,* 1991. *AIDS Dementia; A Guide to the Medical Treatment of HIV-related Diseases,* 1991. *AIDS and Sex Information for Young People,* 1992. *Prison, HIV and AIDS: Risks and Experiences in Custodial Care,* 1991. Report of a survey of 450 prisoners, men and women, about risk behaviour, drug use and sex in prisons, and the response of prisons.

National AIDS Manual

Unit 52
The Eurolink Centre
49 Effra Road
London SW2 1BZ, England

Three-volume guide to topics, treatments and research, and directory of contacts. Mainly about the UK; sections on travel, safer sex, games, legal issues, housing, prisons, insurance, allopathic and alternative treatments and research, STDs and reproductive health, women, and information for people living with HIV/AIDS are widely relevant Loose-leaf holder, updated three times a year.

Finland

The Finnish AIDS Information and Support Center

Linnankatu 2B
00160 Helsinki
Tel: (358-90) 175-822
Fax: (358-90) 656-806

Sex education, condom distribution, HIV testing, counselling, phone helpline, training, research, public education, media campaigns, policy development, self-help groups, legal advice, emotional support, practical help, anti-discrimination and human rights campaigns. Focus on sexual practice. Target population as a whole. Pamphlet (English).

Germany

Deutsche AIDS-Hilfe

Nestorstrasse 8–9
1000 Berlin 31
Tel: (49-30) 896-9060

National AIDS information and services organization, including for women.

Berliner AIDS-Hilfe

Meinekestrasse 12
1000 Berlin 15
Tel: (49-30) 883-3017
Fax: (49-30) 882-5194

Support groups, counselling and referral for HIV-positive people, including women. Leaflet.

Netherlands

Buro Vrouwen en AIDS (Women and AIDS Bureau)

Predikherenkerkhof 2
3512 TK Utrecht
Tel: (31-30) 33-47-08

National coordination centre on women & AIDS issues and secretariat for the Women and AIDS Platform. Promote information, education and prevention activities on women and AIDS. Identify needs of particular sub-groups of women. Develop informational materials. Monitor and encourage projects for quality of care and support for women and children with HIV. Training for primary health care workers. Monitor government policy and research on women; advocacy for these to take account of women's interests; policy development. Resource centre. National and international networking.

Vrouwen en AIDS: Een Overzicht (Women and AIDS: An Overview) Symposium, 1 December 1990. Papers by Dutch and English-speaking authors from this symposium. (Dutch/English)

Women and AIDS Project

Rutgers Stichting
Postbus 17430
2502 CK 's-Gravenhage
Tel: (31-70) 363-1750

Project of the national family planning association in the Netherlands to educate general practitioners and social workers on working with women with HIV. Training manual for this work. The association does work on sexuality, especially with young people. Booklets with drawings and information about safer sex and family planning for young people.

SOA Stichting (Dutch STD Foundation)

Postbus 19061
3501 DB Utrecht
Tel: (31-30) 31-39-20
Fax: (31-30) 33-24-19

Information for women, sex education, condom distribution, public education, media campaigns, policy development. Focus on sexual practice and STDs. Target sex workers, women in the general public, and young women.

Safe Sex: A Magazine about Safe Sex at Work and at Play (Dutch/English/German).
Safe Sex. Cassette tape for sex workers, with music. (Spanish/English/Akan).
Condom case with a condom, lubricant and information.
Two comic strips: one with HIV/AIDS information and one about all STDs, including HIV, with minimal text, using nationally known comic strip characters.
Promoting Safer Sex: Proceedings of an International Workshop on Prevention of Sexual Transmission of AIDS and Other STD, Netherlands, May 1989. Edited by Maria Paalman. Swets Zeitlinger BV, Amsterdam 1990.

Positieve Vrouwen (Positive Women)

HIV-Vereniging Nederland
Postbus 15847
1001 NH Amsterdam
Tel: (31-20) 664-4076
Fax: (31-20) 664-6689

Group for all women living with HIV/AIDS nationally. Information, workshops/meetings, self-help groups, emotional support, including for partners in distress, meeting-cafe for women with HIV/AIDS. Leaflet (Dutch/ English).
Newsletter: *Positieve Vrouwen.*

Schorerstichting (National Agency for Homosexuality)

P.C. Hooftstraat 5
1071 BL Amsterdam
Tel: (31-20) 662-4206
Fax: (31-20) 664-6069

Case management for women with HIV/AIDS. Counselling, training, emotional help. Particularly target lesbians. Book in progress on medical and social aspects of women and HIV/AIDS.

Municipal Health Service

Dept Public Health/Environment
P.O. Box 20244
1000 HE Amsterdam, Netherlands
Tel: (31-20) 5555-384
Fax: (31-20) 5555-533

Epidemiology of HIV Infection among Drug Users in Amsterdam, edited by Anneke van den Hoek. Rodopi, Amsterdam, 1990. Collection of research papers by the editor and others for a thesis on HIV, drug use and sex work.

Norway

Kvinnefronten i Norge (Women's Front of Norway)
Helgesengate 12
0553 Oslo 5
Tel: (47-2) 37-60-54

A feminist organization with groups and members all over Norway. Work against the oppression of women in all areas of society, including women and HIV/AIDS. Information. Leaflet (Norwegian/ English). Magazine.

PLUSS
P.O. Boks 6879, St Olavspl.
0130 Oslo
Tel: (47-2) 211-4900
Fax: (47-2) 236-0269

National organization for people with HIV/ AIDS. Condom distribution, HIV/AIDS counselling, workshops, emotional support. Focus on sexual practice and injection drug use.

Scotland

Women and HIV/AIDS Network
64a Broughton Street
Edinburgh EH1 3SA
Tel: (44-31) 557-5199

Information for women, local seminars, conferences, leaflets, training, public education, policy development, outreach to women in their local areas for needs assessment, advocacy of women's needs. Focus on women affected by HIV/AIDS and workers in the field. Leaflets under production.
Newsletter: *Women & HIV/AIDS Network Update.* Proceedings of Network Conferences for 1988, 1989, 1990, 1991 and 1992. Contain papers by all speakers at each conference.

Women's Reproductive Health Service
Royal Maternity Hospital
Rottenrow
Glasgow G4 0NA
Tel: (44-41) 552-3400

A city-wide multi-disciplinary service providing reproductive health care, and for women with social problems, including drug use, and women affected by HIV/AIDS. Through a single agency approach, help is offered with a wide range of medical and social problems. Drug-using women are offered a range of options during pregnancy, including inpatient and outpatient detoxification, reduction or maintenance therapy. Information, sex education, free condom distribution at clinics and on the wards, HIV testing at all outlets of the service and community clinics with counselling, drugs programme in collaboration with drugs services, research, public education, HIV/AIDS clinical services. Focus on sexual practice, pregnancy-related transmission and injection drug use. Leaflets and videos under production.

Pediatric AIDS Resource Centre
25 Hatton Place
Edinburgh EH9 1UB
Tel: (44-31) 668-4407
Fax: (44-31) 668-3916

Information and enquiry database on services for HIV-infected children, research, sources of support, management issues. Resources: reprints, information leaflets, guidelines. Training for health care and lay workers. Share expertise on working with HIV-affected families, personal care, foster care, adoption, school placement. Focus particularly on children living with HIV/AIDS and their mothers.
Leaflets: *I am HIV positive – what does this mean for my child? Infants and children at risk of HIV infection. Guidance notes for carers.*

Spain

Salud y SIDA: Información, Comunicación y Asesoramiento
Calle Desengaño 18, 10 A
28004 Madrid
Tel: (34-1) 532-2150
Fax: (34-1) 523-3601

Documentation and resource centre with support and services for those working and interested in the health field. Documentation, international medical database, videos and press archive. HIV/AIDS counselling, drugs programme, training, research, meetings, public education, policy development, human rights campaigns. Focus on sexual practice, STDs, injection drug use and pregnancy-related transmission. Pamphlets and range of other publications, research reports.

Switzerland

AG Frau und AIDS (Women and AIDS Society)
Zürcher AIDS Hilfe
Postfach 650
8026 Zurich
Tel: (41-1) 461-1516
Fax: (41-1) 461-4669

Information, sex education, HIV/AIDS counselling, phone help line for women, workshops, public education/media campaigns, self-help groups, emotional support, practical help.

Association Aspasie
10, rue Charles-Cusin
1201 Geneva
Tel: (41-22) 732-6828

Information, outreach, advocacy, sex education, condom distribution, HIV testing, HIV/AIDS counselling, phone helpline, workshops, public education/media campaigns and centre for women sex workers, based on the red light district, set up by a group of women concerned about sex work. Focus on sexual practice.
Newsletter: *Mot de Passe.* A newsletter for and by sex workers which regularly covers HIV/AIDS issues and safer sex.
Stickers: *Reviens me voir! Chez moi c'est toujours 'avec' . . .*

Swiss AIDS Foundation
Postfach
8036 Zurich
Tel: (41-1) 462-3077
Fax: (41-1) 462-3225

Condom cartoon postcards. Pamphlet: *'Chez moi, toujours avec . . .'*

Latin America

Argentina

Fundación para Estudio e Investigación de la Mujer
Paraná 135, 30. '13'
1017 Buenos Aires
Tel: (54-1) 476-2763
Fax: (54-1) 274274

Organized national seminars on women & AIDS for health professionals in Buenos Aires, in 1991 Bahia Blanca, and six others in the interior of the country. Information, sex education, training, advocacy, policy development, workshops for women and adolescents. Focus on sexual practice and STDs. Also active in maternal mortality prevention, primary health care and other women's health issues.
Newsletter about women and prevention of AIDS.
Proceedings of the Symposium on Women & AIDS, Buenos Aires, April 1991.
Training manual: *Women, sexuality and reproduction.*

Brazil

Núcleo de Estudios Para a Prevenção da AIDS
Universidade de São Paulo
Av. Prof. Mello Moraes 1721
Cidade Universitaria-IPUSP
São Paulo
Tel: (55-11) 813-3222 x 2701
Fax: (55-11) 813-8895

Information, sex education, safer sex workshops, HIV/AIDS counselling, training, research, workshops, meetings, public education, media campaigns, policy development, anti-discrimination and human rights campaigns. Focus on sexual practice. Target for 1992/3: poor adolescent girls, college students, bank workers, women's movement leaders.
Book: *Em Tempos de AIDS,* edited by Vera Paiva. In press 1992. About AIDS symbolism, approaches to life and death, psycho-social support, prevention among women, teenagers, drug users and reports of community interventions by sex workers, NGOs and others.

Report: *Io Encontro: AIDS Repercussões Psico-Sociais/1st Meeting: Psycho-Social Repercussions of AIDS* (Portuguese/English).

Grupo Pela Vidda

Caixa Postal 54063
01296 São Paulo SP

Groups for people affected by HIV/AIDS, including for women. Safer sex workshops for gay men and teenagers. Focus on sexual practice and STDs.

Núcleo de Investigação em Saúde de Mulher

Instituto de Saude
Rua San Antonio 590/2º andar
Bela Vista
São Paulo SP CEP 01314
Tel: (55-11) 35-90-47 x 234
Fax: (55-11) 35-27-72

Research in reproductive health issues, including on the risk of HIV infection among women in São Paulo; workshops and seminars on prevention of AIDS and safer sex. Preparation of educational material on women & AIDS, including a video and manual. Focus on sexual practice. Target women leaders working on women's health issues.
Video on women and AIDS, with training manual for community leaders on prevention of AIDS.

Grupo de Apoio a Prevenção a AIDS

R. Barão de Tatui, 376
São Paulo SP 01226
Tel: (55-11) 66-07-55
Fax: (55-11) 825-6003

Information, sex education, safer sex workshops, condom distribution, outreach, HIV/AIDS counselling, phone help line, workshops, public education, policy development, home care, childcare, legal advice, emotional support, financial help, housing, human rights campaigns, psychological services. Focus on sexual practice, injection drug use and blood transfusion. Leaflets.

Associação Brasileira Interdisciplinar de AIDS (ABIA)

Rua Lopes Quintas 576
Jardim Botanico
Rio de Janeiro 22460
Tel: (55-21) 239-5171
Fax: (55-21) 294-5602

Active groups in a number of cities nationally.
Fotonovela: *Que qui e essa tal de AIDS?*

Apoio Religioso Contra a AIDS

Instituto de Estudos da Religião
Ladeira da Glória 98
Glória
Rio de Janeiro 22211
Tel: (55-21) 265-5747   Fax: (55-21) 205-4796

A network of professional health workers, non-governmental organizations, churches, pastors and lay people fighting against the AIDS epidemic, attempting to overcome panic and prejudice. Health education projects, home and hospital visits, telephone counselling and training courses. Producing an epidemiological profile of children with AIDS in Rio de Janeiro and São Paulo. Pamphlet for women, including resources in Rio de Janeiro. *Igrejas e AIDS: Perspectivas biblicas e pastorais,* 1990.

GELEDES – Instituto da Mulher Negra

Praça Carlos Gomes 67
5º andar – CJM
01501 - 040 São Paulo
Tel: (55-11) 35-3869   Fax: (55-11) 36-9901

Information, workshops, outreach on sexual and reproductive health for black women. Video on women and AIDS. Available in English.

Chile

Centro de Educación y Prevención en Salud Social

Casilla 3440
Concepción
Tel: (56-41) 223-447   Fax: (56-41) 233-298

Information for adolescents and sex workers, sex education, safer sex workshops, condom distribution, outreach, networking, HIV testing, counselling, phone help line, training teachers of children, high-school students and social workers, workshops e.g. for gay men and youth, media campaigns, summer campaigns at the seaside, support/solidarity group for people with HIV/AIDS, emotional support, practical help, financial help for expenses related to illness, human rights campaigns, help in obtaining medication. Focus on sexual practice. Sex workers particularly targeted.

Instituto de la Mujer

Claudio Arrau 0211
Santiago
Tel: (56-2) 222-0784   Fax: (56-2) 635-3106

Information; sex education for high school and technical school students, women's and youth groups; condom distribution; training of sex workers to do peer education in the streets and districts where sex is sold; qualitative research on attitudes towards AIDS prevention among youth, and attitudes and practices for prevention by sex workers; workshops, public education, policy development. Focus on sexual practice, STDs and reproductive and sexual rights. Leaflet on AIDS prevention for sex workers, designed jointly with them. Reports, leaflets, comic, training manual, and badge: For safe and responsible sex, use a condom.

Grupo de Investigación y Capacitación en Medicina Social

Concha y Toro 17C
Casilla 53.144
Correo 1
Santiago
Tel/Fax: (56-2) 672-3038

Women professionals in health and social sciences who develop participative research, educational and training courses for women, unpaid women workers, and women health workers and social scientists. Collaborate with the Latin American Association for Human Rights on prevention of unwanted pregnancy among adolescents and reproductive rights in Chile. Information, sex education, safer sex workshops, condom distribution, outreach, research, workshops, anti-discrimination and human rights campaigns. Focus on sexual practice. Target adolescent women, women working without pay, women health workers, housewives. Leaflets.
Mujeres, SIDA y Derechos Humanos by María Isabel Matamala.
Newsletter: *Carta Informativa.*

Asociación Chilena de Prevención del SIDA

Calle Dieciocho 120
Santiago
Tel: (56-2) 697-3711
Fax: (56-2) 698-4127

Phone helpline and referral; HIV/AIDS testing/ counselling, education, condom distribution;

information and documentation centre; workshops, training, lectures and courses. Psycho-social support programme for women with HIV, their children and families; workshops on stress for health personnel; monthly counselling sessions for parents of HIV-positive children; legal advice; practical help. Focus on sexual practice and pregnancy-related transmission. Urban poor and working class women particularly targeted.

Colombia

Pro-Familia

Calle 34, No. 14-52
Bogotá
Tel: (57-1) 287-2100
Fax: (57-1) 287-5530

Among the first family planning associations in Latin America to investigate their potential role in HIV/AIDS education, prevention and diagnosis. Condom education and distribution through community-based distributors in rural areas. Series of messages about HIV, safer sex and condoms on radio. HIV/AIDS information available in family planning clinics. Information, outreach, HIV counselling and testing, phone helpline also gives family planning information. Focus on STDs. The community-based programme targets sex workers. Leaflet and video: *SIDA – Cambiando las reglas.*

México

Salud Integral para la Mujer

Prolong. 5 de febrero 1374-4
Col. San Simón-Portales
C.P. 03600
México, DF
Tel: (52-5) 674-2447

Aim to develop and strengthen women's rights and dignity, especially in the area of health. Active in reproductive health, sexuality, AIDS and health policy. Networking, education, training, assistance, support, workshops, STD and HIV testing and counselling centre, conference participation, media work including regular radio programme, outreach. Leaflets.
Consultative document: *El SIDA y la Mujeres*, 1992.

Communicación, Intercambio y Desarrollo en America Latina (CIDHAL)
Apartado 1-579
Cuernavaca, Morelos 62000
Tel/Fax: (52-73) 18-20-58

Sexuality and safer sex workshops; antenatal and childbirth classes for women. Alternative and holistic treatments. Information, sex education, condom distribution, HIV testing, meetings, clinical services, reproductive health services. New birthing centre. Documentation on reproductive tract infections. Focus on sexuality and STDs.

Coordinadora de Salud, Plenario de Mujeres
Unión Popular Nueva Tenochtitlan
Zapotecos 7 Bis
Col. Obrera
México D.F.
Tel: (52-5) 578-1301
Fax: (52-5) 590-2110

Medical and psychological support counselling; courses, workshops and training for health education promoters; research; lobbying for better government policies; subsidized food; clinical services; support in finding work. Community-based groups a central part of the women's section's work. Training for parents to teach young children about health, sexuality and HIV/AIDS. Newspaper.

Programa Interdisciplinario de Estudios de la Mujer
El Colegio de México
Camino al Ajusco 20
C.P. 01000
10740 México D.F.

Long-term project of research and courses on reproductive health.
Mujer y SIDA: Jornadas 121. Programa Interdisciplinario de Estudios de la Mujer, 1992. Papers from a forum on women and HIV/AIDS organized by PIEM and CONASIDA, covering epidemiology, gender, risk, sexuality, abortion, sex work, safer sex and condoms.

Nicaragua

Centro de Información y Asesoria en Salud
Apartado 3267
Managua

Educational work on women and AIDS. Poster.

Perú

Movimiento Homosexual de Lima
Apartado 11-0289
Lima 11
Tel: (51-14) 224-007
Fax: (51-14) 454-681

Educational and support activities primarily for gay and bisexual men, but increasing attention to women's health issues. Information, sex education, safer sex workshops, condom distribution, helpline, workshops, anti-discrimination and human rights campaigns. Focus on sexual practice. Target women street prostitutes. Leaflets.

Uruguay

Associación Uruguaya de Planificación Familiar
Casilla de Correo 10634
Distrito 1
Montevideo
Tel: (598-2) 78-53-28
Fax: (598-2) 77-16-67

Workshops on quality of care, family planning, sexuality and HIV/AIDS for activists and professionals nationally.
Carpeta de Repaso: Talleres de Orientación/Consejeria sobre Calidad de Atención Sexualidad y SIDA. Ayudas didácticas y material bibliográfico. AUPFIRH, Montevideo, 1990.

Middle East

Israel

Hava'ad Lemilehamah B'AIDS
Israel AIDS Task Force
P.O.B. 33602
Tel Aviv 61336
Tel: (972-3) 566-1639

Information, condom distribution at special events, HIV testing, HIV/AIDS counselling, helpline, buddies and buddy training programme, educational activities, workshops, public education, policy development, parliamentary lobbying, self-help groups, home care, financial help for medicines. Focus on sexual practice. Leaflets.

North America

Canada

Women and AIDS Project
AIDS Committee of Toronto
Box 55, Station F
Toronto, Ontario M4Y 1W9
Tel: (1-416) 926-0063
Fax: (1-416) 926-0386
TTY for the Deaf: (1-416) 926-8295

Information, sex education, safer sex workshops, condom distribution, outreach, HIV/AIDS counselling, helpline, workshops, public education, media campaigns, policy development, self-help groups, emotional support, anti-discrimination and human rights campaigns. Pamphlets (English/French).
Posters: *The woman with AIDS: she's the girl next door. Love is a serious thing.*

Voices of Positive Women
P.O. Box 471, Stn. C
Toronto, Ontario M6J 3P5
Tel: (1-416) 324-8703

Run for and by women living with HIV and AIDS.
Newsletter: *Voices of Positive Women.*
Leaflets: *HIV, Pregnancy and Our Children. Positive Sexuality. So Your Test is Positive.*

Women and AIDS Project – AIDS Vancouver
1107 Seymour Street
Vancouver, BC V6B 5S8
Tel: (1-604) 893-2210

Leaflets: *Lesbians and AIDS; Safer Sex; Does Your Birth Control Protect You against AIDS?*
Women and AIDS: A Resource Guide (with IDERA) 1990. A collection of articles and papers about women and HIV/AIDS in Canada, the USA and internationally, produced for World AIDS Day 1990.

United States

Association for Women's AIDS Research & Education (Project AWARE)
3180 18th Street
Suite 205
San Francisco, California 94110
Tel: (1-415) 476 4091
Fax: (1-415) 476 0362

AIDS research and health promotion for high risk women via heterosexual transmission. Collaborative referral and follow-up for HIV-positive programme study participants. Information flyers, bibliographies of published articles on women and HIV and clinical issues for women with HIV, information on safe sex for lesbians, articles on women, sex workers and HIV.

Latino AIDS Project
2639 24th Street
San Francisco, California 94110
Tel: (1-415) 647-5450
Fax: (1-415) 647-0740

Information, sex education, safer sex and other workshops, condom distribution, outreach, HIV/AIDS counselling, training, self-help groups, emotional support, public education and media campaigns. Focus on sexual practice and pregnancy-related transmission. Target Spanish-speaking women and gay Latino men.
Fotonovela: *Ojos Que No Ven/Eyes That Do Not See.* Story of friends, lovers, and families in the California Latino community confronting drug use, heterosexuality, homosexuality and their lives as AIDS affects them. Based on video of the same name.

Sapphex Learn
Lesbian's Educational AIDS Resource Network
14002 Clubhouse Circle, #206
Tampa, Florida 33624
Tel: (1-813) 962-7643

Educational AIDS resource network for lesbian and bisexual women's communities. Information on diversity of women's sexuality, safer sex workshops, training seminars for safer sex workshops, condom distribution, phone line, media campaigns, self-help groups and information to health care providers. Focus on sexual practice, STDs and injection drug use. Also target male-to-female lesbian transsexuals.

Pamphlet: *Lesbians loving lesbians* (late 1992).
Training manual for workshops: *Lesbian HIV Primer Notebook.*
Newsletter: *Sexual Health Enlightenment (SHE).* Sexual issues pertinent to lesbians and bisexual women, including the latest information on AIDS, STDs and other immune disorders.
Safer sexuality kit and lesbian safer sexuality menu.

Sisterlove: Women's AIDS Project
1132 West Peachtree Street
Atlanta, Georgia 30310
Tel: (1-404) 872-0600
Fax: (1-404) 755-5221

Safer sex parties for women with follow-up meetings. Training sessions to teach other women to run the parties locally, and training for other groups interested in running parties.
Is Your Love healthy? Facilitator's Guide to the Healthy Love Party – An AIDS Education Workshop for Women Only, 1990.

Chicago Women's AIDS Project
5249 North Kenmore
Chicago, Illinois 60640
Tel: (1-312) 271-2070

Health education, support services, patient advocacy, case management.
Girls Night Out: A Safer Sex Workshop for Women – Manual for Peer Leaders.

Women & Children with HIV Program
Cook County Hospital
CCSN- Room 912
1835 West Harrison Street
Chicago, Illinois 60612
Tel: (1-312) 633-5080
Fax: (1-312) 633-8333

Education, counselling, HIV testing, comprehensive medical treatment, health services and care, drug abuse prevention and treatment, support services, help with basic needs, financial assistance, housing referrals, childcare for HIV-positive children, childcare for children of people with AIDS, advocacy, legal services, peer education, training. Focus on sexual practice, STDs, injection drugs and pregnancy-related transmission.

Multicultural AIDS Coalition
566 Columbus Avenue
Boston, MA 02118, USA
Tel: (1-617) 536-8610

Searching for Women: A Literature Review on Women, HIV and AIDS in the United States, 1991. Comprehensive summary of medical and social research findings and an extensive bibliography.

New Jersey Women and AIDS Network
5 Elm Row, Suite 112
New Brunswick, New Jersey 08901
Tel: (1-908) 846-4462
Fax: (1-908) 846-2674

Advocacy for appropriate legislation and public health policy on HIV/AIDS for women; promotion education and information which is culturally sensitive and gender specific; safer sex and other workshops; media, human rights and anti-discrimination campaigns; mobilization to ensure adequate resources and services for women who have HIV or AIDS or are at risk of infection.
Leaflet and pamphlet: *Me First: Medical Manifestations of HIV in Women* (English/Spanish).
Newsletter: *NJWAN News.*

Community Family Planning Council
92–94 Ludlow Street
New York, NY 10002
Tel: (1-212) 979-9014
Fax: (1-212) 477-8957

Community-based HIV testing, support and counselling in the context of health care for women, pregnancy and family planning needs, including homeless and single mothers and particularly black and Hispanic women. Clinical services for family planning, antenatal care, STDs, and primary health care. Advocacy and anti-discrimination work.

New York City Commission on Human Rights
40 Rector Street
New York, NY 10006
Tel: (1-212) 306-7057
Fax: (1-212) 306-7514

HIV-Related Discrimination in Abortion Clinics in New York City, by Katherine M. Franke, AIDS Discrimination Division, 1989.

Video: *The Second Epidemic*, by Amber Hollibaugh. New York, 1989. Portraits of people with AIDS who have fought discrimination with help from the NYC Human Rights Commission, including a young Puerto Rican woman.

AIDS Counseling and Education
Bedford Hills Correctional Facility
247 Harris Road
Bedford Hills, New York 10507
Tel: (1-914) 241-3100 x 275

Safer sex and other workshops, outreach, HIV counselling, training, self-help groups, emotional support. Model project for women in prison, provide peer education and counselling, inmate and staff education, workshops for general public. Focus on sexual practice, STDs, injection drug use, pregnancy-related transmission and blood transfusion. Leaflet: *Break through the wall of fear. Once Upon a Virus Coloring Book*, for children.

Pediatric and Pregnancy AIDS Hotline
Comprehensive AIDS Family Care Centre
Albert Einstein College of Medicine
1300 Morris Park Avenue MN19
Bronx, NY 10462
Tel: (1-212) 430-2940

Information, sex education, safer sex workshops, condom distribution, outreach, HIV testing, counselling, phone helpline, drugs programme, training, research, public education, policy development, self-help groups, home care, childcare, legal advice, emotional support, practical and financial help, housing, human rights campaigning, HIV/AIDS and other clinical services, reproductive health services. Support groups for mothers, bereavement groups for families and children. Particularly target injection drug users and their partners.
Pamphlets: *Children can get AIDS too.* Recommended precautions for caretakers of children.

Brown University AIDS Program
The Miriam Hospital
164 Summit Avenue
Providence, Rhode Island 02906
Tel: (1-401) 331-8500

Major research on the natural history of HIV in women in the state of Rhode Island. Comprehensive care for women with HIV infection in southwestern New England. Information, outreach, HIV testing and counselling, phone helpline, training, research, workshops, public education, self-help groups, home care, practical help, human rights campaigns, HIV/AIDS and other clinical services. Leaflets, pamphlets, videos, newsletters, reports, regularly updated.

South Carolina AIDS Education Network
2768 Decker Boulevard, Suite 98
Columbia, South Carolina 29206
Tel: (1-803) 736-1171

Education for women about AIDS in a beauty salon, called DiAna's Hair Ego. Information, sex education, safer sex workshops, condom distribution, HIV/AIDS counselling, phone helpline, meetings, public education, self-help groups, emotional support, community education, peer training. Culturally sensitive materials for the black community, low literacy educational materials. Outreach to adolescents through safer sex parties and plays. Focus on sexual practice, STDs, and injection drug use. Safer Sex Packets; Condom Love Basket; Safer Sex Get Acquainted Kit; Dancing Condom Nightshirt and T-Shirt.
Videos: *DiAna's Hair Ego AIDS Info UpFront*. A straight-talking video about sexuality for grassroots education among adolescents and adults, aimed at southern USA black communities.
Party safe with DiAna and Bambi (for adults – no nudity).
What if you gave a kid a condom? For children, this video was made by 9- to 14-year-olds who are not sexually active. Also a workbook for school and home, in press.

Native American Women's Health Education Resource Center
P.O. Box 572
Lake Andes, South Dakota 57356
Tel: (1-605) 487-7097
Fax: (1-605) 487-7964

Information, sex education, women-only workshops for obstetrics and gynaecology patients, short-term counselling, self-help support groups, child development and parenting classes, domestic abuse and sexual assault shelters, tutoring for pregnant teens, prenatal care and birthing classes, HIV/AIDS counselling, public education, policy development, human rights campaigns. Focus on sexual practice and STDs.

Posters:
Traditional values can stamp out the AIDS virus. Ina Ka Hoksiyopa.
Native Americans can get the AIDS virus.
How well do you know your partner?
What do you do when your partner won't use a condom.
How can reading the package save your life?
Videos:
It Could Happen to Anybody. 'Mom and Son' series, with comics.
Report: *The Impact of AIDS in the Native American Community.*

National Hispanic Education and Communications Projects

1000 16th Street NW, Suite 504
Washington DC 20036, USA
Tel: (1-202) 452-0092
Fax: (1-202) 452-0086

Latina AIDS Action Plan and Resource Guide, 1990. Critical issues for successful programmes and policies for women, model programmes, bibliographies (English/Spanish).

National Women's Health Network

1325 G Street NW
Lower Level B
Washington DC 20005
Tel: (1-202) 347-1140   Fax: (1-202) 347-1168

Information and documentation centre on all women's health issues, training, policy development and lobbying, raising awareness of AIDS among women health activists and reproductive health service providers, workshops and conferences, networking, advocacy.
Guidelines on testing and counselling women at high risk for HIV infection.
Women, AIDS and Public Health Policies, 1990.
AIDS and Women Information Packet (updated regularly).
AIDS Education Workshop by and for Women in their 20s. Training manual.

Center for Women Policy Studies

Suite 508
2000 P Street NW
Washington DC 20036
Tel: (1-202) 872-1770
Fax: (1-202) 296-8962

Information, outreach, training, research, workshops, meetings, public education, policy development, human rights campaigns.
More Harm Than Help: The Ramifications for Rape Survivors of Mandatory HIV Testing of Rapists, by Lisa Bowleg and Kathleen D. Stoll, 1991.
Women and the Definition of AIDS: focus points for frustration, by Kathleen D. Stoll, 1992.
The Guide to Resources on Women and AIDS, 2nd edition 1991. Contains ten detailed case studies of groups active in women and HIV/AIDS work in the USA, papers on current issues, and a state-by-state directory of HIV/AIDS programmes in the USA. New editions planned annually.
Video: *Fighting for Our Lives: Women Confronting AIDS,* 1990, and Action Kit. Portrays the strengths and strategies of women of colour who are leaders in confronting HIV disease. Features six projects, as described by the women who shape them, to meet women's needs in the struggle against AIDS. The Action Kit aims to help groups to use the video effectively in AIDS education programmes.

The Pacific

Regional Network

South Pacific Commission

AIDS & STD Prevention Project
B.P. D5
Noumea Cedex, New Caledonia
Tel: (687) 26-20-00
Fax: (687) 26-38-18

A network of everyone in the Pacific region who produces or wants to receive HIV/AIDS education materials and is involved in project work/service provision related to HIV/AIDS. Organization of meetings and consultations regionally. The SPC also have an extensive Health Documentation Centre, a Pacific Women's Resource Bureau, Community Health Services, and a Regional Media Centre.

Newsletter: *Pacific AIDS Alert Bulletin*. Contains examples of leaflets, slogans, stickers, posters and activities for AIDS education work from the Pacific region and many other countries. Also monthly newssheet.

AIDS and STD Prevention Report: First Sub-Regional Caucus for Melanesian Women, Noumea, 14–18 October 1991.

Video: *Charlotte's Story*, by the SPC Regional Media Centre. Interview with a Samoan woman about her experience of losing her son to AIDS.

Dramatized radio plays on AIDS. Comics on AIDS for school students.

T-shirt: Captain Condom.

Australia

Positive Women
P.O. Box 1546
Collingwood 3066

Self-help support group for HIV-positive women.

Prostitutes Collective of Victoria, Inc.
10 Inkerman Street
St Kilda
Melbourne 3182
Tel: (61-3) 534-8319

Information on sex industry skills, safer sex workshops including negotiation skills, condom distribution to sex workers and their clients, outreach to sex workers on local streets, needle exchange, harm minimization education, human rights campaigning, methadone self-help group, policy development, emotional help, housing referrals, emergency housing relief. Promote condom-only sex establishments and safe sex for prostitutes in Victoria. Member of the Scarlet Alliance, a coalition since 1988 of six Australian sex workers' organizations. Now making links with similar organizations in southeast Asia and Oceania, for staff exchanges and meetings. Focus on sexual practice, STDs, and injection drug use. Target women sex workers, young and male sex workers.

Leaflet: *HIV/AIDS and other sexually transmitted diseases*.

Sticker: *This House is Endorsed as a Safe Sex House*.

Newsletter: *Working Girl Magazine*.

Family Planning Association of Western Australia
70 Roe Street
Northbridge, Perth 6003
Tel: (61-9) 227-6177

Information, sex education, safer sex workshops, HIV testing, counselling and referrals, phone line help, training, workshops, public education, policy development, reproductive health services. Focus on sexual practice and STDs. Library with books, journals, videos, evaluations of training programmes. Newsletter. Pamphlets on HIV/AIDS, safer sex, contraception.

Women Talking about AIDS Project
Women in Industry, Community & Health
83 Johnston Street
Fitzroy 3065
Tel: (61-3) 416-3999
Fax: (61-3) 416-3749

Information, sex education, meetings, public education, policy development, human rights campaigns, safer sex workshops, information on contraception and women's health issues for migrant women in their workplaces. Resource development. Training for bilingual and bicultural women community workers to take HIV/AIDS education to industrial worksites. Focus on sexual practice and STDs. Target migrant women of non-English speaking background, particularly Vietnamese, Spanish-speaking and Arabic-speaking women.

Booklet: *Women Talk about AIDS, Sex and Sexual Health*, 1992 (Arabic/English). Audio cassette of same title for use of leaders of women's groups to start discussions (Arabic).

Women Talking About AIDS Project Report. June 1992. Evaluation of a community development project on HIV/AIDS with women of Arabic and Islamic communities.

Social Biology Resources Centre
139 Bouverie Street
Carlton, Victoria 3053
Tel: (61-3) 347-8700
Fax: (61-3) 347-5892

Education in health and human sexuality for those working in health, education and welfare. HIV education programmes within a sexual health context for health professionals, local government staff, drug treatment agencies, refuge workers, teachers and students, sex workers, police, prison officers, church representatives, employers and others. Ongoing working group for those doing community AIDS education. Started an AIDS counsellors group which is now a national, independent association. Public meetings about AIDS and STDs. Policy development, training in communication skills for working with intellectually disabled people, educational resources, education on how HIV affects homelessness. Library.

New Zealand

Positive Women
76 Grafton Road
Auckland
Tel: (64-9) 309-5560
Fax: (64-9) 302-2338

Support group run by and for women with HIV/AIDS with a centre for meeting, getting information on treatments and access to supportive health professionals. Outreach to HIV-positive women, public education, interviews for media, and work with Area Health Board on education programmes for health workers, social workers and schools.

International Non-Government Organizations

International Planned Parenthood Federation
AIDS Prevention Unit
Regents College
Inner Circle, Regents Park
London NW1 4NS, England
Tel: (44-71) 486-0741
Fax: (44-71) 487-7950

International federation of national family planning associations. Education for member associations and others on the relationship between AIDS, sexuality, and family planning work. Focus on sexual practice and STDs.

All about AIDS: A Workbook. Developed in the Caribbean.
Dangerous Love. A story developed and printed in Zimbabwe about a married man living apart from his wife who infects her and their first child with HIV.
Protect Yourself and Your Clients. A durable plastic wall chart for health workers (English/French/Arabic/Spanish).
Preventing a Crisis: AIDS and Family Planning Work, 1989. (English/French/Spanish/Arabic). Originally intended for family planning clinics but used by a much wider audience, this manual covers planning, services, education, counselling, empowerment, training, young people, and discussion starters.
Training Manuals:
AIDS Education for Family Planning Clinic Service Providers. Self-study modules using real-life situations to stimulate discussion and learning about HIV/AIDS, counselling of clients, and prevention of infection in the workplace.
Videos:
Unmasking AIDS. Plus detailed guides for training in experiential group work approaches and the use of story telling, drama, and puppetry in HIV education.
Caring about AIDS: The Common Ground. Shows four NGOs – in California, Brazil, Zambia and Sweden – in action (English/French/Spanish).
Counselling and Sexuality: Training Resources. A set of videos and a comprehensive training manual for counselling on sexuality, including STDs, sexual problems and pre-marital counselling.

Appropriate Health Resources & Technologies Action Group (AHRTAG)
1 London Bridge Street
London SE1 9SG, England
Tel: (44-71) 378-1403
Fax: (44-71) 403-6003

Information and enquiry service using databases. Technical support for regional networks, partner support for HIV/AIDS resource centres in developing countries; international and regional networking; resource centre on HIV/AIDS as an international health and development issue. Also work on primary health care issues.
Newsletter: *AIDS Action*. Covers one main topic per issue, e.g. sexuality, blood transfusion, human

rights, with articles from a range of countries (English/French/Spanish/Portuguese).
Let's Teach about AIDS. Series of booklets on participatory learning techniques.

The Panos Institute
AIDS Unit
9 White Lion Street
London N1 9PD, England
Tel: (44-71) 278-1111
Fax: (44-71) 278-0345

Newsletter: *WorldAIDS*. (English/Spanish/French).
AIDS & Children: A Family Disease, 1989. Dossier.
Books:
The Third Epidemic: Repercussions of the Fear of AIDS.
AIDS and the Third World.
Blaming Others: Prejudice, Race and Worldwide AIDS, by Renee Sabatier *et al.*
Triple Jeopardy: Women and AIDS, 1990.

World Council of Churches
AIDS Working Group
P.O. Box 2100
1211 Geneva 2, Switzerland
Tel: (41-22) 791-6111
Fax: (41-22) 791 0361

Programmes addressed to member churches.
Guide to HIV/AIDS Pastoral Counselling, 1990. Handbook on giving compassionate care, counselling and support to people with HIV/AIDS, their families and loved ones (English/Spanish/Portuguese).

Consejo Latinoamericano de Iglesias
Pastoral de Familia, Mujeres y Niños
Casilla 85-22
Quito, Ecuador
Tel: (593-2) 561-539
Fax: (593-2) 504-377

An ecumenical organization that views AIDS as a family disease. Education and prevention of AIDS in church populations, workshops for pastoral care of people with HIV/AIDS. Especially interested in involving church women and health professionals in campaigns and training workshops.
Caminando con VIH/SIDA/Caminhando com HIV/AIDS. Workbook about living with HIV/AIDS,

facing death, and acknowledging loss. Notes for using the workbook and working with children with AIDS in the Latin American context. Also English, from the World Council of Churches, Geneva.

International Federation of Red Cross and Red Crescent Societies
P.O. Box 372
17, Chemin des Crets
Petit Saconnex
1211 Geneva 19, Switzerland
Tel: (41-22) 730-4222
Fax: (41-22) 733-0395

Federation of national Red Cross and Red Crescent societies, who have been instrumental in making national blood supplies safe from HIV. Range of projects and policy development with national members. Focus on blood transfusion and sexual practice. Action for youth project. Training manuals for youth work and workplace training, video, media pack.

UK NGO AIDS Consortium for the Third World
Fenner Brockway House
37/39 Great Guildford Street
London SE1 0ES, England
Tel: (44-71) 401-8231
Fax: (44-71) 401-2124

Consortium of UK-based NGOs whose work focuses on developing countries. Activities include information sharing, networking, lobbying.
Directory of European Funders of AIDS/HIV Projects in Developing Countries, 1991.
Women & AIDS in the Developing World, Conference Report, November 1990.

Royal Tropical Institute
Department of Information & Documentation
Mauritskade 63
1092 AD Amsterdam, Netherlands
Tel: (31-20) 568-8298
Fax: (31-20) 568-8444

Newsletter: *AIDS Health Promotion Exchange*. Illustrates and describes HIV/AIDS health education projects. (English/French/Spanish)
Also AIDS Coordination Bureau – secretariat/information centre for a consortium of Dutch NGOs

who support health care programmes in developing countries. International resource centre.

Program on Critical Issues in Reproductive Health and Population
The Population Council
1 Dag Hammarskjold Plaza
New York, NY 10017, USA

Workshops, seminars, social and behavioural research, publications, design and evaluation of programmes that integrate STD diagnostic, treatment and referral services within family planning and reproductive health services. Work on quality of care, unwanted pregnancy, consequences of unsafe abortions and post-partum care. AIDS in context of reproductive health. Research on woman-controlled technology for protection against sexual transmission of STDs/HIV, e.g. virucides.
Meeting Male Reproductive Health Care Needs in Latin America, by Debbie Rogow. Quality/Calidad/Qualité No. 2, 1990.
Sexually transmitted diseases and the reproductive health of women, by Christopher Elias. Working Paper No. 5, 1991.

Global AIDS Policy Coalition
Harvard School of Public Health
677 Huntington Avenue
Boston, MA 02115, USA
Tel: (1-617) 432-4311
Fax: (1-617) 432-4310

Building a network of professionals internationally to promote independent analysis, advocacy and socially committed and relevant programmes for HIV/AIDS prevention and control, including those with a focus on women.
AIDS in the World 1992, edited by Jonathan Mann *et al*, Harvard University Press, Cambridge, in press.

Center for Communications Programs
Johns Hopkins University
527 St Paul Place
Baltimore, MD 21202, USA
Tel: (1-410) 659-6300
Fax: (1-410) 659-6266

International HIV/AIDS media/materials collection. Popline, on-line databases on reproductive health programmes, family planning, AIDS and child survival programmes, with emphasis on developing countries. Population Reports: Periodical with in-depth coverage of one topic per issue, on family planning, reproductive health, AIDS or population policy.

AIDS Control and Prevention Project (AIDSCAP)
Family Health International
2101 Wilson Blvd STE 710
Arlington, VA 22201, USA
Tel: (1-703) 516-9779
Fax: (1-703) 516-9781

Information, condom distribution, outreach, HIV/AIDS counselling, workshops, public education/media campaigns, policy development/campaigns, HIV/AIDS clinical services. Focus on sexual practice and STDs. Aim to support developing country programmes.

International Governmental Organizations

World Health Organization
WHO Global Programme on AIDS (GPA)
1211 Geneva 27
Switzerland
Tel: (41-22) 791-2106/3187
Fax: (41-22) 791-0746

Main UN agency for planning and coordination of national AIDS programmes with national governments globally.
Women and AIDS: An Annotated Bibliography of Work Done by the WHO GPA. Prepared by Angela Trenton, February 1992.
The Care and Support of Children of HIV-Infected Parents, May 1991.
Management of patients with sexually transmitted diseases: Report of a WHO Study Group. WHO Technical Report Series 810. WHO, Geneva, 1991. Detailed guidelines on topics such as partner notification, counselling and health education, STD management protocols, case reporting and surveillance.
AIDS and Maternal and Child Health.
AIDS and Family Planning; Guidelines for Nursing Management of People infected with HIV (with the International Council of Nurses).

Instructions for Adapting the Condom Flier and Prototype Condom. Leaflet.
Report of the Meeting on Research Priorities Relating to Women and HIV/AIDS, Geneva, 19–20 November 1990.
Report of the Consultation with International Women's Non-Governmental Organizations, Geneva, December 1989. Proposals by women's organizations of what the GPA should be doing for women.

WHO Africa Region
P.O. Box 6
Brazzaville, Congo
Tel: (242-83) 3860
Fax: (242-83) 1879

WHO Eastern Mediterranean Region
P.O. Box 1517
Alexandria 21511, Egypt
Tel: (20-3) 483-0090
Fax: (20-3) 483-8916

Training for nurses in HIV/AIDS care, education aimed at women, WHO materials in Arabic, e.g. for nurses and on AIDS/MCH and on breastfeeding.

WHO Europe Region
8 Scherfigsvej
2100 Copenhagen, Denmark
Tel: (45-31) 29-01-11
Fax: (45-31) 18-11-20

Many reports with recommendations for policy and examples of services, on a range of topics about all European countries, including: nursing, counselling, care, drug use, youth, travel, self-help, psycho-social and cultural issues, and AIDS telephone hotlines.
Women living with HIV: Report of a future workshop, 1991.
Taking up the challenge in the '90s. Contains list of all their publications to end 1991.

WHO Southeast Asia Region
World Health House
Indraprastha Estate
New Delhi 110 002, India

Health promotion materials for prevention and control of AIDS in South East Asia region.
Mobilization of Women's Organizations/NGOs in the Prevention and Control of HIV Infection/AIDS: Report of an Intercountry Consultation. New Delhi, May 1990.

Pan American Health Organization
525 23rd Street NW
Washington DC 20037-2895, USA
Tel: (1-202) 861-3200
Fax: (1-202) 223-5971

Organized the 1st Regional Meeting on AIDS and Maternal and Child Health in the Latin American Region in São Paulo, November 1990 and the 1st Latin American and Caribbean Symposium on Women and AIDS in Buenos Aires, Argentina, December, 1990, with the collaboration of the Latin American and Caribbean Women's Health Network/Isis International. Journal: *Bulletin of PAHO*.

STD/AIDS Education
P.O. Box 113
Suva, Fiji

Health education office on STDs and AIDS. Media training and materials production. Serving all Pacific islands/countries. In cooperation with the WHO Western Pacific Region.
Education to prevent AIDS/STD in the Pacific: A teaching guide for secondary schools, UNESCO/WHO 1989. Widely used by secondary schools in the Pacific region and elsewhere.

WHO Regional Office for the Western Pacific
United Nations Avenue
P.O. Box 2932
1099 Manila, Philippines
Tel: (63-2) 521-8421
Fax: (63-2) 521-1036

Information, training, research, workshops, public education, policy development, human rights campaigns, technical support for national programmes on women and AIDS.
Women & AIDS: Text of a Radio Programme for World AIDS Day 1990. Interviews with health workers and activists involved in AIDS work with women from Asia and the Pacific region.

All WHO resources available from:
Distribution and Sales Unit
World Health Organization
1211 Geneva 27, Switzerland

UNICEF
3 United Nations Plaza
New York, NY 10017, USA
Tel: (1-212) 326-7383

Education and information about children, for young people in schools, and for women of childbearing age. Have been involved in development of posters, pamphlets, cartoon strips, videos, radio spots, sex education curricula for schools, health education and training. Work mainly in Africa and developing countries. Newsletter: *Action for Children*.
Pamphlets: *Children and AIDS: An Impending Calamity*, 1990.
AIDS and Orphans in Africa: Report of a Meeting, 1991.

United Nations Development Programme
AIDS Programme
1 UN Plaza
New York, NY 10017, USA
Tel: (1-212) 906-5082
Fax: (1-212) 906-5365

Support for AIDS projects, training research and meetings, particularly as they relate to socio-economic, human rights and development issues, including effects on women and development.

AIDSED Centre
UNESCO Regional Office for Asia and the Pacific
920 Sukhumvit Road
Prakanong
Bangkok 10110, Thailand
Tel: (66-2) 391-0577
Fax: (66-2) 391-0866

Public education and documentation centre. Newsletter: *AIDSED*. Resource kit: *AIDS, women and education*.

AIDS Task Force
European Community
Rue Josef 11 67 A
Brussels 1040, Belgium
Tel: (32-2) 231-1495
Fax: (32-2) 230-5574

Research on STDs and AIDS and support for projects in 21 developing countries for improved and linked STD/AIDS clinical services. Concern about the low uptake by women of STD clinic services and how this can be changed in women's favour.

Publications

Women and AIDS: The Role of Women in the Prevention and Control of AIDS/HIV Infection in Nine Sub-Saharan African Countries and in the Care and Support of Those Affected by the Epidemic: Report of a workshop held in Malawi, 10–12 December 1991.

From:
Commonwealth Medical Association
c/o BMA House
Tavistock Square
London WC1H 9JP, England

Positive Women: Voices of Women Living with AIDS, Edited by Andrea Rudd and Darien Taylor, 1992. Women from 14 countries express their experience of living with HIV and AIDS through personal histories, art and poetry.

From:
Second Story Press
760 Bathurst Street
Toronto, Ontario M5S 2R6, Canada

AIDS: The Women, edited by Ines Rieder and Patricia Ruppelt, 1988.
Writings by women with HIV and AIDS, friends, family, lovers and spouses of people with HIV/AIDS, caregivers and professionals working with people with HIV/AIDS, lesbians, sex workers, educators and community organizers, mainly from the USA, Europe, and Latin America.

From:
Cleis Press
P.O. Box 8933
Pittsburgh, PA 15221, USA

Canadian Women and AIDS: Beyond the Statistics. Edited by Jacquie Manthorne, November 1990. (French/English). More than 50 women with HIV and activists and professionals in HIV/AIDS work talk about their lives and their work. Includes the issues for women; personal histories of young women, black women, lesbians, women using drugs, sex workers and women in prison; educating ourselves and each other; organizing our communities; a bibliography and groups in Canada.

From:
Les Editions Communiqu'Elles
3585 St-Urbain
Montreal, Quebec H2X 2N6, Canada
Tel: (1-514) 844-1761
Fax: (1-514) 842-1067

Positively Women: Living with AIDS. Edited by Kate Thomson and Sue O'Sullivan, 1992.
Personal testimonies, and information on medical treatments, holistic health practices, HIV and pregnancy, legal issues, research, housing, drugs, safer sex and healthy living in the UK.

From:
Sheba Feminist Press
10A Bradbury Street
London N16 8JN, England
Tel: (44-71) 254-1590
Fax: (44-71) 249-5351

Don't die of ignorance – I nearly died of embarrassment: condoms in context, by Janet Holland *et al*, 1990.

From:
Tufnell Press
47 Dalmeny Road
London N7 0DY, England

Making It: A Woman's Guide to Sex in the Age of AIDS, by Cindy Patton and Janis Kelly (English/Spanish).

From:
Firebrand Books
141 The Commons
Ithaca, NY 14850, USA
Tel: (1-607) 272-0000

Safer Sex: The Guide for Women Today, by Diane Richardson, 1990.

Women and the AIDS Crisis, by Diane Richardson, 1989.

From:
Pandora, HarperCollins
77–85 Fulham Palace Road
London W6 8JB, England

Women, AIDS & Activism, edited by the Act-Up NY Women & AIDS Book Group, 1990. Papers by 40 women professionals and activists on epidemiology, transmission, HIV-related illness and treatments, race issues, sexuality and safer sex issues, youth, prison issues, pregnancy and motherhood, sex work, reproductive rights, and translating issues into actions. Extensive section on resources, groups, and videos for and about women in the USA.

From:
South End Press
116 Saint Botolph Street
Boston, MA 02115, USA

Working with Women and AIDS: Medical, Social and Counselling Issues. Edited by Judy Bury, Val Morrison and Sheena McLachlan, 1992. Collection of papers by women in HIV/AIDS work in Scotland.

From:
Routledge
11 New Fetter Lane
London EC4P 4EE, England
Tel: (44-71) 583-9855
Fax: (44-71) 936-2407

Our Lives in the Balance: US Women of Color and the AIDS Epidemic, in press 1992 (English/Spanish).

From:
Kitchen Table Women of Color Press
P.O. Box 908
Latham, NY 12110 USA
Tel/Fax: (1-518) 434-2057

HIV and Human Rights – From Victim to Victor: The Voice of People with HIV and AIDS. Report of the 5th International Conference for People with HIV & AIDS, 11–15 September 1991, London. Conference proceedings, papers, personal statements, resolutions and action proposals.

From:
London Lighthouse
111-117 Lancaster Road
London W11 1QT, England
Tel: (44-71) 792-0936
Fax: (44-71) 229-1258

Sexual Behaviour in Sub-Saharan Africa: A Review and Annotated Bibliography, by Hilary Standing and Mere N. Kisekka, 1989.

From:
Library, Overseas Development Administration
Abercrombie House
Eaglesham House
Eaglesham Road
East Kilbride
Glasgow G75 8EA, Scotland
Tel: (44-3552) 41199

Promoting Sexual Health: Proceedings of the Second International Workshop on Prevention of Sexual Transmission of AIDS and other STDs, Cambridge, 1990. Edited by Hilary Curtis, 1992.

From:
British Medical Association Foundation for AIDS
BMA House
Tavistock Square
London WC1H 9JP, England

Sexualities: An Advanced Training resource, by Ewan McKay Armstrong and Peter Gordon, 1992.

Working with Uncertainty: A Handbook for Those Involved in Training on HIV and AIDS, by Hilary Dixon and Peter Gordon, 1990.

From:
Healthwise Bookshop
Family Planning Association
27–35 Mortimer Street
London W1N 7RJ, England
Tel: (44-71) 636-7866

Socioeconomic Aspects of HIV and AIDS in Developing Countries: A Review and Annotated Bibliography, by Susan Foster and Sue Lucas, 1991.

From:
Department of Public Health and Policy
London School of Hygiene and Tropical Medicine
Keppel Street
London WC1E 7HT, England
Tel: (44-71) 636-8636

AIDS Counselling: A Manual for Primary Health Care Workers on AIDS, 1990.

Guidelines on the Management of HIV-Associated Syndromes: A Simplified Approach. Edited by Ahmed S. Latif, Evaristo Marowa and Robert G. Choto, January 1990. For medical professionals.

From:
AIDS Control Programme
Ministry of Health
P.O. Box 8204
Causeway
Harare, Zimbabwe
Tel: (263-4) 702-446

Strategies for Hope Series. ActionAid, AMREF & World in Need (English/French):
From Fear to Hope: AIDS Care and Prevention at Chikankata Hospital, Zambia, 1990. Describes this rural hospital's home care programme for people with HIV/AIDS.
The AIDS Support Organization (TASO): Living Positively with AIDS, 1991. Describes how health workers and volunteers provide care, counselling and support for people with HIV/AIDS and their families.
AIDS Management: An Integrated Approach, 1992. Describes the organization and management of a comprehensive AIDS control and prevention programme by a rural hospital in Zambia.
Meeting AIDS with Compassion: Care/Prevention in Agomanya, Ghana, 1991. Describes how St Martin's Clinic AIDS programme, which integrates the efforts of the Ministry of Health, the Catholic Church, NGOs, political and women's groups, community leaders and traditional healers, is helping mainly women, who have returned from the Ivory Coast, where they did sex work, with AIDS.
AIDS Orphans: A Community Perspective from Tanzania, 1991. Describes how families, communities, NGOs and government services in Kagera region, with 21,000 orphans, are responding to the impact of AIDS on the family system.
The Caring Community: Coping with AIDS in Urban Uganda, 1992. Describes how members of nine small Christian communities in a low-income neighbourhood of Kampala provide care, support, and comfort to people with AIDS and their families, and also promote safe sexual behaviour.

Videos:
TASO: Living Positively with AIDS, 1991.

The Orphan Generation, 1992. Two videos, one aimed at government ministries, international agencies and donors; the other aimed at voluntary agencies, women's groups, community and religious leaders, health professionals and social workers. Describe the struggle of one Ugandan village to cope with the deepening orphan crisis and how the needs of children can be met by community-based organizations.

Slide sets:
HIV Infection: Virology and Transmission, 1989.
HIV Infection: Clinical Manifestations, 1989.
HIV Infection: Prevention and Counselling, 1989.
HIV Infection: Children, 1992.
For primary health care workers and their trainers.

Flannelgraph:
Family planning, STDs and AIDS, 1988.

From:
TALC
P.O. Box 49
St Albans, Herts AL1 4AX, England
Tel: (44-727) 53869
Fax: (44-727) 46852

Say Yes, Say No, Say Maybe – Safe Sex Magazine.
For adolescents.

From:
Brook Advisory Centres
Education and Publications Unit
24 Albert Street
Birmingham B4 7UD, England
Tel: (44-21) 643-1554

It Can't Happen to Me.
Comic for adolescents on sex, AIDS and HIV.

Leaflets/pamphlets:
AIDS and HIV: Questions & Answers.

STDs: The Facts.
Sex & Disease: What you need to know.
Teensex: It's OK to say no way/Esta bien decir de ningun modo.
A Man's Guide to Sexuality.

From:
Planned Parenthood Federation of America
810 Seventh Avenue
New York, NY 10019, USA
Tel: (1-212) 541-7800

Captain Condom & Lady Latex at War with the Army of Sex Diseases, 1991.
Comic for adolescents on sex, STDs and AIDS.

From:
Program for Appropriate Technology in Health
1990 M Street, NW
Suite 700
Washington, DC 20036, USA
Tel: (1-202) 822-0033

Children and the AIDS Virus: A Book for Children, Parents and Teachers, by Rosmarie Hausherr. New York: Clarion Books, 1989.

From:
Houghton Mifflin
International Division
Wayside Road
Burlington, MA 01803, USA

Does AIDS Hurt?: Educating Young Children about AIDS, by Marcia Quackenbush & Sylvia Villareal, 1988. For teachers, parents and other care providers of children to age 10.

From:
Network Publications
P.O. Box 1830
Santa Cruz, CA 95061-1830, USA

Permissions

Papers

Chapter 1

'Testing positive in Canada', by Darien Taylor. Reprinted in part with kind permission of the author from *Healthsharing*, Spring 1990.

Chapter 2

'The costs of reproductive tract infections in women', by Judith Wasserheit. Excerpts reprinted with kind permission from *Reproductive Tract Infections: Special Challenges in Women's Health*. International Women's Health Coalition, New York, 1991.

'Human Immunodeficiency Virus infection in North American women: experience with 200 cases and a review of the literature', by Charles C. J. Carpenter et al. Summarized with kind permission from: *Medicine*. 1991; 70(5):307–325. © 1991, Williams & Wilkins.

Chapter 3

'HIV/AIDS in women in Puerto Rico', by Carmen Zorrilla. Summarized with kind permission of the author from two papers she presented at the National Conference on Women & HIV Infection, Washington DC, 13–14 December 1990.

'The social epidemiology of women and AIDS in Africa', and 'Women at risk: case studies from Zaïre' (in Chapter 11), by Brooke Grundfest Schoepf.

These form part of a paper originally published as: 'Women, AIDS and economic crisis in Central Africa', *Canadian Journal of African Studies*. 1988; 22(3):225–44. Reprinted in part from a revised/updated version with kind permission from: 'Women at risk: case studies from Zaïre', *The Time of AIDS: Social Analysis, Theory and Method*. Edited by Gilbert Herdt and Shirley Lindenbaum. © Sage Publications Inc., Newbury Park, 1992.

'HIV infection in childbearing women in Kigali, Rwanda', by Susan Allen *et al*. Summarized with kind permission from: 'HIV infection in urban Rwanda: demographic and behavioral correlates in a representative sample of childbearing women'. *Journal of the American Medical Association*. 1991; 266(12):1657–1663. © 1991 American Medical Association.

'The Impact of AIDS on women in Thailand', by Jon Ungphakorn. Reprinted in part with kind permission of the author from a paper presented at the Conference on AIDS in Asia and the Pacific. World Health Organization and the Australian Government. Canberra, 5–8 August 1990.

Chapter 5

'Strategies for prevention of pregnancy-related transmission', by Janet L. Mitchell. Reprinted in part with kind permission of the author from: 'Strategies for prevention of perinatal transmission', paper presented at the 6th International Conference on AIDS, San Francisco, 21 June 1990.

Chapter 6

'A London midwife's experience and recommendations for infection control policy for all pregnant women delivering in hospital', by Sandra Dick. This paper has been written specially for this book. Her permission is required to reprint it.

'Post-partum counselling of HIV infected women and their subsequent reproductive behaviour', by M. Temmerman *et al.* Summarized with kind permission from: 'Impact of single session post-partum counselling of HIV infected women on their subsequent reproductive behaviour.' *AIDS Care.* 1990; 2(3):247–252.

'Reproductive concerns of women at risk for HIV infection', by Ann B. Williams. Reprinted in part with kind permission from: *The Journal of Nurse-Midwifery.* 1990; 35(5):292–98.

'Reflections on the AIDS orphans problem in Uganda', by Christine Obbo. Reprinted in part with kind permission from: *The Courier* (Commission of the European Community). 1991; 126 (March/April):55–57.

The three prototype leaflets have been adapted specially for this book from Sandra Dick's paper in this chapter, and from three leaflets: *Pregnancy and AIDS* (San Francisco AIDS Foundation, 1988), *HIV, Pregnancy and Children* (Positively Women, London, 1991), and *HIV, Pregnancy and Our Children* (Voices of Positive Women, Toronto, 1991). They can be used and adapted without permission.

Chapter 7

'AIDS and sexually transmitted diseases: an important connection', by Mary T. Bassett and Marvellous Mhloyi. Excerpt reprinted with kind permission from: 'Women and AIDS in Zimbabwe: the making of an epidemic', *International Journal of Health Services.* 1991; 21(1):143–56. © 1991 Baywood Publishing Company, Inc.

Chapter 8

'Activity: using sexual language', by John Hubley. Reprinted with kind permission of the author from: *Understanding AIDS: training exercises for developing countries.* Leeds Health Education, Leeds Polytechnic, May 1988.

'Condom etiquette'. Thanks to *Girls Night Out: A Safer Sex Workshop for Women. Manual for Peer Leaders*, Chicago Women's AIDS Project, Chicago, USA, for the inspiration for many of these.

'Women talking about safer sex'. Excerpt reprinted with kind permission of Channel 4 from the pamphlet: *Women, HIV and AIDS: speaking out in the UK*. Produced for Channel 4 Television by Broadcasting Support Services to accompany the documentary of the same name, first televised November 1990.

'Over the dam', by Susie Bright. Reprinted in part with kind permission from: *On Our Backs.* July/August 1989. 6–7/36–37.

Chapter 9

'The female condom', by Barbara James and Patricia Wejr. This paper was written specially for this book. Their permission is required to reprint it.

'Workshops on counselling, quality of care, sexuality and AIDS', by Elvira Lutz. This paper amalgamates translations of two papers with the kind permission of the author: 'Informe de los talleres de orientación/consejeria, calidad de atención, sexualidad y SIDA', 1990; and 'La prevención del SIDA: Un nuevo desafío para las mujeres', paper presented at the 1st Latin American & Caribbean Symposium on Women and AIDS, 16–17 November 1990, Buenos Aires.

Chapter 10

'Don't die of ignorance – I nearly died of embarrassment: condoms in context', by Janet Holland *et al.* Reprinted in part with the kind permission of the WRAP team from the pamphlet of the same title, published by Tufnell Press, London, 1990.

'Sexual insecurity of the boys of today', by Erik Centerwall. Reprinted with kind permission of the International Planned Parenthood Federation Europe Region from: *Planned Parenthood in Europe.* 1990; 19(3):2–3.

'The position of women in our society', by Elvira Lutz. Translated and reprinted in part with kind permission of the author from: 'La condición de la mujer en nuestra sociedad'. Paper presented to the

3rd Uruguayan Conference on Sexology. Montevideo, 25–28 September 1986. In: *Talleres de Orientación/Consejeria sobre Calidad de Atención, Sexualidad y SIDA. Carpeta de Repaso*, AUPFIRH, 1990.

'Issues in women's perception of AIDS risk and risk reduction activities', by Vickie M. Mays and Susan D. Cochran. Excerpts reprinted with kind permission from: 'Issues in the perception of AIDS risk and risk reduction activities by Black and Hispanic/Latina Women'. *American Psychologist*. 1988; 43(11): 949–957. © 1988 The American Psychological Association.

'Condoms, yes, but why?', by Susan D. Cochran. Excerpt reprinted with kind permission from: 'Women and HIV infection: issues in prevention and behaviour change'. *Primary Prevention of AIDS: Psychological Approaches*. Edited by Vickie M. Mays *et al*. Primary Prevention of Psychopathology Series. © Sage Publications Inc., Newbury Park, 1989; 13:309–327.

'Black women and AIDS prevention: a view towards understanding the gender rules', by Mindy Thompson Fullilove *et al*. Reprinted in part with kind permission from: *The Journal of Sex Research*. 1990; 27(1):47–64, published by the Society for the Scientific Study of Sex, PO Box 208, Mount Vernon, IA 52314, USA.

'Sex work and personal life', by Sophie Day and Helen Ward. Excerpt reprinted with kind permission from: 'The Praed Street Project: a cohort of prostitute women in London', *AIDS, Drugs, and Prostitution*. Edited by Martin Plant. Routledge, London. 1990; 61–75.

'Empowerment through risk reduction workshops', by Brooke Grundfest Schoepf *et al*. A more extensive version of this paper is to appear in *AIDS Prevention through Health Promotion: Changing Behaviour*. World Health Organization, Geneva, in collaboration with the Royal Tropical Institute, Amsterdam, in press. Reprinted with kind permission of the World Health Organization.

'Sex work, AIDS and preventive health behaviour', by Carole A. Campbell. Reprinted in part with kind permission of Pergamon Press from: *Social Science & Medicine*, 1991; 32(12):1367–78.

Chapter 11

The prototype leaflet for women about HIV testing was adapted from: *A Brief Guide to the AIDS Antibody Test* (San Francisco AIDS Foundation, 1989), and *AIDS: Should I Have a Blood Test?* (Sussex AIDS Helpline, Brighton, undated). It can be adapted and used without permission.

'The AIDS Information Centre, Uganda', by L. M. Barugahare. Summarized with kind permission from two papers by the author: 'HIV testing as an AIDS prevention strategy in Uganda', and 'What is the AIDS Information Centre', 1991.

Chapter 12

'Personal statement by a woman living with HIV in the South Pacific'. This open letter was read by Mridula Sainath to a workshop on women & AIDS, 6th International Women & Health Meeting, 3–10 November 1990, Manila, and is reprinted here with her permission.

'Black women living with HIV and AIDS in South Africa', by Anna Strebel. From individual interviews in 1991 as part of research to develop appropriate intervention strategies to reduce risk of HIV infection for women in South Africa. Her permission is required to reprint it.

'Reaching within, reaching out', by Marie Marthe Saint Cyr-Delpe. Reprinted in part with kind permission from: *AIDS: The Women*. Edited by Ines Rieder and Patricia Ruppelt. Cleis Press, San Francisco, 1988.

'Personal experiences in the Bahamas', by Rosamae Bain. Reprinted in part with kind permission of the author from a paper presented at Women and AIDS, the 6th National Women's Conference, 30 November 1990, Bahamas.

'The women of Grupo Pela Vidda'. This conversation, recorded in Brazil in 1991, is reprinted in part with kind permission from: *Positive Women: Voices of Women Living with AIDS*. Edited by Andrea Rudd and Darien Taylor. Second Story Press, Toronto, Canada, 1992.

'Proof positive?' Anonymous. Reprinted with kind permission from: First Person, *The Guardian* 21 August 1990, 31. © 1990 The Guardian.

'Witness', by Misha. Translated and reprinted with kind permission of Association Aspasie from: *Mot de Passe*. 89:14.

'In her own words', by Jacqueline Revock. Reprinted with kind permission from: *New Jersey Women and AIDS Network News*. 1992; 2(1):3–4. 'In her own words' is a regular column in this newsletter, written by women living with HIV and caretakers of people with HIV.

Chapter 13

'The Women & AIDS Support Network, Zimbabwe', by Sunanda Ray. This paper was written specially for this book in June 1992. Her permission is required to reprint it.

'WAMATA: People striving to control the spread of AIDS, Tanzania', Theresa Kaijage talks to Sunanda Ray. This paper is based on an interview recorded in November 1991, and was written specially for this book. Their permission is required to reprint it.

'The contribution of churches and other NGOs in Tanzania to AIDS work', by Kari Hartwig. Excerpt reprinted with kind permission of the author from: 'The politics of AIDS in Tanzania: gender perceptions and the challenges for educational strategies'. MA Thesis in International Development. Clark University, Worcester MA, USA, July 1991.

'Approaches to AIDS education for the grassroots in Nigeria', by Adepeju A. Olukoya. Reprinted in part with kind permission from: *Hygie: International Journal of Health Education*. 1990; 9(4):32–33.

'AIDS and sex work: an Indian perspective', by I. S. Gilada. Reprinted in part with kind permission of the author from a paper presented at the 7th Congress of African Union against Venereal Diseases and Trepanomatosis (AUVDT), Lusaka, 17–20 March 1991, and updated July 1992.

'Outreach to bar workers in Bangkok', by Werasit Sittitrai. Reprinted in part with kind permission from: *Hygie: International Journal of Health Education*. 1990; 9:(4), 25–28.

'Positively Women, England', by Kate Thomson. Originally in: *Proceedings of the Third National Conference of the Women and HIV/AIDS Network*. Crieff, 29–30 November 1990. To appear in:

Working with Women and AIDS. Edited by Judy Bury, Val Morrison and Sheena McLachlan. Routledge, London, December 1992. © 1992 Routledge. Reprinted in part with their kind permission.

'Women as carers, Scotland', by Jane Wilson. Originally in: *Proceedings of the Second National Conference of the Women and HIV/AIDS Network*. Edinburgh, October 1989. To appear in: *Working with Women and AIDS*. Edited by Judy Bury, Val Morrison and Sheena McLachlan. Routledge, London, December 1992. © 1992 Routledge. Reprinted in part with their kind permission.

'Salud Integral para la Mujer, Mexico', by Ana María Hernández Cárdenas. Written specially for this book, March 1992. Her permission is required to reprint it.

'Project AWARE: a community study of women at high risk for AIDS', by Judith B. Cohen. Updated and reprinted in part with kind permission from a paper presented at a national meeting on women and AIDS, 1 December 1990, Amsterdam, Netherlands.

'Only your hairdresser knows: South Carolina AIDS Education Network', USA, by Ellen Spiro. Reprinted with kind permission from: *Mother Jones*. 1991; 16(1):44–45.

'AIDS Counseling and Education Organization, USA'. This paper is summarized from: Sue Rochman, 'In an unlikely place, women offer each other AIDS education and love'. *Gay Community News*, 1989; 8–14 October; and Laura Zeyer, '#1 woman and project named'. *Women's News*. 1989; 7(12): 1,4. These were sent to us by ACE in 1992.

'Housing: a critical need for people with AIDS', by Helen Schietinger. Reprinted in part with kind permission of Oxford University Press from: *Community Development Journal*. 1989; 24(3):195–201.

'Some activities in the Pacific Islands', by Karen Heckert. Information about Fiji was provided by Mridula Sainath. Written specially for this book, April 1992. These are their personal experiences and perceptions of some of the work being done in the region. Their permission is required to reprint it.

'Women Talking about AIDS Project Australia', by Di Surgey. The description of the project was written specially for this book in March and July 1992. Excerpts from the booklet reprinted with kind permission of the author from: *Women Talk . . . about AIDS, sex and sexual health* produced by the Women Talking about AIDS Project, Melbourne, Australia, 1992.

Visuals

Chapter 1

'They show all the signs of having HIV' poster, Department of Health and Human Services, Public Health Services, Centers for Disease Control, USA, reproduced with kind permission.

Chapter 2

'AIDS attacks the body, Prejudice attacks the spirit . . .' The text of this poster was in a collection of visual materials, with no indication of its source.

Chapter 3

'What you see is not what you get' poster, Ministry of Health, Kenya. Photo by Rob Cousins, reproduced with kind permission of Panos Pictures, Panos Institute, London.

'She may look clean, but . . .' World War Two poster, courtesy of the National Library of Medicine, USA, reproduced with kind permission.

'Chain of sexual transmission of HIV: an example' adapted from a similar illustration in *Speak Out/Taurai/Khulumani* No. 10, January–March 1990, Zimbabwe.

Chapter 4

Visuals depicting universal precautions, by Petra Röhr-Rouendaal, part of the wallchart for health workers 'Protect yourself and your clients', International Planned Parenthood Federation, 1989, reproduced with kind permission.

Chapter 5

'I'm on the pill. Why should I use a condom? . . .' cartoon by Petra Röhr-Rouendaal, from *Preventing a Crisis: AIDS and Family Planning Work*, International Planned Parenthood Federation, Macmillan, London, 1989, reproduced with kind permission.

Chapter 8

'And five hours later he was still going through his sexual history . . .' cartoon by Cath Jackson, for the pamphlet 'Women and AIDS' by the Terrence Higgins Trust, England, reproduced with kind permission.

'How well do you know your partner . . .' poster by the Native American Women's Health Education Resource Center, USA, reproduced with kind permission.

'They say it's safe to squeeze . . .' cartoon by Cath Jackson, for the pamphlet 'Women and AIDS' by the Terrence Higgins Trust, England, reproduced with kind permission.

'Girls have a right to say no to sex' poster of the AIDS Counselling Trust, Zimbabwe, illustration by Jane Shepherd, reproduced with kind permission.

'No condom, no sex! Play it safe' poster of the AIDS Counselling Trust, Zimbabwe, illustration by Jane Shepherd, reproduced with kind permission.

'Smart girls say no to sex before marriage' poster of the Anti-AIDS Project and the Copperbelt Health Education Project, Zambia, reproduced with kind permission.

'Chez moi: toujours avec' cartoon by Véronik from this booklet for sex workers, by the Swiss AIDS Foundation, Switzerland 1989, reproduced with kind permission.

'Safe house scheme', sticker of the Prostitutes' Collective of Victoria Inc., Australia, reproduced with kind permission.

'Keep to your regular partner' poster, Health Education Division, Ministry of Health, Ghana, reproduced with kind permission.

'Tell him if it's not on, it's not on'. This slogan is found in numerous sources with a variety of visuals. This one was in the *Pacific AIDS Alert Bulletin*, South Pacific Commission, May 1991, reproduced with kind permission as per the cover of the *Bulletin*..

'Pas un pas sans protection', part of a leaflet of the Comité National de Lutte contre le SIDA, Zaïre, we received no reply to our requests for reproduction.

'Por una sexualidad segura y responsable: usa condón', badge of the Instituto de la Mujer, Equipo de Salud Reproductiva, Santiago, Chile, reproduced with kind permission.

'The Straight Talkin' Hot 'n Healthly Menu', re-drawn version of a leaflet by Leeds AIDS Advice, England, reproduced with kind permission.

'Are you wondering how to get your boyfriend to use a rubber?' leaflet of the Women and AIDS Project – AIDS Vancouver, Canada, reproduced with kind permission.

Chapter 9

'Does your birth control protect you against AIDS?' condom instructions packet by the Women and AIDS Project – AIDS Vancouver, Canada, reproduced with kind permission.

'Get it on to get it off . . .' poster of the Women's National Abortion Action Campaign, New Zealand, from *Women's Global Network for Reproductive Rights Newsletter*, Amsterdam, April–June 1986.

'There are a lot of things worth protecting, one of them is your life' poster by HERO (Health Education Resource Organization), 101 West Read St, Baltimore MD 21201-4911, USA, 1990, reproduced with kind permission.

Cartoon figures eyeing a condom, by P. Mayle and A. Robins, from the *Family Planning Association of Western Australia Newsletter*, 1987. We were unable to contact the cartoonists for their permission and seek information on how to contact them.

Prototype condom flyer, World Health Organization, reproduced with kind permission.

'It's not the end of everything . . . condoms because you care' poster of the Caribbean Family Planning Association, Antigua, reproduced with kind permission.

'This condom fits like a glove', cartoon by David, from the *Family Planning Association of Western Australia Newsletter*, 1987. We were unable to contact the cartoonist for his permission, and seek information on how to contact him.

Condoms hanging on clothesline, by Charles Papavoine 1987/Concept, on a postcard by Art Unlimited, Amsterdam, Netherlands, reproduced with kind permission.

Condoms from the past, illustration by Marc Terstroet, from *De Groene Amsterdammer,* 1987, Netherlands, reproduced with kind permission.

Femidom press kit photographs, Chartex International, 1991, reproduced with kind permission.

Chapter 10

'Human sexual relations can best be understood . . .', cartoon by Neil Phillips, from the *Family Planning Association of Western Australia Newsletter*, 8(1), 1987. We were unable to contact the cartoonist for his permission, and seek information on how to contact him.

'If you think sex education is dangerous . . . try ignorance', mailing wrapper logo of the *Pacific AIDS Alert Bulletin*, South Pacific Commission, reproduced with kind permission as per the cover of the *Bulletin*.

Condom as butterfly net, postcard by the Swiss AIDS Foundation, Switzerland, reproduced with kind permission.

'Stop older men having sex with schoolgirls', from *Speak* No. 34, 1991. We received no reply to our requests to reproduce it.

'Lads night out' postcard cartoon by Clara Vulliamy for the Family Planning Association, UK, 1991, reproduced with kind permission.

'Not bad, but not as good as Chris' from the pamphlet 'AIDS on campus', Queensland Department of Health/Queensland AIDS Council, Australia, in *Pacific AIDS Alert Bulletin*, October–December 1991, reproduced with kind permission as per the cover of the *Bulletin*.

'We are professional about preventing AIDS. Are You?', poster of the New Zealand Prostitutes Collective, reproduced with kind permission.

Chapter 11

'Moi, je préfére savoir', poster of Médécins du Monde, photograph by the World Health Organization, in *World Health*, November-December 1990, reproduced with kind permission.

Illustration by Jonathan Muchemwa in *AIDS Counselling: A Manual for Primary Health Care*

Workers, p.18, Ministry of Health (AIDS Control Programme), Zimbabwe, 1990, reproduced with kind permission.

Groups/Organizations/Resources

Photograph of a collage of leaflets about women and HIV/AIDS, received mainly from women's groups and non-governmental organizations, and some governmental programmes, as credited, reproduced with kind permission.

References

Chapter 1 (pages 5–13)

1. Gerald Corbitt *et al., Lancet* 336 (1990):51.
2. Clue to earlier appearance of the syndrome in the USA, *New Scientist,* 12 September 1987.
3. S. S. Froland *et al.,* 'HIV-1 infection in a Norwegian family before 1970', *Lancet* (1988) p. 1344.
4. Alan F. Fleming, 'AIDS in Africa', *Ballière's Clinical Haematology* 3(1) (1990):177.
5. Helen Jackson, *AIDS Action Now: Information, Prevention and Support in Zimbabwe* (Harare: AIDS Counselling Trust, 1988), pp. 6–7.
6. Jo Calluy and Helen Jones, 'AIDS: How to answer the hard questions', *Healthright* 9(3) (1990):14.
7. Stephen J. Clark *et al.,* 'High titers of cytopathic virus in plasma of patients with symptomatic primary HIV-1 infection', *New England Journal of Medicine* 324:14 (1991):954–60.
8. Jay A. Levy, 'Changing concepts of HIV infection: challenges for the 1990s', *AIDS* 4 (1990):1051–8.
9. Deborah Anderson *et al.,* 'Prevalence and temporal variation of HIV-1 in semen', 6th International Conference on AIDS, San Francisco, 1990, Abstract No. Th.C.553.
10. Bruce D. Forrest, 'Women, HIV and mucosal immunity', *Lancet* 337 (1991):835–6.
11. Baccio Baccetti *et al.,* 'HIV particles detected in spermatozoa of patients with AIDS', 7th International Conference on AIDS, Florence, 1991, Abstract No. W.B.2010.
12. See papers and discussion by Miller and Scofield, Bagasra and Freund, Whenhao *et al.,* Dym and Orenstein, Pudney, Witkin and Bernstein, 1990. 'Part III: Mechanics of heterosexual transmission', in Nancy J. Alexander *et al., Heterosexual Transmission of AIDS* (New York: Wiley-Liss), 147–224.
13. Virginia Scofield *et al.,* 'Sperm as activating co-factors in AIDS transmission'. 7th International Conference on AIDS, Florence, 1991, Abstract No. W.C.50.
14. S. P. Donegan *et al.,* 'HIV-1 infection of the lower female genital tract', 6th International Conference on AIDS, San Francisco, 1990, Abstract No. F.C.750. This study in six women found evidence of HIV in the lining of the cervix but not of the vagina.
15. Markus W. Vogt *et al.,* 'Isolation patterns of HIV from cervical secretions during the menstrual cycle of women at risk for AIDS', *Annals of Internal Medicine.* 106 (1987):380–82.
16. Constance Wofsy *et al.,* 'Isolation of AIDS-associated retrovirus from genital secretions of women with antibodies to the virus', *Lancet* (1986):527–9.
17. Y. Henin *et al.,* 'Prevalence of HIV in the cervico-vaginal secretions of women sero-positive for HIV: correlation with the clinical status and implications for heterosexual transmission', 6th International Conference on AIDS, San Francisco, 1990, Abstract No. Th.C.554.
18. Phyllida Brown, 'How does HIV cause AIDS', *New Scientist,* 18 July 1992, 31–5.

19. Kenneth M. Mayer, 'Natural history and current therapy'. In Lawrence O. Gostin (ed.), *AIDS and the Health Care System* (New Haven: Yale University Press, 1990), 21–31.
20. Joseph K. Konde-Lule, 'The progression of HIV infection in a Uganda cohort', 6th International Conference on AIDS in Africa, Dakar, 16–19 December 1991, Abstract No. T.A.113.
21. Charles C. J. Carpenter *et al.,* 'Distinctive features of HIV infection in 200 North American women', 7th International Conference on AIDS, Florence, 1991, Abstract No. M.C.3000.
22. George F. Lemp, 'Survival trends for patients with AIDS', *Journal of American Medical Association* 263(3) (1990):402–06.
23. Pedro Chequer *et al.,* 'Survival in adult AIDS cases, Brazil 1980–1989', 6th International Conference on AIDS, San Francisco, 1990, Abstract No. Th.C.40.
24. Aggrey Anzala *et al.,* 'The rate of development of HIV-1 related illness in women with a known duration of infection', 6th International Conference on AIDS, San Francisco, 1990, Abstract No. Th.C.37.
25. Rainer Weber *et al.,* 'Progression of HIV infection in misusers of injected drugs who stop injecting or follow a programme of maintenance treatment with methadone', *British Medical Journal* 301 (1990):1362–5.
26. George W. Rutherford *et al.,* 'Course of HIV-1 infection in a cohort of homosexual and bisexual men: an 11-year follow-up study', *British Medical Journal.* 301 (1990):1183–8.
27. Rachel Royce *et al.,* 'Cigarette smoking and incidence of AIDS', 6th International Conference on AIDS, San Francisco, 1990, Abstract No. Th.C.39.
28. P. Kloser *et al.,* 'Women's clinic: A full service clinic for women with HIV disease', 7th International Conference on AIDS, Florence, 1991, Abstract No. S.D.816.

Chapter 2 (pages 14–37)

1. James Chin, 'Public health surveillance of AIDS and HIV infection', *Bulletin of WHO.* 68(5) (1990):529–36.
2. Centers for Disease Control, 1992 revised classification system for HIV infection and expanded AIDS surveillance case definition for adolescents and adults', US Department of Public Health, November 1991.
3. *Searching for Women: a literature review on women, HIV and AIDS in the United States* (Boston: College of Public and Community Service (Univ Mass) and Multicultural AIDS Coalition, 2nd edition, 1991), 15–16.
4. Naiyer Imam *et al.,* 'Hierarchical pattern of mucosal candida infections in HIV-seropositive women', *American Journal of Medicine* 89 (August 1990):142–6.
5. Risa Denenberg, 'Unique aspects of HIV infection in women: women and symptoms'. In Cynthia Chris, Monica Pearl and ACT-UP/New York Women & Book Group (eds), *Women, AIDS and Activism* (Boston: South End Press, 1990), 31–43.
6. Women from the national activist network Act-Up in the USA interrupted plenary speakers from the US Centers for Disease Control and the National Institutes of Health, who fund most AIDS research in the USA, during National Conference on Women and HIV Infection, 13–14 December 1990, Washington DC. They demanded answers about when large research studies on women were going to be done and when the CDC case definition for AIDS was to be changed to include manifestations of HIV disease in women.
7. Michael Merson, Report of the meeting on research priorities relating to women and HIV/AIDS, Geneva, World Health Organization Global Programme on AIDS, 19–20 November 1990, 3.
8. David. From a presentation at HIV regional forum in Central New York, *Women and AIDS Project Newsletter,* Winter 1991:2.
9. David Miller, *Living with AIDS and HIV* (London: Macmillan, 1987).
10. Graeme Moyle, 'A guide to the medical treatment of HIV related diseases', *AVERT,* Horsham, UK (January 1992):7.
11. Helen Jackson, *AIDS action now: information, prevention and support in Zimbabwe* (Harare: AIDS Counselling Trust, 1988), 25.
12. Sam Kalibala, 'Skin conditions common to people with HIV infection or AIDS' and 'The WHO Report: What does adult AIDS look like?', *AIDS Action* 10 (1990):2–3.
13. Patricia Warne *et al.,* 'Menstrual abnormalities

in HIV+ and HIV− women with a history of intravenous drug use', 7th International Conference on AIDS, Florence, 1991, Abstract No. M.C.3113.

14. Olaf Muller *et al.,* 'The presentation of adult HIV-1 disease in Kampala hospitals', *AIDS* 4(6) (1990):601–02.

15. Susan Allen *et al.,* 'HIV and malaria in a representative sample of childbearing women in Kigali, Rwanda', *Journal of Infectious Diseases* 164 (July 1991):67–71.

16. Robert W. Ryder *et al.,* 'Fertility rates in 238 HIV-1 seropositive women in Zaïre followed for three years postpartum', *AIDS* 5(12) (1991):1521–7.

17. U. Familiari *et al.,* 'Premenopausal cytomegalovirus oophritis in a patient with AIDS', *AIDS* 5(4) (1991):458–9.

18. See papers and discussion by Miller and Scofield, Bagasra and Freund, Whenhao *et al.,* Dym and Orenstein, Pudney, Witkin and Bernstein, 'Part III: Mechanics of heterosexual transmission', in Nancy J. Alexander *et al.,* (eds), *Heterosexual Transmission of AIDS* (New York: Wiley-Liss, 1990), 147–224.

19. J. R. Smith *et al.,* 'Infertility management in HIV-positive couples: a dilemma', *British Medical Journal* 302 (15 June 1991):1447–50.

20. Sebastian Lucas, personal communication, February 1992.

21. A. Terragna *et al.,* 'Influence of pregnancy on disease progression in 31 HIV-infected patients', International Conference on the Implications of AIDS for Mothers and Children, Paris, November 1989, Abstract No. E2. Summarized in Lindgren [23] below.

22. Jacqueline Mok, 'Children and HIV infection', paper presented to Third National Conference of the Women & HIV/AIDS Network, Crieff, Scotland, 29–30 November 1990.

23. Susanne Lindgren *et al.,* 'HIV and child-bearing clinical outcome and aspects of mother-to-infant transmission', *AIDS* 5(9) (1991):1111–16.

24. Edison Morozi *et al.,* 'Five-year follow-up of HIV-infected mothers and their children', 7th International Conference on AIDS, Florence, 1991, Abstract No. W.B.2011.

25. Alan F. Fleming, 'AIDS in Africa', *Ballière's Clinical Haematology* 3(1) (1990):187.

26. Janet Mitchell, paper to the National Conference on Women and HIV Infection, Washington, DC, 13–14 December 1990.

27. S. K. Hira *et al.,* 'Perinatal transmission of HIV-1 in Zambia', *British Medical Journal* 299 (1989):1250–52.

28. J. F. Delfraissy *et al.,* 'Does pregnancy influence disease progression in HIV-positive women', International Conference on the Implications of AIDS for Mothers and Children, Paris, November 1989, Abstract No. E7. Summarized in Lindgren [23].

29. G. B. Scott *et al.,* 'Mothers of infants with AIDS: evidence for both symptomatic and asymptomatic carriers', *Journal of American Medical Association* 253 (1985):363–6.

30. Paolo Miotti *et al.,* 'Infant and childhood mortality in children of HIV-infected mothers in Malawi', 6th International Conference on AIDS, San Francisco, 1990, Abstract No. F.C.101.

31. M. Temmerman *et al.,* 'Infection with HIV as a risk factor for adverse obstetrical outcome', *AIDS* 4 (1990):1087–93.

32. Judith Wasserheit and Ruth Dixon-Mueller, *The Culture of Silence: Reproductive Tract Infections among Women in the Third World* (New York, International Women's Health Coalition, 1991).

33. Rani Bang *et al.,* 'High prevalence of gynaecological diseases in rural Indian women', *Lancet* 335 (14 January 1989):85–8. Re the men: Rani Bang, personal communication, July 1991.

34. Judith Wasserheit, 'Epidemiological synergy: inter-relationships between HIV infection and other STDs'. Unpublished paper, 1990.

35. Mary Beth Caschetta, 'Clinical manifestations of HIV in women', *AIDS Treatment News* 5(1) (1991):3–5.

36. Charles C. J. Carpenter *et al.,* 'HIV infection in North American women: experience with 200 cases and a review of the literature', *Medicine* 70(5) (1991):307–25. See also Bente Hoegsberg *et al.,* 'Sexually transmitted diseases and HIV infection among women with pelvic inflammatory disease', *American Journal of Obstetrics and Gynecology* 163(4) (1992): 1135–9, which found an insignificant trend towards more surgery in HIV-positive women with PID than HIV-negative women.

37. Ahmed S. Latif *et al.,* 'Genital ulcers and transmission of HIV among couples in Zimbabwe', *AIDS* 3(8) (1989):519–23.

38. New Jersey Women and AIDS Network, *Me First! Medical Manifestations of HIV in Women* (New Brunswick, 1990).

39. S. Foster *et al.*, 'Impact of the HIV Epidemic on Essential Drugs and Supplies: Visit to the Republic of Zambia'. World Health Organization, Geneva, 14–25 November 1988. Unpublished.

40. Ahmed S. Latif *et al.*, 'Factors associated with progression of HIV-1 infection', 6th International Conference on AIDS in Africa, Dakar, 16–19 December 1991, Abstract No. T.O.130.

41. Judith Wasserheit, 'Reproductive tract infections'. *Special challenges in Third World Women's Health* (New York: International Women's Health Coalition, March 1990).

42. Joel M. Palefsky *et al.*, 'Anal intraepithelial neoplasia and anal papilloma virus infection among homosexual males with group IV HIV disease', *Journal of American Medical Association* 263(21) (1990):2911–16.

43. Anthony R. Dixon *et al.*, letter to *Lancet* 25 November 1989: 1285.

44. See, for example, Micheline A. Byrne *et al.*, 'The common occurrence of HPV infection and intraepithelial neoplasia in women infected by HIV', *AIDS* 3 (1989):379–82.

45. *International Family Planning Perspectives* 14(2) (1988):43. Full report in *Bulletin of WHO* 64 (1986), 607.

46. Ralph M. Richart, 'Cervical cancer in developing countries.' *Special Challenges in Third World Women's Health* (New York: International Women's Health Coalition, 1990).

47. Ann Williams *et al.*, 'Association of HIV-1, cervical/anal cytological abnormalities and HPV in female injection drug users in San Francisco', 7th International Conference on AIDS, Florence, 1991, Abstract No. M.C.3116.

48. Howard L. Minkoff and Jack A. DeHovitz, 'Care of women infected with HIV', *Journal of American Medical Association* 266(16) (1991):2253–8. The study of 114 women quoted was from Michael Maiman, oral communication to the authors, April 1991.

49. A. M. Nelson *et al.*, 'Increased rates of cervical dysplasia associated with clinical and immunological evidence of immuno-deficiency', 6th International Conference on AIDS in Africa, Dakar, 16–19 December 1991, Abstract No. W.A.209.

50. IARC Working Group on Evaluation of Cervical Screening Programmes, 'Screening for squamous cervical cancer: duration of low risk after negative results of cervical cancer: cytology and its implications for screening policies', *British Medical Journal* 293 (13 September 1986):659–64.

51. Editorial, 'Oral candidosis in HIV infection', *Lancet,* 23/30 December 1989: 1491–2.

52. Melanie Thompson *et al.*, 'Gender differences in the spectrum of HIV diseases in Atlanta', 7th International Conference on AIDS, Florence, 1991, Abstract No. M.C.3115.

53. Charles F. Gilks *et al.*, 'Life-threatening bacteraemia in HIV-1 seropositive adults admitted to hospital in Nairobi', *Lancet* 336 (1990):545–9. Also Anthony J. Pinching and C. U. Perera *et al.*, letters to *Lancet* 336 (1990):877.

54. Sunanda Ray, personal communication, February 1992.

55. See paper by Darien Taylor, 'Testing positive in Canada', in *Women and AIDS: A Resource Guide* (Vancouver Women & AIDS Network and International Development Resources Association, 1990). Also reported at a workshop of the London Women & HIV/AIDS Network on medical manifestations of HIV/AIDS in women, 29 May 1991.

56. Christopher J. L. Murray, letter to *Lancet* 335 (1990):1043–4.

57. Richard H. Morrow *et al.*, 'Interactions of HIV infection with endemic tropical diseases', *AIDS* 3 (Supplement 1) (1989):S79–S87.

58. Susan E. Jones, letter to *British Medical Journal* 301 (1990):608.

59. Alison M. Elliott *et al.*, 'Impact of HIV on TB in Zambia', *British Medical Journal* 301 (1990):412–15.

60. Richard W. Goodgame, 'AIDS in Uganda: Clinical and social features', *New England Journal of Medicine* 323(6) (1990):383–8.

61. Stephen Norman *et al.*, 'HIV infection in women', *British Medical Journal* 301 (1990):1231–2.

62. John M. Watson and O. Noel Gill, 'HIV infection and tuberculosis', *British Medical Journal* 300 (1990):63–4.

63. Giovanni Di Perri *et al.*, 'Nosocomial epidemic

of active TB among HIV-infected patients', *Lancet,* 23/30 December 1989: 1503.

64. Michael Tan, personal communication, February 1992.

65. Goesch *et al.,* letter to *Lancet,* 23/30 December 1990, 1503.

66. Sebastian Lucas, 'The clinical face of HIV disease', *AIDS Watch* 12 (1990):5.

67. Sarah Gill, 'Treatments: progress with opportunistic infections', *AIDS Watch* 12 (1990):4–5.

68. Editorial, 'Pneumocystis carinii pneumonia', *British Medical Journal* 300 (1990):211–12.

69. G. N. Fuller *et al.,* letter to *Lancet* 335 (1990):48–9.

70. *AIDS-related Dementia* (Horsham: AVERT, 1989).

71. Henry Purcell, 'Heart disease in AIDS patients', *British Journal of Sexual Medicine,* April 1990: 111–13.

72. S. D. Desmond-Hellman *et al.,* 'The epidemiology and clinical features of KS in African women with HIV infection', 6th International Conference on AIDS, San Francisco, 1990, Abstract No. S.B.508.

73. Valerie Beral *et al.,* 'Kaposi's sarcoma among persons with AIDS: a sexually transmitted infection?', *Lancet* 335 (1990):123–8. See also letters to *Lancet* responding to this suggestion by Couterier *et al.,* 335 (1990):1105; Stein-Werblowsky and Ablin, 336 (1990):627; France, 336 (1990):1329; and Bary *et al.,* 337 (1991):234.

74. Kaiss Lassoued *et al.,* 'AIDS-associated Karposi's sarcoma in female patients', *AIDS* 5(7) (1991):877–80.

75. A. D. A. Dalton *et al.,* 'Synovium in AIDS: a postmortem study', *British Medical Journal* 300 (1990):1239–40.

76. P. D. Kell *et al.,* 'The clinical presentation of women with HIV infection', *British Journal of Obstetrics & Gynaecology* 98 (1991):103–04.

77. Women and AIDS Support Network, personal communication from Sunanda Ray, Chair, February 1992.

78. Claudia Garcia Moreno, 'AIDS: Women are not just transmitters'. Unpublished paper, 5 July 1990.

79. Mardge Cohen, 'A service delivery model', paper presented to National Conference on Women and HIV Infection, Washington, DC, 13–14 December 1990.

80. Janie Hampton, *Meeting AIDS with compassion: AIDS care and prevention in Agomanya, Ghana* (London: ActionAid, AMREF and World in Need, Strategies for Hope Series No. 4, 1991).

81. Noerine Kaleeba with Sunanda Ray and Brigid Willmore, *We miss you all; Noerine Kaleeba: AIDS in the family* (Harare: Women and AIDS Support Network, 1991).

82. Carola Burroughs, 'Holistic treatment for HIV/AIDS: an overview'. From a paper written specially for this book, December 1991.

83. Michel Nyst *et al.,* 'Prospective comparative study of gentian violet, ketoconazole and nystatin to treat oral and oesophageal candidiasis in AIDS patients', 6th International Conference on AIDS, San Francisco, 1990, Abstract No. Th.B.465.

84. Sunanda Ray, personal communication, 7 March 1991. She recommends these for HIV-positive patients in Harare.

85. 'Nutritional guidelines for people with HIV', *AIDS Letter* 17 (February/March 1990):6–7. Source: *Focus,* January 1990.

86. Hazel Ross, *Taking control of your diet if you are HIV-positive* (Horsham: AVERT, April 1992).

87. *Memorandum: In vitro screening of traditional medicines for anti-HIV activity, based on an informal WHO consultation on traditional medicines and AIDS,* Doc. No. WHO/GPA/BMP/89.5, in *Bulletin of WHO* 67(6) (1989):613–18. Quoted in Burroughs [82].

88. Results of this study and two others in the Ivory Coast and Belgium were presented at the Advanced Immune Discoveries Symposium, San Francisco, 1990. They were conducted by Bernard Marichal and Maurice Janaer, principal investigators for Immujem/In'pact, Belgium. Quoted in Burroughs [82].

89. See also S. Dharmananda, Chinese herbal therapies for the treatment of immune deficiency syndromes', *Oriental Healing Arts International Bulletin* 12(1) (1987):24–38; and Nancy Rabinowitz, 'Acupuncture and the AIDS epidemic: Reflections on the treatment of 200 patients in four years', *American Journal of Acupuncture* 15(1) (1987). Quoted in Burroughs [82].

90. Nordic Medical Research Councils' HIV

Therapy Group, 'Double blind dose-response study of zidovudine in AIDS and advanced HIV infection', *British Medical Journal* 304 (1992):13–17.

91. Information for this section came from Gerald H. Friedland, 'Early treatment for HIV: the time has come', *New England Journal of Medicine* 322(14) (1990):1000–02; and Ann Marie Swart *et al.*, 'Early HIV infection: to treat or not to treat', *British Medical Journal* 301 (1990):825–6.

92. John D. Hamilton *et al.*, 'A controlled trial of early vs late treatment with zidovudine in symptomatic HIV infection', *New England Journal of Medicine* 326(7) (1991):437–43.

93. Neil M. H. Graham *et al.*, 'Effect of zidovudine and PCP prophylaxis on progression of HIV-1 infection to AIDS', *Lancet* 338(8762) (1991):265–9.

94. Richard D. Moore *et al.*, 'Zidovudine and the natural history of AIDS', *New England Journal of Medicine* 324(20) (1991):1412–16.

95. Charles C. J. Carpenter, personal communication, March 1992.

96. Carlo Carcassi *et al.*, 'A study of 9 infants born from HIV-1 positive mothers who continued treatment with AZT during pregnancy', 1991, and Antonio Ferrezin *et al.*, 'Zidovudine therapy of HIV infection during pregnancy: assessment of the effect on the newborns.' 7th International Conference on AIDS, Florence, 1991, Abstract Nos W.C.3228 and M.C.3023.

97. Reported in a plenary discussion at National Conference on Women and HIV Infection, Washington, DC, 13–14 December 1990.

Chapter 3 (pages 38–57)

1. Jonathan Mann, 'How AIDS has changed epidemiology', *New Scientist,* 9 February 1991, 1755:16.

2. F. I. D. Konotey-Ahulu, 'Clinical epidemiology, not seroepidemiology, is the answer to Africa's AIDS problem', *British Medical Journal* 294 (1987):1593–4.

3. Vickie Alexander, 'Women and AIDS: Overlooked and undercounted'. Unpublished paper, 1990.

4. Susan Y. Chu *et al.*, 'Impact of the HIV epidemic on mortality in women of reproductive age, United States', *Journal of American Medical Association* 264 (1990):225–6.

5. Owais Tohid, 'Life with AIDS', *Newsline,* January 1992: 218–24.

6. Julia Hausermann, 'Effects of AIDS on the advancement of women', *Report to the Commission on the Status of Women,* UN Economic and Social Council, 33rd session, 29 March–7 April 1989, Vienna, 5.

7. 'DOH to test more males for AIDS', *Health Alert* 103 (1990):116.

8. Michael Tan, personal communication, February 1992.

9. J. Bugnicourt, 'Femmes et enfants d'Afrique frappés de plein fouet par le SIDA'. Unpublished paper for ENDA (Environment and Development in the Third World), Dakar, 1989.

10. *Searching for Women: a literature review on women, HIV and AIDS in the US* (Boston: College of Public and Community Service (Univ Mass) and the Multicultural AIDS Coalition, second edition 1991), 14.

11. Rachel Anderson, 'Differences in stated behaviour of female and male IVDUs', 6th International Conference on AIDS, San Francisco, 1990, Abstract No. 3001.

12. Alan F. Fleming, 'AIDS in Africa', *Ballière's Clinical Haematology* 3(1) (1990):177–205.

13. Marcia Quackenbush and Sylvia Villareal, *'Does AIDS hurt?': Educating young children about AIDS* (Santa Cruz: Network Publications, 1988).

14. Ann Marie Kimball *et al.*, 'AIDS among women in Latin America and the Caribbean', *Bulletin of Pan American Health Organization* 25(4) (1991):367–73.

15. Act-Up London, *Women, HIV and AIDS: Speaking Out in the UK* (London: Broadcasting Support Services for Channel 4 TV, 1990).

16. Warren Johnson, quoted in Chris Norwood, *Advice for Life: A Woman's Guide to AIDS Risks and Prevention* (New York: Pantheon, 1987), 145.

17. Oakland Ross, 'Fatal disease moving quickly to Haiti's female population', *Globe & Mail,* 25 May 1987.

18. *Women & AIDS Project Newsletter,* Winter 1991: 16–17. Full report: 'Epidemiology of reported cases of AIDS in lesbians: US 1980–89', *American Journal of Public Health* 80(11) (1990):1380–81.

19. Nancy J. Schmidt, 'African press reports on the social impact of AIDS on women and children

in sub-Saharan Africa', paper presented to Symposium: Impact of AIDS on maternal-child health care delivery in Africa', University of Illinois, 4-6 May 1990, 6.

20. Judith Mariasy and Marty Radlett, 'Women: the vulnerable sex', *AIDS Watch* 10 (1990), 2-3.

21. See posters in *New Scientist*, 21/28 December 1991, 56.

22. James Chin, 'Current and future dimensions of the HIV/AIDS pandemic in women and children', *Lancet* 336 (1990), 221-4.

23. World Health Organization press release, 'AIDS, over a million new infections in 8 months', Geneva, 12 February 1992.

24. Figures from Chin [22], except for New York City, which is from '80,000 women have AIDS virus, study finds', *New York Times*, 4 March 1991.

25. World Health Organization Global Programme on AIDS, 'Current and future dimensions of the HIV/AIDS pandemic: A capsule summary', September 1990, No. WHO/GPA/SFI/90.2 Rev. 1

26. H. Brenner *et al.*, 'AIDS among drug abusers in Europe: review of recent developments'. WHO Global Programme on AIDS, Regional Office for Europe, Copenhagen, 3.

27. David Miller, *Living with AIDS and HIV* (London: Macmillan, 1987).

28. AIDS Control Programme, Ministry of Health, Uganda, *AIDS Surveillance Report* (third quarter 1989). From Noerine Kaleeba, keynote address presented to Women & AIDS Support Network Conference, 23 November 1989, Harare, in *AIDS: An Issue for Every Woman* (Harare: Women & AIDS Support Network, 1990).

29. Seth Berkley *et al.*, 'AIDS and HIV infection in Uganda: are more women infected than men?', *AIDS* 4(12) (1990):1237-42.

30. Jai Narain, 'Epidemiology: Caribbean', *AIDS Action*, 10 (1990):7.

31. Mavis Johnson, introductory remarks for the National Women's Advisory Council, Women and AIDS: Sixth National Women's Conference, Bahamas, November 1990.

32. Lair Rodiques *et al.*, 'The AIDS epidemic in Brazil 1980-1989', 6th International Conference on AIDS, San Francisco, 1990, Abstract No. F.C.98.

33. Diana G. Smith, 'Thailand: AIDS crisis looms', *Lancet* 335 (1990):781-2.

34. J. A. Wortman *et al.*, 'The AIDS pattern among Canadian aboriginals', 6th International Conference on AIDS, San Francisco, 1990, Abstract No. Th.C.709.

35. Jackie Wilson, 'AIDS, Black women and the Black community in Toronto', in Jacquie Manthorne (ed.), *Canadian Women and AIDS: Beyond the Statistics* (Montreal: Éditions Communiqu'Elles, 1990).

36. Lyle Petersen *et al.*, 'Sentinel surveillance for HIV infection in primary care outpatients in the United States', 6th International Conference on AIDS, San Francisco, 1990, Abstract No. Th.C.754.

37. Vickie Alexander, 'Black women and AIDS', *Siecus Report* (1990), 3.

38. R. Ancelle, 'Female AIDS cases in Europe', WHO Collaborating Centre on AIDS, Paris, for WHO Global Programme on AIDS, Europe Region, press packet for World AIDS Day, 1 December, 1990.

39. Sunanda Ray, 'An overview of the epidemiology of HIV infection in women in Africa' and Noerine Kaleeba, keynote address, papers presented to Women and AIDS Support Network Conference, 23-24 November 1989, Harare, in *AIDS: An Issue for Every Woman* (Harare: Women & Aids Support Network, 1990). And 1992 figures from National AIDS Control Programme, Zimbabwe, for first quarter of 1992, reported in *Herald*, 13 May 1992.

40. Mary T. Bassett and Marvellous Mhloyi, 'Women and AIDS in Zimbabwe: the making of an epidemic', *International Journal of Health Services* 21(1) (1991):143-56.

41. James Chin, personal communication, May 1992.

42. Nicola Low *et al.*, 'AIDS and migrant populations in Nicaragua', *Lancet* 336 (1990):1593-4.

43. Ann Larson, 'The social epidemiology of Africa's AIDS epidemic', *African Affairs* 89(35) (1990):5-25.

44. Catherine Hankins, 'An overview of women and AIDS in Canada', in Jacquie Manthorne (ed.), *Canadian Women and AIDS: Beyond the Statistics* (Montreal: Éditions Communiqu'Elles, 1990).

45. Enrique Bravo *et al.,* 'Distribution and trends of AIDS cases by socio-economic strata in Mexico', 6th International Conference on AIDS, San Francisco, 1990, Abstract No. Th.C.715.

46. Mauro Schechter, 'Brazil: activists take on AIDS', *Women's Health Journal* 17 (1990):56.

47. Debrework Zewdie *et al.,* 'Seroprevalence of HIV and syphilis infections among childbearing age women of central Ethiopia', 6th International Conference on AIDS, San Francisco, 1990, Abstract No. F.C.600.

48. World Health Organization, 'The Global AIDS Situation', *In Point of Fact* 68 (June 1990):1.

49. James Chin, 'Present and future dimensions of the HIV/AIDS pandemic', lecture presented to 7th International Conference on Aids, Florence, 1991. In *Science Challenging AIDS* (Basel: Karger, 1992), 33–50.

50. Simon Chapman, 'Dogma disputed: potential endemic heterosexual transmission of HIV in Australia', *Australian Journal of Public Health* 16(2) (1992):128–41. See also commentaries that follow by Alex Wodak and Peter Karmel, which dispute his position, 141–4.

Chapter 4 (58–70)

1. Alan F. Fleming, 'AIDS in Africa', *Ballière's Clinical Haematology* 3(1) (1990):177–205.

2. Herbert Daniel, 'Brazil: breaking the blood mafia', *AIDS Action* 14 (1991):4.

3. Walter Almeida, 'The face of AIDS in Brazil', *AIDS Action* 4 (1988):4.

4. 'Latest health news from Brazil', *Living Conditions* 3 (Masta Ltd, London), 4 June 1991. Data approved by London School of Hygiene and Tropical Medicine.

5. Barbara Goldoftas, 'Hazards of taking blood from private blood banks', *Manila Times,* 29 January 1992.

6. Alan F. Fleming, 'Prevention of transmission of HIV by blood transfusion in developing countries', paper presented to Global Impact of AIDS Conference, London, 10 March 1988.

7. E. J. Watson-Williams *et al.,* 'Selection of low-risk HIV-1 negative blood donors in Uganda: an economic necessity', 3rd Conference on AIDS and Associated Cancers in Africa, 1989. Abstract, quoted in Strang and Farrell [33].

8. Francisco Galvan Díaz and Rodolfo N. Morales, 'Epidemiology: HIV/AIDS in Mexico', *AIDS Action* 10 (1990):6.

9. A. J. Sepulveda, 'Prevention of HIV transmission through blood and blood products: experience in Mexico', *Bulletin of Pan American Health Organization* 23 (1989):1–2. Summary in Strang and Farrell [33].

10. Kenneth B. Noble, 'Nigeria is spared the worst of AIDS, but experts wonder for how long', *New York Times,* 18 November 1990, 10L.

11. Nancy Romero Berrios, personal communication, March 1991.

12. Personal communication from African and Asian activists.

13. Khorshed M. Pavri, 'Safety of blood supply', *CARC Calling: Bulletin of Centre for AIDS Research and Control, New Delhi* 3(4) (1990):26.

14. Georg Gossius, 'HIV/AIDS in Children in Institutions in Romania: Report from Cariova/Dolj'. Unpublished paper, 19–27 December 1990.

15. Marge Berer, 'Blood transfusion, AIDS and maternal deaths', *Maternal Mortality: A Call to Women for Action* (Amsterdam: WGNRR and ISIS, 1988), 34–5.

16. Judith Mariasy and Marty Radlett, 'Women: the vulnerable sex', *AIDS Watch* 10 (1990):2–3.

17. Fernando Samuel Sion *et al.,* 'Risk factors for HIV-2 infection in Guinea Bissau', 6th International Conference on AIDS, San Francisco, 1990, Abstract No. Th.C.565.

18. Susan Allen *et al.,* 'HIV and malaria in a representative sample of childbearing women in Kigali, Rwanda', *Journal of Infectious Diseases* 164 (July 1991):67–71.

19. Ann Marie Kimball *et al.,* 'AIDS among women in Latin America and the Caribbean', *PAHO Bulletin* 25(4) (1991):367–73.

20. Chris Norwood, *Advice for Life: A Woman's Guide to AIDS Risks and Prevention* (New York: Pantheon, 1987).

21. Helmut Jager *et al.,* 'Prevention of transfusion-associated HIV transmission in Kinshasa: HIV screening is not enough', *AIDS* 4 (1991):571–4.

22. National Blood Transfusion Service, Harare, Zimbabwe, annual report for year ending June 1991.

23. Alan F. Fleming, 'Antimalarial prophylaxis in pregnant Nigerian women', letter to *Lancet* 335 (1990):45.

24. W. N. Gibbs, 'Appropriate use of blood and blood products', *Essential Drugs Monitor* 9 (1990):18. More detailed information is contained in WHO documents 'Use of plasma substitutes and plasma in developing countries', WHO/LAB/89.9, and 'Guidelines for the appropriate use of blood', WHO/LAB/89.10, available from: Health Laboratory Technology and Blood Safety Unit, WHO, 1211 Geneva 27, Switzerland.

25. Anneke van den Hoek, 'Epidemiology of HIV infection among drug users in Amsterdam', *Rodopi,* Amsterdam (1990).

26. Nicholas Ford and Suporn Koetsawang, 'The socio-cultural context of the transmission of HIV in Thailand', *Social Science and Medicine* 33(4) (1991):405–14.

27. Edna Roland, contribution in a discussion on women and HIV/AIDS. Meeting of grantees of the MacArthur Foundation, Teresopolis, Brazil, 1–3 July 1991.

28. Vickie M. Mays and Susan D. Cochran, 'Issues in the perception of AIDS risk and risk reduction activities by black and Hispanic/Latina women', *American Psychologist* 43(11) (1991):949–57.

29. Charles P. Wallace, 'The AIDS fuse is ignited in Asia', *Los Angeles Times,* 7 January 1992.

30. Aart Hendriks, 'AIDS and mobility', WHO Global Programme on AIDS, Europe Region, Copenhagen, April 1991.

31. Working group, 'Strategy for HIV/AIDS prevention and control in drug users', WHO Regional Office for Europe Global Programme on AIDS' 1991, EUR/ICP/GPA 076(A), 9054s.

32. Don Nutbeam *et al.,* 'The prevention of HIV infection from injecting drug use: a review of health promotion approaches', *Social Science and Medicine* 33(9) (1991):977–83.

33. J. Strang and M. Farrell, 'Harm minimisation for drug misusers: when second best may be best first', *British Medical Journal* 304(6835) (1992):1127–8.

34. Mary Hepburn, paper presented to workshop Women, HIV/AIDS and Medical Issues, London, 29 May 1991.

35. H. Brenner *et al.,* 'AIDS among drug abusers in Europe: review of recent developments'. WHO Global Programme on AIDS, Regional Office for Europe, Copenhagen, 1991.

36. Duncan Campbell, 'Syringe vending machine ready', *Guardian,* 14 January 1991.

37. Hilary Kinnell, 'Effects of needle and syringe provision on the injecting behaviour of drug users in Birmingham, England', paper presented to 1st International Conference on the Reduction of Drug-Related Harm, Liverpool, 9 April 1990.

38. Alexandre Gromyko, 'The case of Elista', *Entre Nous* 14/15 June 1990: 10.

39. Susan Foster and Sue Lucas, 'Socio-economic aspects of HIV and AIDS in developing countries', London School of Hygiene and Tropical Medicine, PHP Departmental Publication No. 3, 1991, 18.

40. Anne Vibeke Reeler, 'Injections: A fatal attraction?', *Social Science and Medicine* 31(10) (1990):1119–25.

41. Hans Veeken *et al.,* 'Occupational HIV infection and health care workers in the tropics', *Tropical Doctor,* January 1991: 28–31.

42. Felicity Barringer, 'Doctor's AIDS death renews debate on who should know', *New York Times,* 8 December 1990, 1/11. Also Lawrence K. Altman, 'Tests set for patients of surgeon who had AIDS', *New York Times,* 15 December 1990, 10; and 'HIV and the dentist', *AIDS Letter* 26, August–September 1991.

43. Inter-African Committee, Report on a Consultative Expert Group Meeting on the Possible Link between Traditional Practices and the Transmission of the AIDS Virus, 9–11 May 1989, Addis Ababa.

44. Hailu Kefenie, 'Traditional practices and their possible link to the spread of AIDS: A survey as first part of an in-depth study in Ethiopia', Report of Regional Conference on Traditional Practices Affecting the Health of Women and Children in Africa, Addis Ababa, 19–24 November 1990, Inter-African Committee, 75–86.

45. Fadel Kane *et al.,* 'Penetration of HIV-1 in a rural area of Senegal', 6th International Conference on AIDS, San Francisco, 1990, Abstract No. F.C.603.

46. Elisabete Inglesi *et al.,* 'Working together with Afro-Brazilian religious leaders in AIDS prevention and control in São Paulo', 6th International Conference on AIDS, San Francisco, 1990, Abstract No. 4067.

47. Kendra Sundquist, 'Healthworkers and AIDS', *Healthright* 9(2) (1990):10–12.
48. Patrick Francioli *et al.,* 'Exposure of health care workers to blood during various procedures: Results of two surveys before and after the implementation of universal precautions', 6th International Conference on AIDS, San Francisco, 1990, Abstract No. Th.C.602.
49. 'Safe injections with versatile portable sterilizer', *Essential Drugs Monitor* 9 (1990):18. The equipment is available from UNICEF or the manufacturer Prestige Medical.
50. M. F. Fathalla, personal communication, 30 August 1991.
51. Chris Foy *et al.,* 'HIV and measures to control infection in general practice', *British Medical Journal* 300 (1990):1048–9.
52. Adelisa Panlilio *et al.,* 'Blood and amniotic fluid contact during obstetrical procedures', 6th International Conference on AIDS, San Francisco, 1990, Abstract No. Th.C.603.
53. Sr Maura O'Donohue, *AIDS Action* 5 (1989):8 in *WGNRR Newsletter* 31 (1989):41.
54. F. Staugaard, 'Role of traditional health workers in prevention and control of AIDS in Africa', *Tropical Doctor* 21 (1991):22–4.
55. *HIV and Overseas Employment: A Guide for Employers* (London: UK NGO AIDS Consortium for the Third World, update, January 1990).

Chapter 5 (pages 71–88)

1. G. J. Stewart *et al.,* 'Transmission of HTLV-III by artificial insemination by donor', *Lancet,* 14 September 1985: 581.
2. Ann Marie Kimball *et al.,* 'AIDS among women in Latin America and the Caribbean', *PAHO Bulletin* 25(4) (1991):367–73.
3. Jacqueline Mok, 'HIV infection in children', *British Medical Journal* 302 (1991):921–2.
4. Gwendolyn B. Scott *et al.,* 'Survival in children with perinatally acquired HIV-1 infection', *New England Journal of Medicine* 321(26) (1989):1791–6.
5. European Collaborative Study, 'Children born to women with HIV-1 infection: natural history and risk of transmission', *Lancet* 337 (1991):253–60.
6. Alan F. Fleming, 'AIDS in Africa', *Ballière's Clinical Haematology* 3(1) (1990):187.

7. WHO Report, 'Paediatric HIV infection/AIDS', *AIDS Action* 9 (1989):2–3.
8. Valerie Beral *et al.,* 'Kaposi's sarcoma among persons with AIDS: a sexually transmitted infection?', *Lancet* 335 (1990):123–8.
9. Helen Jackson, *AIDS Action Now: information, prevention and support in Zimbabwe* (Harare: AIDS Counselling Trust, 1988), 31–2.
10. S. K. Hira *et al.,* 'Perinatal transmission of HIV-1 in Zambia', *British Medical Journal* 299 (1989):1250–52.
11. Edison Morozi *et al.,* 'Five-year follow-up of HIV-infected mothers and their children', 7th International Conference on AIDS, Florence, 1991, Abstract No. W.B.2011.
12. Italian Multicentre Study, 'Epidemiology, clinical features, and prognostic factors of pediatric HIV infection', *Lancet,* 5 November 1988: 1043–6.
13. Susanne Lindgren *et al.,* 'HIV and child-bearing: clinical outcome and aspects of mother-to-infant transmission', *AIDS* 5(9) (1991):1111–16.
14. R. A. Hague *et al.,* 'Do maternal factors influence the risk of vertical transmission of HIV?', 7th International Conference on AIDS, Florence, 1991, Abstract No. W.C.3237.
15. R. Pradinaud *et al.,* 'HIV infection in mother and child in French Guiana: Epidemiological case work on 44 mothers giving birth to 55 children', *Médécine Tropicale* 49(1) (1989):51–7. From 1990 abstract in *Current AIDS Literature* 3(2):40.
16. Virginia Ladeda *et al.,* 'Vertical transmission of HIV in Buenos Aires: Serologic followup in children born from seropositive mothers', 7th International Conference on AIDS, Florence, 1991, Abstract No. M.C.3075.
17. Alan F. Fleming, 'Counselling HIV-positive women about pregnancy'. Unpublished paper, February 1992.
18. Ruy Soeiro *et al.,* 'The incidence of human fetal HIV-1 infection as determined by the presence of HIV-1 DNA in abortus tissues', 7th International Conference on AIDS, Florence, 1991, Abstract No. W.C.3250.
19. A. Ehrnst *et al.,* 'HIV in pregnant women and their offspring: evidence for late transmission', *Lancet* 338 (1991):203–07.
20. James J. Goedert *et al.,* 'High risk of HIV-1

infection for first-born twins', *Lancet* 338 (14 December 1991):1471–5. Data presented at 8th International Conference on AIDS, Amsterdam, 1992, from this group on additional sets of twins continues to show this trend.

21. European Collaborative Study, 'Risk factors for mother-to-child transmission of HIV-1', *Lancet* 339 (25 April 1992):1007–12.

22. *AIDS and artificial insemination: Guidance for doctors and AI clinics,* CMO(86)12 (London: Department of Health and Social Security, 1986).

23. James J. Goedert, 'Mother to infant transmission of HIV-1: Association with prematurity or low anti-gp 120', *Lancet,* 9 December 1989: 1351–4. From 1990 abstract in *Current AIDS Literature* 3(2):40.

24. Uwa Kabagabo *et al.,* 'Maternal factors associated with perinatal HIV transmission', 7th International Conference on AIDS, Florence, 1991, Abstract No. M.C.3027.

25. Marc Lallemant *et al.,* 'Assessing the risk for mother-infant HIV-1 transmission: A challenge in developing countries', 7th International Conference on AIDS, Florence, 1991, Abstract No. M.C.3078.

26. Preliminary data reported at 8th International Conference on AIDS by Marc Bulterys *et al.,* 'Detection of HIV-1 in breastmilk, multiple sexual partners, and mother-to-child transmission of HIV-1: a cohort study', 1992, Abstract No. Th.C.1524.

27. Janet L. Mitchell, 'Strategies for prevention of perinatal transmission', 6th International Conference on AIDS, San Francisco, 1990.

28. 'HIV-1 infection and artificial insemination with processed semen', *Mortality & Morbidity Weekly Report* 39 (249) (1990):255–6. And Simon Rozendaal, 'Help for seropositive partners', *World AIDS News: Newspaper of the Harvard–Amsterdam 8th International Conference on AIDS*, July 1992. Research by Ulrike Sonnenberg-Schwan of the KIS-Curatorium for Immunodeficiency in Munich.

29. See Lisa Saffron, *Alternative Beginnings: A Guide to Getting Pregnant by Self-Insemination* (London: Sheba, in press), for up-to-date AIDS-aware information on donor insemination.

30. Cheri Pies, 'Insemination: Something more to consider', in Ines Rieder (ed.), *AIDS: The Women* (San Francisco: Cleis Press, 1988), 142.

31. WHO/UNICEF consultation on HIV transmission and breastfeeding. Consensus statement and press release, Geneva, 4 May 1992.

32. Jane Cottingham, 'Transmission of HIV through breastfeeding: practical and policy issues'. Unpublished term paper, Harvard School of Public Health, Cambridge, USA, March 1990.

33. A. O. Osoba *et al.,* 'Maternal transmission of HIV', *Saudi Medical Journal* 11(2) (1990):125–9.

34. Philippe Van de Perre *et al.,* 'Postnatal transmission of HIV-1 from mother to infant: A prospective cohort study in Kigali, Rwanda', *New England Journal of Medicine* 325(9) (1991):593–8.

35. Caroline S. Bradbeer, 'Mothers with HIV: risks to baby need to be balanced against benefits of breast feeding', *British Medical Journal* 299 (1989):806.

36. C. Hutto *et al.,* 'A hospital-based prospective study of perinatal infection with HIV-1', *Journal of Pediatrics* 118 (1991):347–53.

37. Robert H. Yolken, 'Human milk may inhibit HIV infection, say Hopkins physicians', press release, Johns Hopkins Children's Center, Baltimore, USA, 8 May 1990.

38. David S. Newburg *et al.,* 'A human milk factor inhibits binding of HIV to the CD4 receptor', *Pediatric Research* 31 (1991):22–8.

39. Alberto Eugenio Tozzi *et al.,* 'Does breast-feeding delay progression to AIDS in HIV-infected children?', *AIDS* 4 (1990):1293–4.

40. Department of Health and Social Security, London, *HIV infection, breastfeeding and human milk banking in the UK,* PL/CMO (88)13 & PL/CNO (88)7, 27 April 1988.

41. Philippa Braidwood, 'Make breast milk safe', *Observer* (UK), 29 March 1987, reprinted in *MIDIRS Information Pack* No. 4, April 1987.

42. Department of Health and Social Security, London, *HIV infection, breastfeeding and human milk banking in the UK,* PL/CMO 89(4) and PL/CNO 89(3), 4 July 1989.

43. Percy Gomez, paper for 6th National Women's Conference, Bahamas, 30 November 1990.

44. Kristi Baker, personal communication, March 1991.

45. Kristi Baker and Vivien Nakawala, 'Breast-

feeding and AIDS Survey', *NGO AIDS Newsletter* (Family Health Trust, Lusaka) 4 (April 1991):2.

46. D. J. Hu and B. M. Nkowane, 'Risks of HIV transmission from breastfeeding: Research design issues and policy implications', 7th International Conference on AIDS, Florence, 1991, Abstract No. W.C.3071.

47. Kathy I. Kennedy *et al.,* 'Breastfeeding and AIDS: A health policy analysis', 7th International Conference on AIDS, Florence, 1991, Abstract No. W.C.3223.

48. World Health Organization, Statement on breastfeeding and HIV, Geneva, 13 September 1991.

49. Nel Druce, personal communication, May 1992.

50. Sunanda Ray, personal communication, May 1992.

Chapter 6 (pages 89–115)

1. American College of Obstetrics and Gyne- cology, quoted in *Searching for Women: A literature review on women, HIV and AIDS in the United States* (Boston: College of Public and Community Service (Univ Mass) and Multicultural AIDS Coalition, 2nd edn May 1990), 99–100.

2. Jane Perlez, 'AIDS outweighed by the desire to have a child', *New York Times,* 20 April 1991.

3. Sunanda Ray, 'Women and AIDS in Zimbabwe'. In Mary Anne Mercer and Sally Scott, *Tradition and transition: NGOs respond to AIDS in Africa* (Baltimore: Johns Hopkins University School of Hygiene and Public Health, Institute for International Programs, 1991), 15–22.

4. Ann B. Williams, 'Reproductive concerns of women at risk for HIV infection', *Journal of Nurse-Midwifery* 35:5 (1990), 292–8.

5. John D. Arras, 'Having children in fear and trembling', *Millbank Quarterly* 68(3) (1990):353–82.

6. Sandra Dick, 'A London midwife's experience and recommendations for infection control policy for all pregnant women delivering in hospital', paper written for this book, 1992.

7. S. Lindgren *et al.,* 'An antenatal programme for HIV-infected pregnant women', in *The Free Woman: Women's Health in the 1990s* Eylard V. van Hall and Walter Everaerd (eds.) (Amsterdam: Parthenon, 1990), 750–55.

8. M. E. Kreyenbroek *et al.,* 'Pregnancy, drugs and HIV: an interdisciplinary approach', in *The Free Woman: Women's Health in the 1990s* Eylard V. van Hall and Walter Everaerd (eds.) (Amsterdam: Parthenon, 1990).

9. Frank D. Johnstone *et al.,* 'Women's knowledge of their HIV antibody state: its effect on their decision whether to continue the pregnancy', *British Medical Journal* 300(6716) (1990):23–4.

10. Carole Levine and Nancy Neveloff Dubler, 'Uncertain risks and bitter realities: the reproductive choices of HIV-infected women', *Millbank Quarterly* 68(3) (1990):321–51.

11. M. Temmerman *et al.,* 'Post-partum counselling of HIV-infected women and their subsequent reproductive behaviour', *AIDS Care* 2(3) (1990), 247–52.

12. Robert W. Ryder *et al.,* 'Fertility rates in 238 HIV-1 seropositive women in Zaïre followed for three years postpartum', *AIDS* 5(12) (1991), 1521–7.

13. Ann Sunderland *et al.,* 'Influence of HIV infection on pregnancy decisions', paper presented to 4th International Conference on AIDS, Stockholm, June 1988.

14. *Tabular information on legal instruments dealing with AIDS and HIV infection: Part I,* WHO Global Programme on AIDS, Geneva, May 1989.

15. Stated by public health official from Mexico during a workshop at Global Impact of AIDS Conference, London, 1988.

16. From a discussion at first WHO Global Programme on AIDS consultation with international women's organizations, Geneva, December 1989.

17. Carola Marte and Kathryn Anastos, 'Women: the missing persons in the AIDS epidemic. Part II', *Health/PAC Bulletin* (Spring 1990):11–18.

18. Linda McCallum, quoted in article by Aileen Ballantyne, 'Doctors "forced AIDS virus women to have abortions"', *Guardian,* 17 August 1988.

19. Reported at a women's pre-conference meeting, 8th International Conference on AIDS, Amsterdam, July 1992.

20. 'HIV infection & pregnancy', *Women & HIV/AIDS Network Update,* May 1991:3.

21. Summarized from an article by Ellen Bilofsky, *Health/PAC Bulletin* (Spring 1990):16–17.

22. J. R. Smith *et al.*, 'Infertility management in HIV positive couples: a dilemma', *British Medical Journal* 302 (15 June 1991), 1447–50.
23. M. Huengsberg and C. Bradbeer, 'Routine testing for HIV at infertility clinics', *British Medical Journal* 303 (14 September 1991):645.
24. Carmen Torres, 'Isabel and her son; healthy for now', *Women's Health Journal* 2 (April–June 1991), 57–60.
25. Janet Mitchell, 'Provision of care for women: challenges and opportunities', paper presented to National Conference on Women and HIV Infection, Washington, DC, 13–14 December 1990.
26. Margarita Cordero, 'Fear of HIV/AIDS in childbirth', *Mujer/Fempress* (October 1989):4.
27. 'Lunch against AIDS', *Health Alert* 90 (1989):74.
28. Deborah Pugh, 'The Arab Middle East', *WorldAIDS* 13 (1991):15.
29. Indira Kapoor, 'Women and AIDS: education and counselling for prevention', *CARC Calling* 3(4) (1990):2–10.
30. Denis McClean, 'Sri Lanka launches an intensive education programme', *AIDS Watch* 12 (1990):8.
31. S. Bond and T. Rhodes, 'HIV infection and community midwives', *Midwifery* 6(1) (1990):86–92. From abstract by Heather Bower in *MIDIRS Information Pack* 15, December 1990.
32. Katherine M. Franke, 'HIV-related discrimination in abortion clinics in New York City'. Report by AIDS Discrimination Division, Law Enforcement Bureau, NYC Commission on Human Rights, NY. Excerpted from the report.
33. Comité National de Lutte contre le SIDA, *Réponses à vos questions sur le SIDA* (Zaïre, undated).
34. Positively Women leaflet *HIV, Pregnancy and Children* (London, 1991).
35. John Cosgrove, 'Children affected by HIV', *Proceedings of the Third National Conference, Women and HIV/AIDS Network, Crieff, Scotland, 29–30 November 1990*, 27–8.
36. Ofelia Ceja and Ofelia Osorio, 'Proteje a tus hijos del SIDA', *Las Buenas Ideas* 2(14) (1990):2.
37. Mary Hepburn, 'Pregnancy and HIV', paper to Second National Conference of the Women & HIV/AIDS Network, Scotland, 23 October 1989.
38. Ana Louisa Liguori, 'El SIDA también se presenta en las mujeres', *Gaceta CONASIDA* 3(4) (1990):12–15.
39. June E. Osborn, 'Women and HIV/AIDS: The silent epidemic', *Siecus Report* 19(2) (1990–91):1–4.
40. Sandra Neville, 'The social and economic impact of AIDS on our society', paper presented to 6th National Women's Conference, whose theme was Women and AIDS, Bahamas, 30 November 1990.
41. Gabriele Schwarz, 'Problems in caring for children with HIV-infected parents', 7th International Conference on AIDS, Florence, 1991, Abstract No. W.C.3273.
42. Christine Obbo, 'Reflections on the AIDS orphans problem in Uganda', *Courier* 126 (March/April 1991):55–7.
43. *The care and support of children of HIV-infected parents,* WHO Global Programme on AIDS, Geneva, May 1991.

Chapter 7 (pages 116–128)

1. R. Fitzpatrick *et al.*, 'Heterosexual sexual behaviour in a sample of homosexually active men', *Genitourinary Medicine* 65 (1989): 259–62.
2. Brad Bartholow *et al.*, 'Contrasting HIV risk behaviour, attitudes and beliefs among exclusively homosexual and behaviorally bisexual men', 7th International Conference on AIDS, Florence, 1991, Abstract No. M.D.4014.
3. Leslie R. Jaffe *et al.*, 'Anal intercourse and knowledge of AIDS among minority-group female adolescents', *Journal of Pediatrics* 112(6) (1988):1005–07.
4. Maria de Bruyn, 'Women and AIDS in developing countries', *Social Science and Medicine* 34(3) (1992):249–62.
5. J. G. McKenna *et al.*, 'Cold sores and safer sex', *Lancet* 338 (7 September 1991):632
6. *'Searching for women: A literature review on women, HIV and AIDS in the United States* (Boston: College of Public and Community Service (Univ Mass) and Multicultural AIDS Coalition, second edn May 1991).
7. Ruth Perry, 'Lesbians and AIDS'. Unpublished paper, 1990.
8. Risa Denenberg, 'A decade of denial: lesbians and HIV', *On Our Backs* (July/August 1991):21–2, 38–42.
9. D. Rowen and C. A. Carne, 'Heterosexual

transmission of HIV', *International Journal of STDs and AIDS* 1 (1990):240.

10. P. J. Feldblum, 'Results from prospective studies of HIV-discordant couples', *AIDS* 5(10) (1991):1265–6.

11. Ahmed S. Latif *et al.,* 'Genital ulcers and transmission of HIV among couples in Zimbabwe', *AIDS* 3(8) (1989):519–23.

12. D. Clemetson *et al.,* 'Incidence of HIV transmission within HIV-1 discordant hetero-sexual partnerships in Nairobi, Kenya', 6th International Conference on AIDS, San Francisco, 1990, Abstract No. 3187. See also Wykoff *et al.,* 'Contact tracing to identify HIV infection in a rural USA community', *Journal of American Medical Association* 259(24) (1988) and N. Merino *et al.,* 'HIV-1, sexual practices and contact with foreigners in homosexual men in Colombia', *Journal of AIDS* 3(4) (1990):330–34, regarding similar insertive-receptive differentials among gay men.

13. Bruce D. Forrest, 'Women, HIV and mucosal immunity', *Lancet* 337 (1991):835–6. These include macrophages, epithelial cells and lymphocytes.

14. Judith K. Bury, 'HIV-positive women and contraception', *British Journal of Family Planning* 14 (1988):50–54.

15. Judith Wasserheit, 'Reproductive tract infections', *Special Challenges in Third World Women's Health* (New York: International Women's Health Coalition, March 1990).

16. Nicholas S. Helmann *et al.,* 'Genital trauma during sex is a risk factor for HIV infection', 7th International Conference on AIDS, Florence, 1991, Abstract No. M.C.3079.

17. M. Elizabeth Duncan *et al.,* 'First coitus before menarche and risk of STD', *Lancet* 335 (1990):338–40.

18. Risa Denenberg, 'Unique aspects of HIV infection in women: women and symptoms', in Cynthia Chris and Monica Pearl, ACT-UP/New York Women & Book Group (Boston: South End Press, 1990), 31–43.

19. Kristina D. Bird, 'The use of spermicide containing nonoxynol-9 in the prevention of HIV infection', *AIDS* 5(7) (1991):791–96.

20. Michael J. Rosenberg *et al.,* 'Barrier contraceptives and STDs in women: a comparison of female-dependent methods and condoms', *American Journal of Public Health* 82(5) (1992):669–74.

21. Somchai Niruthisard *et al.,* 'Use of nonoxynol-9 and reduction in rate of gonoccocal and chlamydial cervical infections', *Lancet* 339 (6 June 1992):1371–75.

22. Questions raised about nonoxynol-9, *Women & AIDS Project Newsletter,* Fall 1990, 11, research reported by British Columbia Centre for Disease Control 6th International Conference on AIDS, San Francisco, 1990.

23. S. Niruthisard *et al.,* 'The effects of frequent nonoxynol-9 use on the vaginal and cervical mucosa', *Sexually Transmitted Diseases* 18(3) (1991):176–79.

24. J. A. Fortney *et al.,* paper to 6th International Conference on AIDS, San Francisco. Referred to in summary of proceedings of 7th International Conference on AIDS, Florence, in *AIDS Newsletter* (August 1991), 5–6.

25. 'AIDS education: A beginning.' *Population Reports,* Series L, 8:16 (1989).

26. Joan Kreiss *et al.,* 'Efficacy of nonoxynol-9 contraceptive sponge use in preventing heterosexual acquisition of HIV in Nairobi prostitutes', *Journal of American Medical Association* 268(4) (1992):477–82. See also editorial by Katherine M. Stone and Herbert B. Peterson in the same issue, 521–23.

27. From discussions with Kristina Bird, Sunanda Ray, Edna Roland, Mabel Bianco, Claudia Garcia Moreno, Barbara James, Toni Belfield and Jane Urwin during and after the 8th International Conference on AIDS, July 1992. The roundtable on 'Intravaginal STD/HIV prevention technology controllable by women' at the conference indicated widespread confusion and varying degrees of informaion among both panelists and audience on this issue, but also generated a great deal of useful debate and discussion.

28. Sara Townsend, 'Many women can use IUDs without increasing risk of PID', *Network* 12(2) (1991):10–12.

29. Caroline Bradbeer, 'AIDS and family planning', *British Journal of Family Planning* 13(4) (1988):26–7.

30. International Medical Advisory Panel, 'Statement on contraception for clients who are HIV-positive', *IPPF Medical Bulletin* 25(6) (1991):1–2.

31. European Study Group, 'Risk factors for male to female transmission of HIV', *British Medical Journal* 298 (1989):411–15.

32. Massimo Musicco, 'Oral contraception, IUD, condom use and man-to-woman sexual transmission of HIV infection', 6th International Conference on AIDS, San Francisco, 1990, Abstract No. Th.C.584.

33. Mary Hepburn, personal communication, June 1991.

34. 'Oral Contraceptives and AIDS: No link established,' *Population Reports,* Series A, 7 (1988):20.

35. Deborah J. Anderson, 'White blood cells and HIV-1 in semen from vasectomised seropositive men', *Lancet* 388 (31 August 1991):573–4.

36. Edgar J. Schoen, 'The status of circumcision of newborns', *New England Journal of Medicine* 322(18) (1990):1308–12.

37. Swapna S. Sengupta and Hemant A. Kamat, 'Preventing the sexual transmission of HIV', *CARC Calling: Bulletin of Center for AIDS Research and Control,* Indian Council of Medical Research, 3(4) (1990):14–16.

38. See for example J. Neil Simonsen *et al.,* 'HIV infection among men with STDs', *New England Journal of Medicine* 319(5) (1988):274–8.

39. Ronald L. Poland, 'The question of routine neonatal circumcision', *New England Journal of Medicine* 322(18) (1990):1312–15.

40. Agathe Lawson, paper presented to meeting on Traditional Practices and the Possible Links to AIDS Transmission, Inter-African Committee, Addis Ababa, 9–11 May 1989.

41. Olayinka Koso-Thomas, 'Female circumcision', Report of the Regional Conference on Traditional Practices Affecting the Health of Women and Children in Africa, Addis Ababa, 19–24 November 1990, Inter-African Committee, 55–6.

42. Olayinka Koso-Thomas, 'Epidemiology of AIDS in relation to female circumcision', paper presented to meeting on Traditional Practices and the Possible Links to AIDS Transmission, Inter-African Committee, Addis Ababa, 9–11 May 1989.

43. Richard C. Brown and J. E. Brown, 'The use of intravaginal irritants as a risk factor for the transmission of HIV infection in Zaïrean prostitutes', 7th International Conference on AIDS, Florence, 1991, Abstract No. M.C.3006.

44. Ernesto Guerrero *et al.,* 'Sexual practices and STDs in female Dominican sex workers', 6th International Conference on AIDS, San Francisco, 1990, Abstract No. F.C.736.

45. Agnes Runganga *et al.,* 'The use of herbal and other agents to enhance sexual experience'. Unpublished paper, 1991, accepted for publication in *Social Science and Medicine.*

46. Gina Dallabetta *et al.,* 'Vaginal agents as a risk factor for acquisition of HIV-1', Fifth International Conference on HIV/AIDS in Africa, 12 October 1990, Abstract No. F.O.A.2. and also their report 'Vaginal tightening agents as risk factors for acquisition of HIV', 6th International Conference on AIDS, San Francisco, 1990, Abstract No. Th.C.754.

47. Vinit Sharma, 'India's poor tribes stick to their traditions', *Entre Nous: European Family Planning Magazine* 19 (December 1991):18.

48. M. R. Chacko, 'Vaginal douching in teenagers attending a family planning clinic', *Journal of Adolescent Health Care* 10 (1989):217. Reported in *Family Planning Perspectives* 21(4) (1989):150.

49. Michael Tan, personal communication, February 1992.

50. S. M. Murphy, 'Rape, STDs and HIV', *International Journal of STDs and AIDS* 1 (1990):79–82.

51. Upton Allen *et al.,* 'Post-exposure management of rape victims: A decision analysis', 7th International Conference on AIDS, Florence, 1991, Abstract No. W.C.3067.

52. Elizabeth Reid, 'Placing women at the centre of the analysis'. Unpublished paper, November 1990.

53. WHO Study Group, 'Management of patients with sexually transmitted diseases', WHO Technical Report Series, Geneva, 1991.

54. C. R. Philpot, 'Goals and objectives for STD/AIDS control into the 1990s', *International Journal of STDs and AIDS* 1 (1990):367.

55. Lieve Fransen, 'Gaps in control of sexual transmission of STDs/AIDS among women', 7th International Conference on AIDS, Florence, 1991, Pre-conference abstract.

Chapter 8 (pages 129–146)

1. Michael Tan, personal communication, February 1992.
2. Sunny Rumsey, 'Communities under siege', in Ines Rieder and Patricia Ruppelt (eds.), *AIDS: The Women* (San Francisco: Cleis Books, 1988), 189.
3. Elizabeth Reid, 'Placing women at the centre of the analysis'. Unpublished paper, Nov. 1990.
4. Zena A. Stein, 'HIV transmission to women: a barrier method urgently needed'. Unpublished paper, 1989.
5. Susan D. Cochran and Vickie M. Mays, 'Women and AIDS-related concerns: roles for psychologists in helping the worried well', *American Psychologist* 44(3) (1989):529–35.
6. Jo Setters, 'Safer sex guidelines for heterosexuals', *Health Education Journal* 47(2/3) (1988):61.
7. Susan D. Cochran, 'Women and HIV infection: issues in prevention and behavior change', in Vickie M. Mays *et al.,* (eds.) *Primary Prevention of AIDS: Psychological Approaches* (Newbury Park: Sage Publications, 1989).
8. P. J. Feldblum, 'Results from prospective studies of HIV-discordant couples', *AIDS* 5(10) (1991):1265–6.
9. Ivana Markova, quoted in 'Fear of discovery deters AIDS victims from using condoms', *Guardian*, 21 August 1990.
10. Mere Kisekka, 'Social and sexual practices related to the epidemiology of STDs', paper for Inter-African Committee Meeting on Traditional Practices Affecting the Health of Women and Children, Addis Ababa, 9–11 May 1989.
11. Fernando Lado, 'Camisinha por favor; entrevista con Nana', *Diaro de República,* 26 October 1990.
12. Project AWARE, San Francisco General Hospital, 'Women at risk of AIDS more likely to switch partners than sex practices', press release at 5th International Conference on AIDS, Montréal, 7 June 1989.
13. Project AWARE, San Francisco General Hospital, 'HIV-positive women changing behavior to reduce transmission', press release at 5th International Conference on AIDS, Montréal, 7 June 1989.
14. Susan Robbins *et al.,* 'A description of HIV risk factors among 17,655 women', 6th International Conference on AIDS, San Francisco, 1990, Abstract No. F.C.746.
15. Mere Kisekka, reported in a discussion on women and AIDS, meeting of grantees of the MacArthur Foundation, Teresopolis, Brazil, 1–3 July, 1991.
16. Adapted from: draft for leaflet on lesbians and AIDS by San Francisco Women's AIDS Network, 1990; *Women Talk . . . about AIDS, sex and sexual health* by Di Surgey, Women Talking about AIDS Project, Melbourne, 1992; and other sources.

Chapter 9 (pages 147–170)

1. World Health Organization, *Research in Human Reproduction,* Biennial Report 1988–9, Geneva, 1990.
2. Sharon L. Camp, 'Limited access: Contraceptive costs may impede use', *Conscience* 12(6) (1992):12–13.
3. Axel Mundigo, 'Behavioural aspects of condom acceptability', *Progress* 13 (1990):3. Extracted from 'Condom promotion and use: family planning versus HIV protection', *IPPF Medical Bulletin* 23(6) (1989):1–3.
4. 'Condoms, now more than ever', *Population Reports,* H8 (September 1990).
5. Gill Shepherd, 'Attitudes to family planning in Kenya: an anthropological approach', *Health Policy and Planning* 2(1) (1987):80–89.
6. From an exchange between Nancy Williamson and Jeffrey R. Harris following his paper 'The role of condoms in preventing HIV transmission in developing countries', in Nancy J. Alexander *et al.,* (eds), *Heterosexual Transmission of AIDS, Proceedings of the Second Contraceptive Research and Development Program International Workshop, Norfolk, USA, 1–3 February 1989* (New York: Wiley-Liss, 1990), 399–413.
7. Frank Johnstone *et al.,* 'Contraceptive use in HIV-infected women', *British Journal of Family Planning* 16 (1990):106–08.
8. Sandra Azevedo, reported in a discussion on women and AIDS, meeting of grantees of the MacArthur Foundation, Teresopolis, Brazil, 1–3 July 1991.
9. Kay Armstrong *et al.,* 'Reducing the perinatal transmission of AIDS by providing family planning services in drug treatment centres',

6th International Conference on AIDS, San Francisco, 1990, Abstract No. 4098.

10. Elizabeth B. Younger and Patrick Friel, 'How to develop culturally appropriate condom instructions', *AIDS Health Promotion Exchange* 3 (1990):11–13.

11. W. Woods *et al.*, 'Interventions for condom use skill development in the eastern Caribbean', 6th International Conference on AIDS, San Francisco, 1990, Abstract No. SC.693.

12. Jeffrey R. Harris, 'The role of condoms in preventing HIV transmission in developing countries', in Nancy J. Alexander *et al.* (eds), *Heterosexual Transmission of AIDS, Proceedings of the Second Contraceptive Research and Development Program International Workshop, Norfolk, USA, 1–3 February 1989* (New York: Wiley-Liss, 1990), 399–413.

13. Population Council, 'Actitudes sobre el uso del condón en el Caribe', *Alternativas* (March 1990):8–9.

14. Toni Belfield, personal communication, May 1992.

15. International Medical Advisory Panel, 'Statement on contraception for clients who are HIV positive', *IPPF Medical Bulletin* 25(6) (1991):1–2.

16. From an interview with Arletty Pinel of Brazil, in *Health Alert* 98 (October 1989):166.

17. Judith Bury, 'Heterosexual transmission', *Women and HIV/AIDS Network: Proceedings of Second National Conference, Edinburgh, October 1989,* 5–10.

18. Vickie M. Mays and Susan D. Cochran, 'Issues in the perception of AIDS risk and risk reduction activities by black and Hispanic/Latina women', *American Psychologist* 43(11) (1988):949–57.

19. Christopher C. Taylor, 'Condoms and cosmology: the fractal person and sexual risk in Rwanda', *Social Science and Medicine* 31(9) (1990):1023–8.

20. Brooke Schoepf, Workshop on women and AIDS, 4th International Interdisciplinary Congress on Women, New York, 3–7 June 1990.

21. 'AIDS Education: A Beginning', *Population Reports,* Series L, No. 8, (September 1989): 24.

22. Erica Greathead, 'Sexuality programme benefits AIDS education in a developing community', 6th International Conference on AIDS, San Francisco, 1990, Abstract No. 4097.

23. Joesoef *et al.,* 'Husband's approval of contraceptive use in metropolitan Indonesia', *Studies in Family Planning* 19(3) (1988):162–8.

24. Debbie Rogow, 'Meeting male reproductive health care needs in Latin America', *Quality/Calidad/Qualité Series* No. 2, (New York, Population Council, 1990).

25. Dominique Hauser *et al.,* 'Changes in Switzerland: condom use in occasional relations', 6th International Conference on AIDS, San Francisco, 1990, Abstract No. F.D.892.

26. 'For men only', *WorldAIDS* 12 (November 1990):9.

27. West African Network of Social Scientists in Action Research on Reproductive Health, June 1988. Letter in *Maternal Mortality: A Call to Women for Action, Report of International Activities.* (Amsterdam, Women's Global Network for Reproductive Rights, June 1988), 6.

28. J. M. Ponnighaus and S. M. Oxborrow, 'Construction projects and spread of HIV', letter to *Lancet* 336 (10 November 1990):1198.

29. J. P. Fraser-Mackenzie, 'The commercial farmer against AIDS', Commercial Farmers Union, Zimbabwe. Unpublished paper, 1991.

30. Michael Tan, personal communication, February 1992.

31. Kari Hartwig, 'The politics of AIDS in Tanzania: gender perceptions and the challenges for educational strategies'. Unpublished MA thesis in International Development, Clark University, Worchester, MA, USA, July 1991.

32. Judy Wilson, 'Always use a condom', *Mainliners* 2 (September 1990):10–11.

33. Jane Perlez, 'Condoms official as Uganda faces up to AIDS disaster', *Guardian,* 31 January 1991.

34. Veronica Rossato, 'Con el preservativo en el cartera', *Mujer/Fempress* 120 (October 1991):9.

35. Fernando Lado, 'Camisinha por favor: entrevista con Nana', *Diario de República,* 26 October 1990.

36. Sara Townsend, 'Social marketing of condoms: selling protection and changing behavior', *Network* 12(1) (1991):17–20.

37. Malcolm Potts and Roger V. Short, 'Condoms for the prevention of HIV transmission: cultural dimensions', *AIDS* 3 (Supplement 1) (1989): S259–S263.

38. Marc Ostfield *et al.,* ' "Condoms because you care": a lifestyle approach to condom promotion in the eastern Caribbean', 7th International Conference on AIDS, Florence, 1991, Abstract No. W.D.4003.

39. 'Japan: selling condoms to housewives', *Progress* 13 (1990):2.

40. Maria Elena Vega, 'Condón para fin de semana', *La Nación,* Chile, undated.

41. Christopher J. Castle, 'Trip report: Indonesia, Malaysia and the Philippines, 20 August–19 September 1991', Appropriate Health Resources and Technologies Action Group (AHRTAG), London 1991.

42. Juliet Richters *et al.,* 'In search of the perfect condom', *Healthright* 9(1) (1989):16–19.

43. 'A female condom?', *Progress* 13 (1990):3.

44. Mahmoud F. Fathalla, personal communication, June 1991.

45. Mahmoud F. Fathalla, personal communication, August 1991.

46. Mahmoud F. Fathalla, personal communication, July 1991.

47. *The Standard,* Switzerland, 21 February 1992, 5.

48. 'FDA panel recommends approval of female condom', press release, Grayling Company, London, 31 January 1992.

49. Stephen L. Coulter *et al.,* 'Low particle transmission across polyurethane condoms', 7th International Conference on AIDS, Florence, 1991, Abstract No. M.C.3022.

50. Susan Muska *et al.,* 'The WPC-333 female condom: perceptions of male and female drug users', 7th International Conference on AIDS, Florence, 1991, Abstract No. M.D.4257.

51. Jeannette Parisot, *Johnny Come Lately: A short history of the condom* (London: Journeyman Press, 1987).

52. Walli Bounds *et al.,* 'Female condom (Femidom TM). A clinical study of its use – effectiveness and patient acceptability', *British Journal of Family Planning* 18 (1992):36–41.

Chapter 10 (pages 171–228)

1. R. W. Connell and Susan Kippax, 'Sexuality in the AIDS crisis: patterns of sexual practice and pleasure in a sample of Australian gay and bisexual men', *Journal of Sex Research* 27(2) (1990):167–98.

2. Hilary Standing and Mere Kisekka, 'Sexual behaviour in sub-Saharan Africa: a review and annotated bibliography', Overseas Development Administration, April 1989.

3. Mere Kisekka, 'Social and sexual practices related to the epidemiology of STDs', paper for the Inter-African Committee Meeting on Traditional Practices Affecting the Health of Women and Children, Addis Ababa, 9–11 May 1989.

4. Nancy Gibbs, 'Teens: the rising risk of AIDS', *Time*, 2 September 1991, 60.

5. *USP Bulletin* 23(42) (1990), in *Tok Blong SPPF* 34 (January 1991):14–15.

6. Glenda Maynard, 'AIDS: the facts, the reality and the challenges', paper presented to 6th National Women's Conference, on Women and AIDS, Bahamas, 30 November 1990.

7. Ed Hooper, *Slim* (London: Bodley Head, 1990), 253.

8. Dázon Dixon, personal communication, 1991.

9. Dázon Dixon, 'Facilitators' guide to The Healthy Love Party', SisterLove: Women's AIDS Project, Atlanta, October 1990.

10. Chicago Women's AIDS Project, *Girls Night Out: A safer sex workshop for women: Manual for peer leaders,* undated.

11. Alma Aldana, 'Safer sex workshops in Mexico', *Women's Health Journal* 20 (1990):26–7.

12. Sharon Thompson, 'Putting a big thing into a little hole: teenage girls' accounts of sexual initiation', *Journal of Sex Research* 27(3) (1990):341–61. Summarized. The list of questions about sexual feelings is quoted, with several additions, with permission of Society for the Scientific Study of Sex, P.O. Box 208, Mount Vernon, IA 52134, USA.

13. AIDS and STD prevention report, first sub-regional caucus for Melanesian women, Noumea, 14–18 October 1991.

14. Clement Malau, 'Support more women', *Pacific STD/AIDS Alert* 6 (October 1991):1.

15. Norma Valle, 'Esperán las feministas un principe azúl?', *Mujer/Fempress* 119 (September 1991):11.

16. See Janet Holland et al, pages 197–202. And: Cathie Wright, 'Young women and safer sex', *Proceedings of the Third National Conference of the Women & HIV/AIDS Network, Edinburgh, Scotland, November 1990,* 39–43.

17. Purnima Mane, 'Taboos against sex education in India and implications for women in the

context of AIDS'. Unpublished paper, 1992.

18. Nema Mdoe, 'Three steps forward: interview by Liz Kelly', *Trouble and Strife* 21 (Summer 1991):47–52.

19. Kari Hartwig, 'The politics of AIDS in Tanzania: gender perceptions and the challenges for educational strategies'. Unpublished MA thesis in International Development, Clark University, Worcester, MA, USA, July 1991.

20. Janie Hampton, *Meeting AIDS with compassion: AIDS care and prevention in Agomanya, Ghana,* Strategies for Hope Series No. 4 (London: ActionAid, AMREF and World in Need).

21. Beth Maina Ahlberg, 'African culture and development: the changing sexuality in sub-Saharan Africa and its impact on women's reproductive health', paper presented to Expert Group on Women and HIV/AIDS and the Role of National Machinery for the Advancement of Women, Vienna, 24–28 September 1990.

22. Brenda Spencer, 'From kisses to coitus', 7th International Conference on AIDS, Florence, 1991, Abstract No. M.D.4064.

23. Aida Iris Cruz Alicea, 'La violencia contra la mujer y el SIDA', Casa Pensamiento de Mujer del Centro, Puerto Rico. Unpublished paper, 1991.

24. Daniela Butler *et al.,* 'Même une fois "sans" c'est trop: bases pour une prévention du sida auprès des clients des prostituées'. Unpublished thesis, École de Service Social à Soleure, at the request of Aide Suisse contre le Sida, Zürich, February 1990.

25. Hansje Verbeek, 'AIDS and sex work'. Unpublished paper for De Rode Draad, April 1988.

26. Nell Rasmussen, 'Sexual abuse and incest in Europe', *Planned Parenthood in Europe* 21(1) (1992):15–18.

27. I. S. Gilada, 'AIDS and prostitution: an Indian perspective', paper presented to 7th Congress of African Union against Venereal Diseases and Trepanomatosis (AUVDT), Lusaka, Zambia, 17–20 March 1991.

28. Ruth Morgan-Thomas, 'The sex industry', *AIDS Action* 15 (September 1991):1.

29. Mizuho Matsuda, 'Child prostitution in Asia; Koson Srisang, Campaign to end child prostitution launched'; and Mayuree Rattana-wannathip, 'Prostitution: necessity or greed',

Friends of Women Newsletter 1(1) (1990):18–21.

30. Women's Resource and Research Center, 'Towards a preliminary viewing of child prostitution and tourism', *Flights* 4(2) (1990):3–5.

31. Mere Kisekka and Bernadette Otesanya, 'STDs as a gender issue: examples from Nigeria and Uganda', paper presented at AAWORD Seminar, Dakar, 8–14 August 1988.

32. Dooley Worth *et al.,* 'Sexual and physical abuse as factors in continued risk behavior of women injection drug users in a South Bronx methadone clinic', 6th International Conference on AIDS, San Francisco, 1990. Abstract in *Women & AIDS Project Newsletter,* Winter 1991, 11.

33. Karen Heckert, personal communication, April 1992.

34. Sunanda Ray, 'Women and AIDS in Zimbabwe', in Mary Anne Mercer and Sally Scott (eds), *Tradition and Transition: NGOs respond to AIDS in Africa* (Baltimore: Johns Hopkins University School of Hygiene and Public Health, Institute for International Programs, 1992).

35. Merrill Singer *et al.,* 'SIDA: the economic social and cultural context of AIDS among Latinos', *Medical Anthropological Quarterly* 4(1) (1990):92–101.

36. P. Kraft, 'Age at first experience of intercourse among Norwegian adolescents: a lifestyle perspective', *Social Science and Medicine* 33(2) (1991):207–13.

37. Leslie R. Jaffe *et al.,* 'Anal intercourse and knowledge of AIDS among minority-group female adolescents', *Journal of Pediatrics* 112(6) (1988):1005–07.

38. I. O. Orubuloye, 'Patterns of female sexuality in the Ekiti district of Ondo State, Nigeria', paper presented to the Expert Group on Women and HIV/AIDS and the Role of National Machinery for the Advancement of Women, Vienna, 24–28 September 1990.

39. Rani Bang, 'High prevalence of gynaecological diseases in rural Indian women', *Lancet* 335 (14 January 1989):85–8.

40. M. Elizabeth Duncan *et al.,* 'First coitus before menarche and risk of STD', *Lancet* 335 (1990):338–40.

41. Mary T. Bassett and Marvellous Mhloyi, 'Women

and AIDS in Zimbabwe: the making of an epidemic', *International Journal of Health Services* 21(1) (1991):143-56.

42. Priscilla Ulin, 'African women and AIDS: negotiating behavioural change', *Social Science and Medicine* 34(1) (1992):63-73.

43. Maria de Bruyn, 'Women and AIDS in developing countries', *Social Science and Medicine* 34(3) (1992):249-62.

44. Jane Perlez, 'Toll of AIDS on Uganda's women puts their roles and rights in question', *New York Times,* 28 October 1990: 11.

45. Eva Magambo, 'Women responding to AIDS', Experiment in International Living, School for International Training, Kampala, Uganda. Paper written specially for this book, 1991.

46. Society for Women and AIDS in Africa, summary report of 3rd International Conference on Women and AIDS in Africa, Yaoundé, 19-22 November 1991.

47. Christopher J. Castle, 'Trip report: Indonesia, Malaysia and the Philippines, 20 August-19 September 1991', AHRTAG, London, 1991: 21.

48. Okako Bibi Ayowa, with the collaboration of La Condition Feminine et Famille, 'Les femmes à partenaires multiples face au SIDA: cas des femmes de Kananga'. Unpublished paper, L'Institut Médical Chrétien du Kasai, Centre d'Études, December 1989.

49. John Tierney, 'AIDS tears lives of the African family', *New York Times,* 17 September 1990.

50. Sofi Ospina *et al.,* 'The concept of fidelity in different cultures: implications for AIDS prevention campaigns', 7th International Conference on AIDS, Florence, 1991, Abstract No. M.D.4115.

51. Karen Jochelson *et al.,* 'HIV and migrant labor in South Africa', *International Journal of Health Services* 21(1) (1991):157-73.

52. Michael Tan, personal communication, February 1992.

53. Werasit Sittitrai *et al.,* 'Survey of partner relations and risk of HIV infection in Thailand', 7th International Conference on AIDS, Florence, 1991, Abstract No. M.D.4113.

54. Fernando Lado, 'Camisinha, por favor: entrevista con Nana', Diario del República, Uruguay. 26 October 1990.

55. Rani Bang, personal communication, July 1991.

56. Christina Lindan *et al.,* 'Knowledge, attitudes, and perceived risk of AIDS among urban Rwandan women: relationship to HIV infection and behaviour change', *AIDS* 5(8) (1991): 993-1002.

57. Marvellous Mhloyi, 'Perceptions in communication and sexuality in marriage in Zimbabwe', in E. D. Rothblum and Ellen Cote, *Women's Mental Health in Africa* (New York: Haworth Press, 1990).

58. 'Brazil: sex and self-worth', *AIDS Action* 15 (September 1991):5.

59. Else Smith *et al.,* 'Heterosexually acquired HIV infection in women in Copenhagen: sexual behaviour and other risk factors', *International Journal of STDs and AIDS* 1 (1990):416-21.

60. Else Smith, personal communication, 6 January 1992.

61. Augusta Del Zotto, 'Latinas with AIDS', *Women and AIDS: A Resource Guide* (IDERA & Vancouver Women and AIDS Project, 1990), 22-3.

62. R. E. Fullilove *et al.,* 'Risk of STD among black adolescent crack users in Oakland and San Francisco', *Journal of American Medical Association* 263(6) (1990):851-5.

63. Judi Wilson, 'Women, drugs and HIV', *Mainliners* 2 (September 1990):2.

64. Susan Allen *et al.,* 'HIV infection in urban Rwanda: demographic and behavioural correlates in a representative sample of childbearing women', *Journal of American Medical Association* 266(12) (1991):1657-63.

65. Brenda Stolzfus *et al., Hospitality – what price? The US Navy at Subic Bay and the women's response* (Olongapo City, Philippines: Buklod Center, 1990).

66. Aart Hendriks, 'AIDS and mobility', WHO Global Programme on AIDS, Europe Region, Copenhagen, April 1991.

67. Charles P. Wallace, 'The AIDS fuse is ignited in Asia', *Los Angeles Times,* 7 January 1992.

68. Ellen R. Koenig, 'International prostitutes and transmission of HIV', *Lancet* (8 April 1989):782-3.

69. Aart Hendriks, personal communication, 19 September 1991.

70. Martin Wilke and Dieter Kleiber, 'AIDS and sex tourism', 7th International Conference on AIDS, Florence, 1991, Abstract No. M.D.4037.

71. Hilary Kinnell, 'Prostitutes, their clients, and

risks of HIV infection in Birmingham'. Occasional paper, Department of Public Health Medicine, Central Birmingham Health Authority, UK, August 1989.

72. Julie Hamblin and Elizabeth Reid, 'Women, the HIV epidemic and human rights: a tragic imperative', paper presented to International Workshop on AIDS: A Question of Rights and Humanity, International Court of Justice, Den Haag, May 1991.

73. Ann Larson, 'The social epidemiology of Africa's AIDS epidemic', *African Affairs* 89(35) (1990):5-25.

74. Never Gadaga, 'AIDS: What others say', *Sunday Mail,* 15 September 1991.

75. Everjoice Win, 'AIDS: empowering women is one of the solutions', *Sunday Mail*, 22 September 1991.

76. Marsha F. Goldsmith, 'As AIDS epidemic approaches second decade, report examines what has been learned', *Journal of American Medical Association* 264(4) (1990):431-2.

77. Taweesap Siraprapasiri, 'Risk factors for HIV among prostitutes in Chiangmai, Thailand', *AIDS* 5(5) (1991):579-82.

78. Rudolph P. Mak and Jean Plum, 'Do prostitutes need more health education regarding STDs and HIV infection: experience in a Belgian city', *Social Science and Medicine* 33(8) (1991):963-6.

79. Jon Ungphakorn, 'The impact of AIDS on women in Thailand', paper presented to Conference on AIDS in Asia and the Pacific, Canberra, Australia, 5-8 August 1990.

80. 'Women speak out about AIDS: an interview', *Critical Health* 34 (June 1991):48-53.

81. Richard Rhodes, 'Death in the candy store; the prostitution capital of the world, Thailand is committing sexual suicide by HIV infection', *Rolling Stone,* 28 November 1991: 62-70.

82. 'Prostitutas buscan frenar epidemia del SIDA a travès de mensajes por radio', *Mujer/Fempress* 119 (September 1991):21. Source: *El Heraldo,* Honduras, 19 June 1991.

83. Edna Roland, reported in a discussion on women and AIDS, meeting of grantees of the MacArthur Foundation, Teresopolis, Brazil, 1-3 July 1991.

84. Agnete Strom, personal communication, August 1991.

85. From Isis WICCE, *Women's World,* 1988, quoted in Roberta Cohen and Laurie Wiseberg, *Double Jeopardy – Threat to Life and Human Rights: Discrimination against Persons with AIDS* (Human Rights Internet, March 1990), 30.

86. Shyamala Nataraj, three untitled papers about this case for Panos Institute and the UN Development Forum, 1990-91. She personally initiated the court case.

87. Christopher Peterson, 'Prostitutes and public health services cooperate on AIDS prevention in Brazil', *Hygie: International Journal of Health Education* 9(4) (1990):29-31.

88. Carole Campbell, 'Prostitutes, AIDS and preventive health behavior', *Social Science and Medicine* 32(12) (1991):1367-78.

89. Werasit Sittritai, 'Outreach to bar workers in Bangkok', *Hygie: International Journal of Health Education* 9(4) (1990):25-8.

90. Chuanchom Sacondhavat, 'Promoting condom-only brothels through solidarity and support for brothel managers'. Unpublished paper for 6th International Conference on AIDS, San Francisco, 1990. See Abstract No. W.D.53.

91. Cheryl Overs, 'How to sell safer sex', *AIDS Action* 15 (September 1991):2-3.

Chapter 11 (pages 229–247)

1. Zoë Leonard, 'HIV-antibody testing and legal issues for HIV-positive people', in Act Up New York Women & AIDS Book Group (eds), *Women, AIDS and Activism* (Boston: South End Press, 1990), 58-9.

2. J. Chin, 'Public health surveillance of AIDS and HIV infection', *Bulletin of WHO* 68(5) (1990):529-36.

3. R. L. Colebunders and W. L. Heyward, 'Surveillance of AIDS and HIV infection: opportunities and challenges', *Health Policy and Planning* 15(1) (1990):1-11.

4. Mary Ann Benitez, 'Experts propose testing pregnant women for AIDS', *SCMP* 27 October 1989. In *Women's News Digest* 18 (January 1990):12.

5. 'HIV dipstick: A low-cost screening test for AIDS' leaflet (Program for Appropriate Technology in Health, 1991).

6. See J. A. Connell *et al.,* 'Preliminary report: accurate assays for anti-HIV in urine', *Lancet* 335 (1990):1366-9.

7. Reported at meeting of the UK NGO AIDS Consortium for the Third World, London, 22 January 1991.

8. Reported at meeting of the UK NGO AIDS Consortium for the Third World, London, October 1990.

9. 'Veronica', 'You're straight and think you won't get it? Better think again!' In Jacquie Manthorne (ed.), *Canadian Women and AIDS: Beyond the Statistics* (Montréal: Éditions Communiqu' Elles, 1990), 51–9.

10. K. Peltzer *et al.,* 'Psychosocial counselling of patients infected with HIV in Lusaka, Zambia', *Tropical Doctor* (October 1989):164–8.

11. F. I. D. Konotey-Ahulu, 'Clinical epidemiology, not seroepidemiology, is the answer to Africa's AIDS problem', *British Medical Journal* 294 (20 June 1987):1593–4.

12. Doreen Boyd, from a workshop discussion on women and AIDS, YWCA International Training Workshops on Technology, Zeist, September 1989.

13. Bernard M. Dickens, 'Legal limits of AIDS confidentiality', *Journal of American Medical Association* 259(23) (1988):3449–51.

14. 'Confidentiality and blackmail in Canada', *Connexions* 33 (1990):25. Originally in *Rites,* April 1990.

15. M. L. Rekart, 'Patient referral or provider referral partner notification: Which do patients prefer?', 6th International Conference on AIDS, San Francisco, 1990, Abstract No. S.C.103.

16. Guadalupe Ramirez, 'The impact of partner notification on sexual behaviour among a heterosexual population', 6th International Conference on AIDS, San Francisco, 1990, Abstract No. S.C.104.

17. Chris Norwood, 'Drugs, prostitution, and the heterosexual connection' *Advice for Life: A woman's guide to AIDS risks and prevention* (New York: Pantheon, 1987), 109.

18. Susan M. Rubin *et al.,* 'Partner notification may deter HIV+ drug users from treatment', 7th International Conference on AIDS, Florence, 1991, Abstract No. M.C.3331.

19. L. M. Barugahare, 'HIV testing as an AIDS prevention strategy in Uganda', AIDS Information Centre, Kampala. Unpublished paper, 1991.

20. World Health Organization, 'Consensus statements on HIV transmission', *Lancet* (18 February 1989):396.

21. Allan M. Brandt *et al.,* 'Routine hospital testing for HIV: health policy considerations', in Lawrence O. Gostin (ed.), *AIDS and the Health Care System* (New Haven: Yale University Press, 1990).

22. Chris Mihill, 'Surgeons back AIDS test without consent: Royal College advice for staff injured in operations' *Guardian* 11 January 1991.

23. H. Brenner *et al.,* 'AIDS among drug abusers in Europe: review of recent developments', WHO Regional Office for Europe Global Programme on AIDS, Copenhagen, 1991.

24. Anastasia Roumeliotou *et al.,* 'Prevention of HIV infection in Greek registered prostitutes, a five-year study', 6th International Conference on AIDS, San Francisco, 1990, Abstract No. S.C.100.

25. Philip Kell *et al.,* 'Why don't heterosexuals have HIV antibody tests?', 7th International Conference on AIDS, Florence, 1991, Abstract No. M.D.4151.

26. Christine Ogu and Nancy Yamaguchi, *More harm than help: the ramifications for rape survivors of mandatory HIV testing of rapists,* Center for Women Policy Studies, Washington, DC, 1991.

27. Fiona Boag *et al.,* 'Rape, STDs and HIV', letter to *International Journal of STDs and AIDS* 1 (1990):291.

28. C. S. Peckham *et al.,* 'Prevalence of maternal HIV infection based on unlinked anonymous testing of newborn babies', *Lancet* 335 (1990):516–19.

29. Elisabeth Couturier *et al.,* 'HIV-1 and HIV-2 seroprevalence in childbearing women at outcome of pregnancy in the Paris Area, France', 7th International Conference on AIDS, Florence, 1991, Abstract No. W.C.3246.

30. Susanne Lindgren *et al.,* 'Swedish national antenatal screening program for HIV-1: three years' experience', 7th International Conference on AIDS, Florence, 1991, Abstract No. W.C.3278.

31. Helvi Holm Samdal, 'HIV infection among pregnant women in Norway', 7th International Conference on AIDS, Florence, 1991, Abstract No. W.C.3279.

32. L. Salvaggio *et al.,* 'Seroprevalence of HIV-1 infection in pregnant women in Milan, Italy', 7th International Conference on AIDS, Florence, 1991, Abstract No. W.C.3242.

33. Sybille Wieser, 'Is voluntary HIV testing during pregnancy voluntary?', 7th International Conference on AIDS, Florence, 1991, Abstract No. M.C.3333.
34. M. Denayer *et al.,* 'Antenatal testing for HIV', letter to *Lancet* 335 (3 February 1990):292.
35. C. F. Davison, 'Antenatal testing for HIV', *Lancet* (16 December 1989):1442–4.
36. Christoph Rudin *et al.,* 'HIV seroconversion during pregnancy', 7th International Conference on AIDS, Florence, 1991, Abstract No. W.C.3247.
37. A. Stevens *et al.,* letter to *Lancet* 335 (1990):292.
38. *Searching for women: a literature review on women, HIV and AIDS in the United States* (Boston: College of Public and Community Service (Univ Mass) and Multicultural AIDS Coalition, second edn May 1991).
39. William B. Caspe *et al.,* 'HIV testing in a high-risk post-partum population', 6th International Conference on AIDS, San Francisco, 1990, Abstract No. S.C.667.
40. Marie St Cyr, quoted in Gina Kolata, 'Growing movement seeks to help women infected with AIDS virus', *New York Times,* 4 May 1989, B16.
41. 'HIV testing as an integrated activity at a family planning clinic', *Planned Parenthood in Europe* 19(1) (1990):30.
42. Ndugga Maggwa *et al.,* 'Acceptability of screening for HIV infection among women attending family planning clinics in Nairobi, Kenya', 6th International Conference on AIDS, San Francisco, 1990, Abstract No. S.C.668.
43. Patrick Thonneau *et al.,* 'Evaluation by women consulting in a family planning centre of their risk of HIV infection', *AIDS* 5(5) (1991):549–53.
44. Thierry Allegre *et al.,* 'Characteristics of heterosexual couples performing HIV testing before their first sexual intercourse', 7th International Conference on AIDS, Florence, 1991, Abstract No. M.C.3328.
45. Judith Hutterer *et al.,* 'Differences in HIV/AIDS counselling for women and for men', 5th International Conference on AIDS, Montréal, 1989, pre-conference abstract.
46. Manuel Carballo and G. Lloyd, 'Cross-cultural issues in HIV/AIDS counselling', 6th International Conference on AIDS, San Francisco, 1990, Abstract No. S.D.848.
47. 'AIDS hotlines for countries of central and eastern Europe: Report of a WHO workshop, Warsaw, 13–16 December 1991', WHO Europe Region Global Programme on AIDS, Copenhagen, 1992, Doc. EUR/ICP/GPA/116 (Proceedings 11). Very useful on how to organize a hotline.
48. Lydia S. Bond, 'Use of telephone hotlines in counselling in Latin America and Caribbean', 6th International Conference on AIDS, San Francisco, 1990, Abstract No. S.D.821.
49. M. Helquist *et al.,* 'Personal yet confidential use of hotlines to deliver AIDS prevention messages to targeted audiences in the Caribbean', 6th International Conference on AIDS, San Francisco, 1990, Abstract No. S.D.847.
50. Susan D. Cochran and Vickie M. Mays, 'Women and AIDS-related concerns: roles for psychologists in helping the worried well', *American Psychologist* 44 (1989):529–35.
51. This section is adapted from David Miller and Anthony J. Pinching, 'HIV tests and counselling: current issues', *AIDS* 3 (Supplement 1) (1989):S187–S193.
52. Jaklyn Brookman, 'Confessions of an antibody test counsellor', in Ines Rieder and Patricia Ruppelt (eds), *AIDS: The Women* (San Francisco: Cleis Press, 1988), 111–13.
53. Jacquie Manthorne, 'AIDS and feminism', in Jacquie Manthorne (ed.), *Canadian Women and AIDS: Beyond the statistics* (Montréal: Éditions Communiqu'Elles, 1990), 33.
54. Noerine Kaleeba *et al., We miss you all: Noerine Kaleeba: AIDS in the family* (Harare: Women & AIDS Support Network, 1991), 63.
55. *AIDS Counselling: A manual for primary health care workers* (Harare: AIDS Control Programme, Ministry of Health Zimbabwe, 1990).
56. Judy Macks, 'Women and AIDS: counter-transference issues', *Social Casework: Journal of Contemporary Social Work* (June 1988):340–47.
57. Lahire Dutra Carvalho-Neto *et al.,* 'Psychosocial counseling accomplished by male counselors for HIV-infected women in Rio de Janeiro, Brazil', 6th International Conference on AIDS, San Francisco, 1990, Abstract No. S.B.403.

Index

abandonment 96–7, 233
Ablin 352
abortion 37, 46, 60, 70, 74, 76, 90, 92–4, 97–8, 102, 105, 107, 111–12, 123, 126, 147, 150, 155, 196, 236, 239
abuse, sexual 11, 125–6, 179, 180, 198, 235
abusive relationships 22
accidents, infection because of 66
ACOG. *See* American College of Obstetrics and Gynecology
Act-Up 338, 349
acupuncture 29
adoption 78
Advanced Immune Discoveries Symposium 352
advertisements 160, 197, 295
Afghanistan 263
Africa 10, 14, 22–3, 24, 34, 38, 51–2, 72, 74, 105, 108, 123, 128, 134, 162, 163, 165, 185, 189, 223
   Central 36, 51, 52
   East 52
   North 42, 85, 191
   organizations 312–17
   sub-Saharan 42, 49
   traditional healers in 29
   See also individual countries
African medical research Foundation 274
age groups affected 45, 47
AG Frau und Aids (Women and AIDS Society) 324

Agomanya, Ghana 27, 339
Ahlberg, Beth Maina 366
Ahmedabad, India 178
AHRTAG. *See* Appropriate Health resources and Technologies Action Group
AIC. *See* AIDS Information Centre
AIDS Action Committee (Boston) 300
AIDS: A Nation at Risk 279
AIDS and Youth 319
AIDS Control and Prevention Project (AIDSCAP) 335
AIDS Counselling and Education Organization (ACE) 297, 330
AIDS Counselling Trust (Zimbabwe) 269, 317
AIDSED Centre 337
AIDS-Hilfe Wien 320
AIDS Information Centre 246–7
AIDS prevention 227–8
AIDS Research Foundation of India 317
AIDS Resource Foundation for Children (New Jersey, USA) 300
AIDS Resource Network (Broklyn, New York) 238
AIDS Service Organization, The (TASO) 315
AIDS Task Force 337
AIDS Working Group 334
Ajusco, Mexico 290
alcoholism 13, 55, 294, 299

Alexander, Nancy J. 348, 350, 363
Alexander, Vickie 353
Alicea, Aida Iris Cruz 366
Allegre, Thierry 370
Allen, Susan 54, 350, 355
Allen, Upton 362
All Women's Action Society (Malaysia) 185
'Almighty' (condom) 160
alternatives to intercourse 134
alternative treatments 13, 29–30
American College of Obstetrics and Gynecology (ACOG) 89, 90, 359
amniotic fluid 69, 70
Amola, I. 104
amphetamines 63
AMREF (Kenya) 313
Amsterdam, Netherlands 63, 65, 228
anaemia 30, 31, 60, 62, 80, 276
anal intercourse 43, 116, 125, 137
Anastos, Kathryn 359
Ancelle, R. 354
Anderson, Deborah 348, 362
Anderson, Rachel 353
Angola 313
anonymity in screening 102, 229–30, 232, 236
antenatal clinics 105, 127, 230, 233, 238, 303
antenatal screening 235–8
Anyangwe, Stella 313
Anzala, Aggrey 349

Investigación de la Mujer
(FEIM) 324
Fusallah, S. 104

GABRIELA Commission on
Women's Health and
Reproductive Rights
(Philippines) 318
Gadaga, Never 368
gamma globulin 62
Garandy, Roger 207
gay men 9, 24, 39, 79, 116, 157,
170, 172, 175, 189, 190, 208,
210, 298, 302, 307
gender roles 181, 182, 197-8,
202-07, 213-14, 224
Geneva, Switzerland 265
genital herpes 36, 277
genital ulcers 34, 36, 128
genital warts 21
Gentian violet 27, 28
Germain, Adrienne 312
Germany 49, 63, 78, 100, 191,
234
Ghana 27, 178, 191, 228
Gibbs, Nancy 365
Gibbs, W.N. 356
Gilada, I.S. 276, 344, 366
Gilks, Charles F. 351
Gill, O. Noel 351
Gill, Sarah 352
Girls' Brigade 303
Girls Night Out (Chicago
Women's AIDS Project) 142,
174, 329, 342
Global AIDS Policy
Coalition 335
Global Programme on AIDS 15,
48, 151, 303, 354, 356, 359,
369, 370
Goa 191
Goedert, James J. 358
Goesch 352
Goldoftas, Barbara 355
Goldsmith, Marsha F. 368
Gomez, Percy 358
gonorrhoea 118, 119, 120, 121,
214, 215, 225, 234, 277
Goodgame, Richard W. 351
Gordon, Peter 339
Gossius, Georg 355
Gostin, Lawrence O. 369
Graham, Nell M.H. 353
Gram Bharati Samiti 317
Greathead, Erica 364

Greece 234
Gromyko, Alexandre 356
Gross, Shirley 212
groups, organizations and
resources 310-47
Grupo de Apoio a Prevenção
a AIDS 325
Grupo de Investigación y
Capacitación en Medicina
Social 326
Grupo Pela Vidda
(Brazil) 259-63, 325, 343
Guam 304
Guatemala 189
Guerrero, Ernesto 362
Guinea Bissau 61, 312
Gujurat, India 60
Guyana 46

haemophilia 61
Hague, R.A. 357
Haiti 22, 40, 44, 46, 47, 149,
191, 256-7
Hamblin, Julie 368
Hamilton, John D. 353
Hampton, Janie 352, 366
Hankins, Catherine 354
Harare, Zimbabwe 2, 124, 192,
268, 316
Harlem Hospital Center, New
York 18
Harris, Jeffrey R. 363, 364
Hartwig, Kari 273, 344, 364, 366
Hausa, homosexuality
among 189
Hausherr, Rosmarie 340
Hauser, Dominique 364
Hausermann, Julia 353
Hava'ad Lemilebamah
B'AIDS 327
Hayes, Katherine 212
Health Action for Information
Network (Philippines) 318
Health Protection and
Promotion 336
heart disease 24
Heckert, Karen 344, 366
Helmann, Nicholas S. 361
Helquist, M. 370
Hendriks, Aart 367
Henin, Y. 348
hepatitis B 67, 70, 103, 118, 259,
262, 267
Hepburn, Mary 356, 360, 362
herbology 29

Herd, Gilbert 341
'Here Come the Giants'
(condom) 160
Hernández Cárdenas, Ana
María 289
heroin 63
herpes 6, 19, 20, 28, 36, 277
heterosexual transmission 35, 39,
40, 43, 45, 50, 51, 72, 118
Heyward, W.I. 368
Hijras 278
Hira, S.K. 350
Hispanic women 35, 63, 175,
180, 209, 329
Hite, Shere 198
HIV/AIDS:
blood-to-blood
transmission 58-70
and breastfeeding 80-86,
112-13
case definition of 114-15
and contraceptives and
condoms 147-70
diagnosis in women 15, 17
drug treatment for 26-7, 28,
30-31
epidemiology in
women 38-57
gender differences 15, 40
groups, organizations and
resources 310-40
menstruation and fertility,
effects on 17-18
and mental health 15-16
and motherhood 89-115
personal histories of living
with 248-67
pregnancy, interaction
with 18-19
pregnancy-related
transmission 71-88, 105, 220
related illnesses 14-34
and reproductive tract
illnesses 19-21, 32-4
and safer relationships 171-228
and safer sex 129-46
and sexually transmitted
diseases 128
sexual transmission of 76,
116-28
social, economic and political
factors 45-9
survival with 9-10, 37
symptoms of 17

interaction with HIV 19-21,
32-4
resources, groups and
organisations 310-47
Revock, Jacqueline 266, 344
Rhode Island, USA 36
Rhodes, Richard 368
Rhodes, T. 360
Richardson, Diane 338
Richart, Ralph M. 351
Richters, Juliet 365
Rieder, Ines 337, 343, 363
Rio de Janeiro, Brazil 189, 325
risk factors 117-26
risk reduction 50, 64-5, 77-9,
137, 196, 208-10
workshops 219-24
Robbins, Susan 363
Robins, A. 346
Rodriques, Lair 354
Rochman, Sue 344
Rogow, Debbie 335, 364
Röhr-Rouendaal, Petra 345
Roland, Edna 356, 368
role playing 219, 220, 224
Ross, Hazel 352
Ross, Oakland 353
Rossato, Veronica 364
rotation of staff 70
Rough Rider (condom) 160
Roumania 60
Roumeliotou, Anastasia 369
Rowen, D. 360-61
Royce, Rachel 349
Rozendaal, Simon 358
Rubin, Susan M. 369
Rudd, Andrea 337
Rudin, Christoph 370
Rumsey, Sunny 363
Rundle, Amy Chen 54
Runganga, Agnes 362
Ruppelt, Patricia 337, 343, 363
Rutherford, George W. 349
Rwanda 17, 27, 54-6, 61, 81, 90,
122, 151, 155, 187, 313-14
Ryder, Robert W. 350, 359

Sabatier, Renee 334
Sacondhavata, Chuanchom 368
safer relationships 171-228
safer sex 76, 125, 129-46, 148,
181, 199-200, 295-6
education 155, 156, 172-9, 195
parties 296, 329
strategies 130-36

Saffron, Lisa 358
Sainath, Mridula 304, 343, 344
Saint Cyr-Delpe, Marie
Marthe 256, 343, 370
St Lucia 160
St Mary's Hospital, London 102
saliva 70, 103
Salud Integral para la Mujer
(SIPAM) 289-90
Salud y SIDA: Información,
Comunicación y
Asesoramiento 324
Salvaggio, L. 369
Salvation Army Chikankata
Hospital 316
Samdal, Helvi Holm 369
Samoa, Western 301, 302, 303
San Francisco, California 64, 189,
217, 290, 293, 294
São Paulo, Brazil 63, 150, 259,
325
Sapphex Learn 328
Saudi Arabia 81
Save the Children Fund 108
Scandinavia 148, 172
scarification 67, 178
Scarlet Alliance 332
Schechter, Mauro 355
Schietinger, Helen 298, 344
schistosomiasis 60
Schmidt, Nancy J. 353
Schoen, Edgar J. 362
Schoepf, Brooke Grundfest 51,
219, 249, 312, 341, 343, 364
Schoepf, Claude 219
Schorerstichting (National Agency
for Homosexuality) 322
Schwalbe, Joan 54
Schwarz, Gabriele 360
Scofield, Virginia 348, 350
Scotland 18, 64, 92, 94, 98, 154,
287-8, 323
Scott, Gwendolyn B. 250, 357
Scott, Sally 359
Scott, Sue 197
Scottish Women and HIV/AIDS
Network 288
screening, testing and
counselling 21, 229-47
self-care and home care 28
self-insemination 78
semen 8, 70, 78, 79, 103, 117,
154, 229
Senegal 67, 312, 314
Sengupta, Swapna S. 362

'Sensation' (condom) 161
septicaemia 38
Serufilira, Antoine 54
Setters, Jo 363
sexual aids and toys 123-5, 137
sexuality 145, 168, 169, 171-2,
186, 102, 106
male 182, 186-7, 201-05, 107,
257
sex tourism 191
sex work and sex workers 12,
32, 35, 39, 41, 42, 51, 57,
64, 120, 134, 150, 154, 162,
168, 170, 180, 186, 188, 189,
190, 191, 193-6, 210, 217-19,
220, 221, 222-3, 224, 225-8,
233, 234, 264-6, 276-9, 293,
312, 313
legislation and 194, 225-6
sexually transmitted diseases 34,
36, 40, 41, 51, 52, 55, 65,
70, 105, 119, 125-6, 136,
149, 150, 153, 155, 157, 158,
163, 167-8, 190, 214, 217,
218, 220, 222, 223, 224,
234, 277-8, 279, 294
clinics 25, 57, 119, 126, 128,
151, 169, 235
Shanti Project 299
sharing drug equipment 35, 42,
63-4, 90, 174, 294
Sharma, Vinit 362
Sharpe, Sue 197
Shepherd, Gill 363
Shepherd, Jane 345
shingles 11, 17, 19, 25
Short, Roger V. 364
sickle cell anaemia 60, 61, 62
Sierra Leone 314
Simonsen, J. Neil 362
Singapore 148, 162, 191
Singer, Merrill 366
Sion, Fernando Samuel 355
SIPAM. See Salud Integral para la
Mujer
Siraprapasiri, Taweesap 368
Sisterlove: Women's AIDS
Project 174, 329
Sittitrai, Werasit 280, 344, 367,
368
skin infections 17
slavery 51
'slim disease' 275
Smith, Diana G. 354
Smith, Else 367